Basingstoke Healthcare Library
Basingstoke and North Hampshire Hospital
First floor of The Ark
RG24 9NA
Tel: 01256 313169

To be returned on or before the date marked below

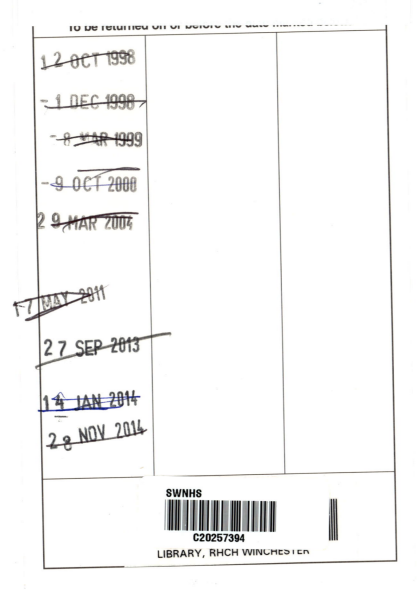

12 OCT 1998

-1 DEC 1998

-8 MAR 1999

-9 OCT 2000

2 9 MAR 2004

17 MAY 2011

2 7 SEP 2013

14 JAN 2014

28 NOV 2014

SWNHS

C20257394

LIBRARY, RHCH WINCHESTER

Atlas of

DENTAL AND MAXILLOFACIAL RADIOLOGY AND IMAGING

Atlas of

DENTAL AND MAXILLOFACIAL RADIOLOGY AND IMAGING

Roger M Browne
BSc, PhD, DDS, FDSRCS, FRCPath.
Professor of Oral Pathology
University of Birmingham, and
Honorary Consultant in Oral Pathology
South Birmingham Health Authority

Hugh D Edmondson
MBChB, BDS, DDS, LDSRCS, FDSRCS, MRCS, LRCP, DA
Professor of Oral Surgery and Oral Medicine
University of Birmingham, and
Honorary Consultant Oral and Maxillofacial Surgeon
South Birmingham Health Authority

P G John Rout
BDS, FDSRCS, MDent.Sc., DDRRCR
Lecturer in Oral Surgery and Dental Radiology
University of Birmingham, and
Honorary Senior Registrar in Oral Surgery
South Birmingham Health Authority

M Mosby-Wolfe

London Baltimore Bogotá Boston Buenos Aires Caracas Carlsbad, CA Chicago Madrid Mexico City Milan Naples, FL New York Philadelphia St. Louis Sydney Tokyo Toronto Wiesbaden

Project Manager   Mike Meakin
Production   Jane Tozer
Publisher   Claire Hooper

Copyright © 1995 Times Mirror International Publishers Limited

Published in 1995 by Mosby-Wolfe, an imprint of Times Mirror International Publishers Limited

Printed by Grafos S.A. arte sobre papel, Barcelona, Spain

ISBN 0 7234 1725 3

All rights reserved. No part of this publication may be reproduced, stored in a retrieval system, copied or transmitted, in any form or by any means, electronic, mechanical, photocopying, recording or otherwise without written permission from the Publisher or in accordance with the provisions of the Copyright Act 1956 (as amended), or under the terms of any licence permitting limited copying issued by the Copyright Licensing Agency, 33–34 Alfred Place, London, WC1E 7DP.

Any person who does any unauthorised act in relation to this publication may be liable to criminal prosecution and civil claims for damages.

Permission to photocopy or reproduce solely for internal or personal use is permitted for libraries or other users registered with the Copyright Clearance Center, provided that the base fee of $4.00 per chapter plus $.10 per page is paid directly to the Copyright Clearance Center, 21 Congress Street, Salem, MA 01970. This consent does not extend to other kinds of copying, such as copying for general distribution, for advertising or promotional purposes, for creating new collected works, or for resale.

For full details of all Times Mirror International Publishers Limited titles, please write to Times Mirror International Publishers Limited, Lynton House, 7–12 Tavistock Square, London WC1H 9LB, England.

A CIP catalogue record for this book is available from the British Library.

Library of Congress Cataloging-in-Publication Data applied for.

TO OUR FAMILIES

for their patience and forbearance
during the compilation of this book

Contents

Acknowledgements

The collection of a number of radiographs such as those presented in this atlas can only be achieved with considerable goodwill and collaboration. The authors were very much aware of this when they commenced the task of compiling this atlas and wish to acknowledge the help and co-operation they have received from colleagues.

Many of the radiographs presented have been selected from those contained within the library of the X-ray Department of the Birmingham Dental Hospital. This collection has been accumulated over the past forty years and the authors are indebted to their predecessors who so painstakingly documented and filed their radiographs. In particular, they would like to acknowledge Mr R.W.H. Tavenner, formerly Senior Lecturer in Dental Surgery, University of Birmingham, and Consultant Dental Surgeon to the General Hospital, Birmingham; Mr J.W. Wheatcroft, formerly Tutor in Dental Radiology, University of Birmingham; Dr D.K.M. Toye, formerly Consultant Radiologist in the Central Birmingham Health Authority; and Mr C.L. Price, formerly Senior Lecturer in Oral Surgery, University of Birmingham. All four provided many radiographs for the collection and the authors have drawn heavily from their contribution.

Grateful thanks are also due to our present colleagues in the Birmingham Dental School and Hospital and to others who have willingly agreed to the use of their radiographs and who have constantly borne our needs in mind, namely: Mr C.L. Brady (**571**, **587**, **604**, **605**); Mr J.G. Burland (**432**, **621**); Mr I. Gorman (**822**); Mr J.M. Harrison (**613**); Mr R. Hensher (**429**); Mr A.D. Hockley (**384**, **385**, **386**, **387**, **388**); Mr K. Horner (**89**, **90**, **688**, **689**, **690**, **691**, **692**, **696**); Mr R. Kendrick (**823**); Mr F. MacCauley (**251**); Mrs J. MacFarlane (**249**, **250**); Mr G.L. Manning (**375**, **591**); Mr I.D.M. Matthew (**330**); Mr C.J. Meryon (**594**); Mr K. Moos (**435**, **449**, **581**); Mr R.R. Nasheed (**743**); Mr L. Oldham (**771**); Mr S.F. Olley (**434**); Dr L. Otis (**91**, **92**, **93**, **94**, **693**, **694**, **695**); Dr P.D. Phelps (**800**, **801**, **802**, **803**); Dr E.B. Rolfe (**799**, **809**, **810**, **811**, **812**); Mr A.J. Sear (**551**); Mr B. Speculand (**521**, **522**); Mr J.R. Totten (**504**); and Mr M.J.C. Wake (**394**, **519**, **520**, **521**, **522**, **548**, **549**).

We wish to thank the staff of the X-ray Department of the Birmingham Dental Hospital for their patience during the preparation of this book and for their ever willing assistance. In particular we would like to thank Miss D. Kelly, Superintendent Radiographer for her invaluable help. We extend our sincere gratitude to Mrs R. McCormack for typing the manuscript.

The diagrams were drawn and prepared by Mr G. O'Grady, Audio Visual Unit, Dental School, University of Birmingham, Mrs C.A. Walker, Radiology Department, Birmingham Dental Hospital, and Mr D. Plester, University of Central England, to all of whom we extend our thanks.

Finally, we should like to thank our publishers, Times Mirror International Publishers Ltd, for their patience during the preparation of this work.

Abbreviations

A(J)	Arthrogram	PZ(F)	Panoramic zonograph (midface programme)
AN	Angiogram	PZ(J)	Panoramic zonograph (temporomandibular joint programme)
BW	Bitewing		
CT	Computerized tomogram	RPA	Rotated postero-anterior skull
CT(SL)	Computerized tomogram (sialography)	S	Soft tissue
DPR	Dental panoramic radiograph	SC	Scintiscan
DPR(J)	Dental panoramic radiograph (temporomandibular joint programme)	SL(L)	Sialogram (lateral skull)
		SL(OLM)	Sialogram (oblique lateral mandible)
DPR(Z)	Dental panoramic radiograph (zonarc)	SL(PA)	Sialogram (postero-anterior skull)
L	Lateral skull	SL(RPA)	Sialogram (rotated postero-anterior skull)
LAO	Lower anterior occlusal	SMV	Submentovertex skull
LC	Lateral skull, cephalometric technique	T	Towne's view
LOO	Lower oblique occlusal	TASC	Time/activity scintiscan
LTO	Lower true occlusal	TG	Tomogram
MRI	Magnetic resonance image/imaging	TLM	True lateral maxilla
OLM	Oblique lateral mandible	TMJ	Transcranial view of the temporomandibular joint
OM	Occipitomental skull	TMJ(Z)	Temporomandibular joint programme (zonarc)
OM30	Occipitomental (30° angle) skull	UOO	Upper oblique occlusal
P	Periapical	US	Ultrasound
PA	Postero-anterior skull	USO	Upper standard occlusal (upper anterior occlusal)
PAC	Postero-anterior condyles	UTO	Upper true occlusal
PZ(D)	Panoramic zonograph (dental programme)	VO	Vertex occlusal

Annotation of the dentition

In this atlas we have used the Zsigmondy system for identifying the teeth. For those more familiar with the system recommended by the Fédération Dentaire Internationale (FDI), the two systems are illustrated diagrammatically in **1**.

PERMANENT DENTITION

(18)	(17)	(16)	(15)	(14)	(13)	(12)	(11)	(21)	(22)	(23)	(24)	(25)	(26)	(27)	(28)
8	7	6	5	4	3	2	1	1	2	3	4	5	6	7	8
8	7	6	5	4	3	2	1	1	2	3	4	5	6	7	8
(48)	(47)	(46)	(45)	(44)	(43)	(42)	(41)	(31)	(32)	(33)	(34)	(35)	(36)	(37)	(38)

PRIMARY DENTITION

(55)	(54)	(53)	(52)	(51)	(61)	(62)	(63)	(64)	(65)
E	D	C	B	A	A	B	C	D	E
E	D	C	B	A	A	B	C	D	E
(85)	(84)	(83)	(82)	(81)	(71)	(72)	(73)	(74)	(75)

1 In the Zsigmondy system, each permanent tooth is represented by a single digit displayed in the appropriate quadrant of the mouth. Thus 6| designates the right mandibular permanent first molar. Above the maxillary teeth and below the mandibular teeth are illustrated the corresponding codes (in brackets) using the FDI system. This is a two digit system in which there is an additional digit for each quadrant of the mouth. Thus 46 designates the right mandibular permanent first molar. The codes in both systems are modified as indicated for the primary dentition.

Introduction

The use of radiographs and other imaging techniques is an essential component of the investigation and treatment of patients with disorders of the face, jaws and teeth. Although the management of such disorders is primarily the responsibility of members of the dental specialties, other groups, such as otorhinolaryngologists, plastic surgeons, neurosurgeons and oncologists, may be involved, particularly with abnormalities of the facial skeleton and neoplasms. This collection of radiographs has, therefore, been compiled with the needs of a wide group of health specialists in mind.

It would take a lifetime of clinical experience, and probably longer, to encounter the whole range of diseases that may affect these tissues and to become familiar with the varied radiographic appearances that may be presented by the same condition. Whereas it is appreciated that there is no real substitute for personal experience, it is hoped that a collection of this sort will help to accelerate the learning process and to some extent provide a reference for some of the less common clinical conditions. We believe that this book will be of particular value to undergraduates (with respect to their preliminary training) and to postgraduate and practising clinicians (in its role as a reference collection). It is, of course, impossible to illustrate the full range of diagnostic images that may be encountered in the investigation of disorders of the face, jaws and teeth, but where possible those most characteristic of the condition described have been chosen. Clearly, with some of the more rare conditions, this choice was not always possible.

Since the majority of patients with disorders of the face, jaws and teeth seek advice in the first instance from a dentist in general practice, particular prominence has been given to the radiographic appearances on radiographs taken in this environment. Dental practitioners are unique among clinicians, in that working in the geographic isolation of their own surgery, they need to have in addition to their clinical skills, an individual competence in radiological interpretation. The use of radiographs plays a crucial role in the diagnosis and follow-up of many diseases treated in the dental surgery, as well as in the monitoring of the techniques used in their treatment. However, more extensive and severe conditions require investigation and management in a hospital environment and here the whole range of modern imaging techniques may be employed. Consequently, where appropriate, examples of the appearances obtained using a variety of these techniques have also been included. Each one has particular advantages, disadvantages and specific applications, which are indicated where appropriate.

The successful employment and interpretation of radiographs and other images of the human body, is dependent upon a number of factors. First, the physico-chemical properties of X-rays and the other imaging modalities, and the factors involved in the production of the resulting image; secondly, the variety of angulations employed in the different radiographic and other imaging techniques; thirdly, the full range of normal appearances that are a consequence of viewing the same anatomical structures by this variety of techniques; and finally, the wide range of disease processes that can affect the tissues.

This book is therefore divided into chapters dealing with each of these topics. Chapter 1 presents a brief discussion on the basic physics of X-rays, together with a simple explanation of the techniques involved in taking the radiographic views illustrated. We have made no attempt to describe in detail the procedures involved and those seeking further technical information are referred to the many texts on the subject (Goaz and White, 1987; Whaites, 1992). Instead, emphasis has been given to the pathway taken by the X-ray beam relative to the tissues of the head and neck, so that a proper understanding of the anatomical structures displayed in each view can be obtained. In addition to conventional X-ray techniques, there are a number of more sophisticated X-ray and other forms of imaging methods and reference has been made to these in a similar manner. Two of these methods, ultrasonography (US) and magnetic resonance imaging (MRI), are of particular value in the investigation of soft tissue lesions in which conventional X-ray techniques play only a small role. They have the added advantage that they lack the potential hazards of X-irradiation. The importance of minimizing the radiation dosage to both patient and operator during the taking of radiographs cannot be overemphasized, and the reader is reminded of the need for such care.

In Chapter 2, a series of films representative of the normal appearances seen in the variety of projections of the jaws, skull and related structures is presented. In each illustration the most important normal anatomical features are highlighted. In addition, some examples of variations in the normal appearances are shown. It is not practical to illustrate the entire range of such variations, but the examples presented have been selected because they may be confused with real abnormalities. One of the keys to successful diagnosis is the ability to relate the abnormal changes displayed to the normal anatomical appearance of the region. In many unilateral lesions, opportunity is readily at hand, as the changes detected in the affected side can be compared with the appearance of the normal side. Most of the human body, including the face, jaws and teeth, is approximately symmetrical and thus provides an ideal basis upon which such comparisons can be made. Where bilateral comparison is not so readily available, reference to the illustrations of normal appearance may be helpful.

Chapter 3 presents a selection of radiographs which show abnormal features arising from errors in technique, introduced during the taking and/or subsequent processing of the different types of radiographs. It is important to have a knowledge of how such abnormal appearances may come about, as they too may be mistaken for some pathological lesion. Deficiences in technique may also reduce, or even preclude, important diagnostic information.

The remaining chapters, which make up the major part of this book, are devoted to presenting illustrations of a wide range of diseases that may affect the face, jaws and teeth. There are separate chapters dealing with the teeth, the periodontium, the facial bones, the temporomandibular joint, the maxillary antrum, the salivary glands and the soft tissues. In each chapter the disorders that may affect each area are presented according to a classification based upon their potential causative mechanisms. The conditions are presented in the following sequence: developmental; microbial and their sequelae; traumatic and their sequelae; regressive; tumorous; and iatrogenic. This allows examples of particular disorders to be referenced more readily and presents the lesions in an order similar to that often used by clinicians to reach a provisional diagnosis. This system of diagnostic analysis is sometimes referred to as the 'surgical sieve'.

For each entity there is a brief summary of the more important pathogenetic features, prior to the descriptions of the radiographs and the other images presented. Reference is made to those components of the tissue changes which contribute to the radiographic images. No attempt, however, has been made to discuss the tissue changes in detail and readers are referred to one of the many texts available for further information (Lucas, 1984; Cawson and Eveson, 1987; Cawson, 1991). The combination of authorship has included an oral radiologist, surgeon and pathologist, with the object of achieving a balanced account of all aspects of the conditions illustrated. It has not been our intention to present the radiological differential diagnosis in all cases, although in some instances reference to those lesions most commonly producing similar changes has been included. With many conditions the space available has allowed us to present only one or two illustrations. However, in clinical practice a number of views of the same lesion, frequently using more than one imaging technique, may be necessary to obtain a detailed picture of all its aspects. Although radiological and other imaging techniques provide only one part of the diagnostic procedures used in the investigation of disease, they are playing an increasingly important role, and it is hoped that this text will add to the process.

References

Cawson, R.A. (1991) *Essentials of Dental Surgery and Pathology*, 4th edn, Churchill Livingstone, Edinburgh.

Cawson, R.A. and Eveson, J.W. (1987) *Oral Pathology and Diagnosis: A colour atlas with integrated text*, Heinemann, London.

Lucas, R.B. (1984) *Pathology of Tumours of the Oral Tissues*, 4th edn, Churchill Livingstone, Edinburgh.

Goaz, P.W. and White, S.C. (1987) *Oral Radiology: Principles and interpretations*, 2nd edn, C.V. Mosby, St Louis.

Whaites, E. (1992) *Essentials of Dental Radiography and Radiology*, Churchill Livingstone, Edinburgh.

1

Radiographic and other imaging techniques

The nature of X-rays

X-rays were discovered by Wilhelm Conrad Roentgen in November 1895 whilst experimenting with a masked cathode ray tube, when he noticed a glow from a fluorescent screen close by. He attributed this phenomenon to an unknown ray, or X-ray, emitted from the tube. It is now known that X-rays form part of the electromagnetic spectrum (2), the properties of which are related to their wavelength and frequencies. They have no mass, travel at the speed of sound, cause certain salts to fluoresce and will darken photographic emulsions. Although electromagnetic radiation demonstrates properties as a wave of energy, X-rays also behave as a stream of finite packets of energy called photons, the unit of photon energy being the electron volt (eV). The X-ray energy (E) is related to its frequency (f) and wavelength (l) according to the following equation:

$$E = hf = hc/l$$

where h is Planck's constant and c is the speed of electromagnetic waves. Thus, as the wavelength reduces, the energy increases.

X-ray formation

For clinical usage, X-rays are produced in an evacuated glass tube containing a filament (or cathode) and a target (or anode), which is made of a button of tungsten set in a block of copper (3). The filament consists of a spiral tungsten wire which, when heated by an electric current, liberates a cloud of electrons. A potential of many thousands of volts is applied between the cathode and the anode which causes the electrons to be attracted at very high speeds to the anode. The stream of electrons is prevented from lateral spread by the negatively-charged focusing hood or cup of the cathode.

When the electrons collide with the tungsten target their kinetic energy is mainly converted into heat which is conducted away by the copper block and dissipated. However, a small percentage (about 1%) is converted into X-rays of various wavelengths and therefore various energies. The higher the kilovoltage, the shorter the wavelength and the greater the ability of the X-rays to penetrate the tissues. The X-rays emerge as a beam via the window in an otherwise shielded X-ray tube, passing through an aluminium filter of appropriate thickness to remove many of the low energy X-rays which would otherwise be absorbed by the soft tissues and not contribute to the formation of the image. The beam is collimated so that the field size involves only the area of clinical interest and conforms to the appropriate safety legislative directives.

Photon energy Electron Volts eV		Wavelength Angstrom Units
10^{+10}	Cosmic Rays Gamma Rays X–Rays Ultra Violet Light Visible Light Infra Red Light	$\overset{\circ}{A}$ 10^{-6}
10^{-8}	Radar and Microwaves Television Radio	10^{+12}

2 A diagram illustrating the position of X-rays in the electromagnetic spectrum relative to photon energy and wavelength.

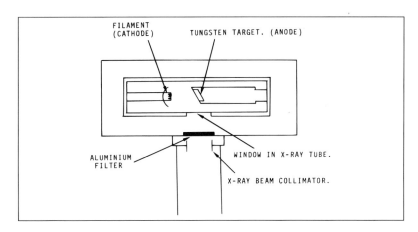

3 The basic components of an X-ray tube.

X-ray interactions

When X-rays interact with matter, their intensity is reduced by the processes of photoelectric absorption and different forms of scatter (**4**).

Photoelectric absorption occurs when an X-ray photon displaces an inner-orbiting or tightly-bound electron from the atom. When this occurs, all the energy of the X-ray is transferred by the process of ejecting the electron, with the remaining energy being imparted to the displaced electron. The atom has now become ionized but regains stability by rearrangement of its remaining electrons which results in the emission of 'characteristic radiation'. The ejected electron interacts with other atoms until all of its energy is lost. Photoelectric absorption depends upon the atomic number of the absorbing material and its density, and is inversely related to the photon energy of the X-ray beam, so these properties are factors which affect the radiographic image.

Compton scatter occurs when the X-ray photon displaces an outer-orbiting or loosely-bound electron from the atom. The X-ray photon loses only part of its energy to the electron and is deflected from its original path—undergoing further interactions—until it has lost all its energy. It is possible for a low-enery X-ray photon to be deflected or scattered by an atom without displacing an electron; this form of scattering is known as the Thompson effect. Scatter may result in image degradation (fogging) and contribute to the radiation exposure of individuals in the proximity of the patient.

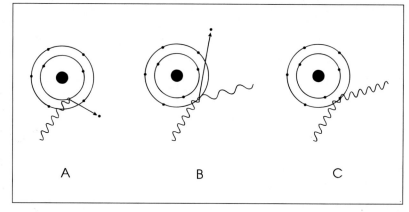

4 The interaction of X-rays with matter: A, photoelectric absorption; B, Compton scatter; C, the Thompson effect.

Hazards of radiation

Soon after Roentgen's discovery, it became evident that X-rays had harmful effects to both the patient and the operator. The first reported effects, such as skin erythema and epilation, were largely due to the excessive dosages being employed, but it was not long before X-rays were linked with tumour induction. The harmful effects depend on many factors such as the dose received, the frequency of exposure and the type of tissue irradiated. In general, tissues whose cells divide frequently are more sensitive to the effects of radiation than are those whose cells are less active. During mitotic division of normal, non-irradiated cells, the deoxyribonucleic acid (DNA) of the two resulting daughter cells often bears minor structural defects due to imperfections in its duplication and splitting, which are both integral to the mitotic process. These defects are only usually temporary, as, in normal circumstances, they undergo repair due to the activity of certain nuclear enzymes. However, radiation has the effect not only of increasing the incidence and the severity of such defects in dividing cells by, for example, causing breaks in the cross-linkages of the DNA molecules, but also of interfering with the normal process of repair. As a consequence, the likelihood of the defects persisting is greatly increased and these may alter the behaviour of the cell and predispose it to malignant change. The damage may arise from the effects of the radiation directly on the DNA and its associated enzymes, or indirectly from the action of free radicals formed in the cytosol.

The effects of radiation can be divided into two types: stochastic (random) and non-stochastic (certainty). In the former, the probability of an effect is related to the dose received and therefore any dose, however small, carries some risk of causing harm. An example of this is the induction of malignant diseases such as carcinomas and leukaemias. For non-stochastic sequelae there is a threshold level below which no apparent effects are observed. These sequelae include cataracts, and erythema and keratosis of the skin and mucous membranes. The dose threshold levels for the non-stochastic effects are above those which occur in the routine use of diagnostic radiography.

It is evident that protective measures are needed to minimize the harmful effects of X-radiation. The risk to both patient and operator has been reduced by progressive improvements to X-ray equipment, the introduction of films of faster speed and the standardization of safe radiographic criteria for patient selection. Other developments include improved collimation, better emulsion characteristics of extra-oral films and more efficient intensifying screens using rare-earth phosphors. Arising from the recommendations of the International Commission for Radiation

Protection (ICRP), many countries have introduced legislation on radiation protection. This is based on the following principles:
• That doses should be kept as low as reasonably achievable (ALARA).
• That there should be a net benefit for the patient from the radiation exposure.

• That radiation doses should not exceed certain limits laid down by the ICRP.

The more recently introduced imaging techniques such as US and MRI do not use ionizing radiation and hence do not carry the risks associated with X-radiation.

Image formation

The most common method of image formation is the exposure of radiographic film to the X-rays after they have passed through the tissues. An X-ray film consists of a flexible transparent plastic base which is coated on either side with an emulsion of silver halide crystals suspended in gelatine. The emulsion is covered by a further protective layer of gelatine.

There are two types of film: direct exposure and screen film. Direct exposure, or non-screen, film is used for intra-oral radiography—the image is formed on the emulsion by the direct action of X-rays. Since it is also sensitive to light, it is sandwiched between two sheets of black paper and contained in a sealed packet to exclude light. Because some of the X-ray photons do not react with the emulsion and pass through the film, a sheet of lead foil is placed on the surface away from the X-ray source to protect the deeper tissue and reduce back scatter. A raised embossed dot on one corner of the film aids correct orientation during viewing. Direct exposure film is used for bitewing, periapical and occlusal radiography.

Screen film, which is used primarily for extra-oral radiography, is placed between two intensifying screens contained within a cassette. The intensifying screens fluoresce when exposed to X-radiation, emitting a blue or green light to which the film is sensitive. The emulsion of screen film contains dyes to increase the absorption of the specific wavelength of light emitted by the intensifying screen. The light is multidirectional and this results in some loss of definition of the image compared with direct

exposure film, but less radiation exposure is required to produce the image. To minimize the loss of definition, it is important that the gap between the film and the intensifying screen is as small as possible.

As the atomic composition and density of the tissues are variable, X-rays are absorbed to different degrees, allowing an image to be recorded on the film. A physicochemical change affects those silver halides which have been irradiated, resulting in the formation of a latent image. This image is made visible by reducing the altered silver halide grains to black metallic silver through the action of a developer solution. This process may be performed either manually or automatically, in accordance with the manufacturer's instructions. Correct temperature and immersion times are essential, after which the film is rinsed in water to wash off the surface alkaline developer before placing it in the acidic fixer solution. This arrests the development process and removes those silver halide crystals that were not affected by the developer solution. The film is then thoroughly washed in running water to remove any remaining processing chemicals absorbed into the emulsion. Because X-ray film is light sensitive, processing must be performed in a darkened room illuminated only by appropriate safe light conditions. Automatic processing is more rapid, and uses a system of rollers to transport the film through a series of solutions at a higher temperature, producing a dry film ready for viewing.

Intra-oral radiographs

The majority of dental radiographs are taken with the film placed in the mouth and consist of bitewing, periapical and occlusal radiographs.

Bitewing radiographs (BW)—so called because the patient stabilizes the film by occluding onto an attached tab or wing (5)—record the images of the crowns and the coronal portion of the roots of maxillary and mandibular posterior teeth and their investing tissues. The film is usually positioned with its long axis horizontal and parallel to the crowns of the teeth. The X-ray beam is directed with a downward angle of approximately 5–10° to the occlusal plane and at right angles to the film, passing between the contact points of the crowns of the teeth being examined so that their images do not overlap.

Periapical radiographs (P) record an image of the whole of the tooth

and its surrounding tissues. There are two techniques commonly used to obtain this image: the paralleling and the bisecting angle. In the paralleling technique (6), the film is placed parallel to the long axis of the teeth but may be some distance from them depending upon the curved shape of the alveolus. To prevent magnification of the image, a less divergent beam of X-rays is used, which is obtained by increasing the film focus distance. A relatively powerful dental X-ray unit is required since the intensity of the X-ray beam decreases as the distance from its source increases, as determined by the inverse square law. It is necessary to position the film by the use of a film holder; most examples incorporate a beam-aiming device to aid the correct alignment of the X-ray tube so that the beam is directed at right angles to the film.

The bisecting angle technique (**7**) is based on the principle of isosceles triangles where AB is the length of the object, BC is the length of the image and BD is the bisector of the triangle ABC. The film is placed in contact with the lingual or palatal aspects of the crowns of the teeth, but inclined away from their roots, according to the shape of the investing tissues. The operator determines the plane of the bisector and directs the X-ray beam at right angles to it, thus the length of the tooth AB will equal the length of its image BC projected onto the film. The image dimensions will alter if the beam is not directed at right angles to the bisector. For example, the image will be elongated if the X-ray beam is directed at right angles to the teeth, and it will be foreshortened if the beam is directed at right angles to the film. The film is placed as parallel as possible to the crowns of the teeth in the horizontal plane and the X-ray beam is directed at right angles to it (**8**).

In occlusal radiography, the film is larger than that used in periapical views and hence records a greater area. The film is placed as far back in the mouth as required and held gently by the patient between the occlusal surfaces of the teeth. Occlusal radiographs can be divided into two groups: those that provide an image similar to that obtained on periapical radiographs; and those on which a plan view is obtained. The first group includes the upper standard (anterior) occlusal (USO), the upper oblique occlusal (UOO), the lower anterior occlusal (LAO) and the lower oblique occlusal (LOO). The second group includes the upper true occlusal (UTO) which provides a plan view of the upper posterior teeth, the vertex occlusal (VO) which demonstrates the upper incisor teeth in plan view, and the lower true occlusal (LTO) which gives a plan view of the lower posterior teeth.

Occlusal radiographs are used, for example, in the assessment of unerupted teeth and in the examination of expansile lesions of the alveolus. In some upper views, structures of the facial skeleton may be superimposed upon the dento-alveolar image. In the case of the vertex occlusal, where the beam passes through much of the anterior facial skeleton, screen film is placed inside a cassette with intensifying screens to minimize the patient dose, although this may result in some loss of definition. Occlusal or periapical films (S) placed intra- or extra-orally may also be used to detect foreign bodies in the perioral soft tissues.

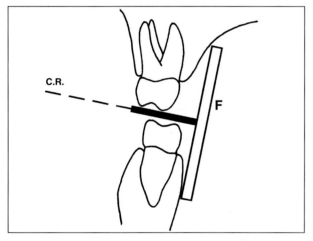

5 The bitewing technique in which the film (**F**) is held in place by occluding on a tab: CR, central ray of the X-ray beam.

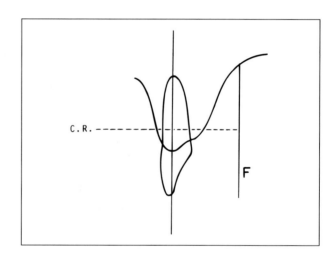

6 The paralleling technique for taking intra-oral radiographs: CR, central ray of the X-ray beam; F, film.

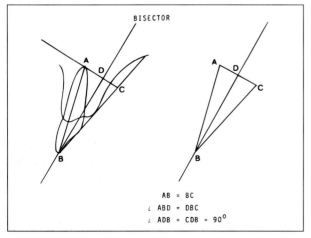

7 The bisecting angle technique for taking intra-oral radiographs (see text).

$$AB = BC$$
$$\angle ABD = DBC$$
$$\angle ADB = CDB = 90°$$

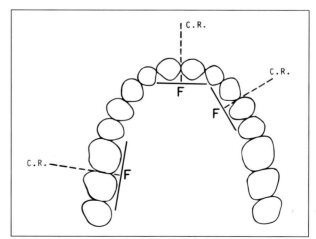

8 The alignment of the X-ray beam relative to the teeth in intra-oral radiographs: CR, central ray of the X-ray beam; F, film.

Parallax

A radiograph demonstrates a three-dimensional object on a flat plane. Therefore, when superimposition of two or more structures occurs, it is not always possible to determine their spatial relationships (**9**). This information can be obtained by employing the principle of parallax, by examining radiographs taken at right angles to one another, or by tomography (see p.[13]), the method of choice being determined by the particular circumstances. The parallax or tube shift technique involves taking two radiographic views of the same area with the film similarly positioned for both exposures, but with either a different horizontal or vertical angulation of the X-ray tube. Structures lying in different planes will appear to move in relation to one another. A structure positioned closer to the X-ray tube moves in the opposite direction to that taken by the tube relative to a structure placed nearer to the film. Conversely, an object lying closer to the film appears to move in the same direction as that taken by the tube, relative to a structure positioned closer to it.

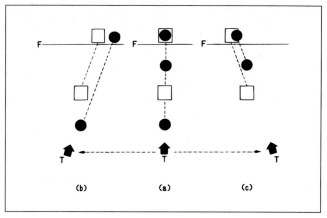

9 The principle of parallax. When two objects are superimposed, it is not possible to be certain if the reference object (✓) is nearer or further from the film (F) than the object of interest (●). If the object of interest is closer to the tube (T), it moves in the opposite direction relative to the reference object. If the object of interest is further from the tube, it moves in the same direction as the reference object.

Extra-oral radiographs

When the area to be examined is larger than can be accommodated on intra-oral radiographs, it is necessary to place the film outside the mouth so that a film of appropriate size can be used. For skull and maxillofacial radiography, X-ray machines which are more powerful and versatile than the dental X-ray set are required. All extra-oral radiographic projections should be performed using screen film in a cassette containing the appropriate intensifying screens. Unlike intra-oral film, screen film does not have a means of identification for correct orientation, thus radio-opaque markers such as lead 'L' or 'R' identification letters are usually placed on the outside of the cassette, the symbol appearing on the processed radiograph. In addition, details of the date and the patient's identification are added to the film by means of actinic markers.

When larger masses of tissue are exposed to X-rays, the amount of scattered radiation arising from them becomes greater. For radiography of the skull and facial bones, therefore, grids are used as the scattered radiation is likely to result in film fogging. The grid, which is placed between the object and the film, consists of a radiolucent plastic base with a series of fine, linear, parallel lead slats which are so angled as to allow the primary beam, but not the scattered radiation, to pass between them (**10**). These grids may be stationary or moveable (e.g. Potter Bucky). The former cast a shadow of fine lines on the film, but this problem is overcome with a moveable grid. Whilst grids prevent loss of contrast from film fogging, the exposure needs to be increased and thus the patient receives a slightly higher dose of radiation.

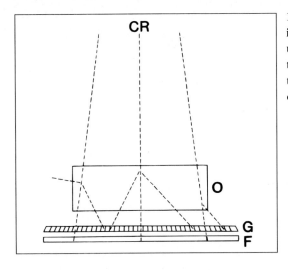

10 A diagram of a grid illustrating how only undeviated rays reach the film: CR, centre of the X-ray beam; O, object; G, grid; F, film.

For accurate positioning of the head and the X-ray tube relative to the film, the radiographer uses visible or palpable anatomical landmarks and planes. These include the interpupillary line, the radiographic base line (orbitomeatal line), the Frankfort plane (the anthropological line) and the median sagittal plane (**11**). The patient is prepared by removing radio-opaque objects such as ear-rings and necklaces. The area of interest is placed closest to the film and the head immobilized by the use of radiolucent sponges when necessary. Whilst it is beyond the scope of this book to cover in detail the full range of extra-oral radiographic views depicted in the following chapters, an outline of some of the more common projections will now be described to assist with the radiological interpretation.

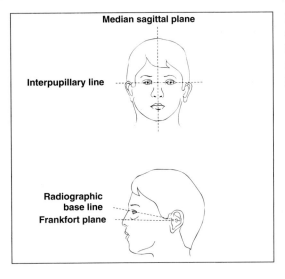

11 Some useful anatomical planes and landmarks used in radiographic positioning.

Dental panoramic radiography

This is shown in **12**. A dental panoramic radiograph displays, on a single film, both sides of the mandible and maxilla, together with a number of other cervicofacial anatomical structures including the maxillary antra. Originally, panoramic radiographs were achieved by placing a curved film lingually within the mouth and rotating an external slit-beam X-ray source in one plane around the patient's jaws. Subsequent development has retained the slit beam source but used two, three and finally continuously moving centres of rotation. The X-ray tube and film holder rotate around the patient's head, and the film moves behind a slit guard so exposing it a portion at a time. This technique produces an image which corresponds to the dental arches; the image layer (or focal trough) is of variable thickness, being narrower anteriorly due to the close proximity of the anterior part of the jaws to the centre of rotation. Objects in the centre of the focal trough will appear sharp, whereas those lying closer to the centre of rotation appear widened and less definite. Objects that are closer to the film, i.e. on the vestibular side of the jaws, appear narrowed and less distinct. Computer driven panoramic machines have increased the range of projections available for imaging the jaws, temporomandibular joints and maxillary sinuses.

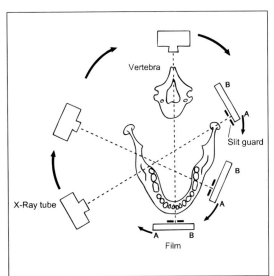

12 Diagrammatic representation of panoramic radiography showing the relative positions of the X-ray tube and the film AB. Note how the slit guard moves across the film during the exposure cycle.

Panoramic zonography (Z)

Zonography uses the principles of panoramic radiography to record an image layer or a number of image layers of bony structures of the head and neck. The Zonarc machine is designed so that the image depth can be varied as well as the image thickness. As a consequence, in addition to a dental panoramic view, it is possible to image other parts of the facial skeleton, the middle ear, the cervical spine, the optic foramina and the temporomandibular joints.

Oblique lateral mandible radiograph (OLM)

This is shown in **13**. This projection demonstrates one side of the body and ramus of the mandible, together with part of the maxilla. The view is 'obliqued' to overcome the problems of superimposition of one side of the mandible upon the other. The film is positioned against the upper and lower jaws, on the side to be examined, the head being turned to bring the area of interest parallel to the film. It is important that the chin is extended to draw the mandible away from the cervical vertebrae. The X-ray tube is centred just below and posterior to the angle of the mandible of the contralateral side and is angled obliquely upwards so that the central ray passes between the ramus of the mandible and the cervical spine to the appropriate part of the mandible on the contralateral side.

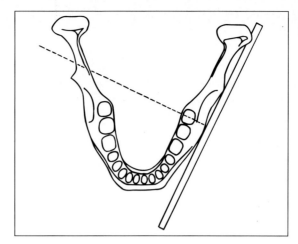

13 Oblique lateral mandible view.

Lateral skull radiograph (L)

This is shown in **14**. In this projection, the patient's head is positioned with the sagittal plane parallel to, and the interpupillary line perpendicular to, the film. The X-ray tube is centred over the ears and directed at right angles to the film. There is, therefore, superimposition of both sides of the skull, facial bones and mandible. For the the lateral facial bones the beam is centred over the infra-orbital margin, as illustrated in the figure.

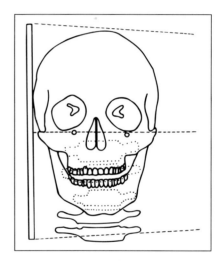

14 Lateral skull view.

Cephalometry (LC)

This is shown in **15**. For the assessment of facial growth, and the planning of orthodontic treatment and maxillofacial surgery, accurate skull measurements are required. These are obtained in a standardized form from cephalometric radiographs, which are taken under reproducible conditions of relationships between the X-ray tube, the patient and the film. The patient's head is located in a specially designed holder—the craniostat—which incorporates an earplug fitting into each external auditory meatus so that the head is correctly centred. The craniostat may also have a calibrated nasal support to assist with head alignment and film analysis. The film holder and the X-ray tube are placed at a fixed distance from the craniostat. By the use of appropriate X-ray beam filtration, the soft tissues (S) of the facial profile may also be demonstrated. It is possible to perform cephalometry in a postero-anterior direction by rotating the craniostat through 90° so that the patient faces the film. The central ray now passes at right angles to the porionic axis.

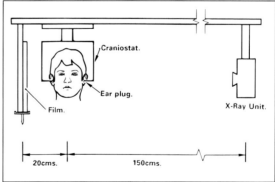

15 Diagrammatic representation of the relative positions of the craniostat, film and X-ray unit used in cephalometry. The figures indicate the standard distances between these elements.

Occipitomental skull radiograph (OM)

This is shown in **16**. In this view the patient's head is inclined upwards so that the image of the base of the skull is projected away from that of the middle third of the face. The patient faces the film with the head adjusted so that the radiographic baseline is at 45° to, and the median sagittal plane at right angles to, the film. The X-ray beam is directed from the external occipital protuberance to the lower orbital margins and is perpendicular to the film.

Modifications of this view direct the beam at 15°, 30° (OM 30°) or 45° caudally to the horizontal.

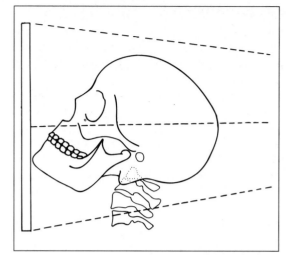

16   Occipitomental view.

Postero-anterior skull radiographs (PA)

This is shown in **17**. In this view the patient's forehead and nose are in contact with the film. The head is adjusted so that the radiographic base line and the midsagittal plane are perpendicular to it. The X-ray beam is directed at right angles to the film, being central just below the nasion. This projection demonstrates the frontal bones, the pituitary fossa, the ethmoid air sinuses and the nasal fossae. There are several modifications of this view, one of which is to angle the tube 12° in a caudal direction so that the petrous ridges partly occlude the orbits. Another, to demonstrate the mandibular condyles, is taken with the mouth open and the beam angled 12° cephalad (PAC). A third modification, to demonstrate parotid duct stones, involves rotation of the patient's head to bring the lateral aspect of the jaws tangential to the direction of the X-ray beam (RPA).

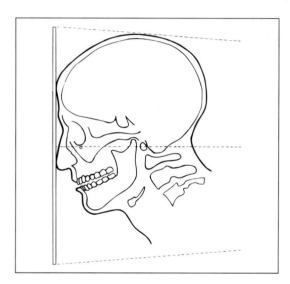

17   Postero-anterior view.

Submentovertex (base view) skull radiograph (SMV)

This is shown in **18**. To obtain this view the neck is fully extended so that the vertex of the head touches the film with the radiographic baseline parallel to, and the median sagittal plane at right angles to, the film. The beam is centred midway between the angles of the mandible and directed 5° in a cephalad direction. This view demonstrates the base of the skull, the petrous ridges and the sphenoidal sinuses. A modification of the technique employing a reduction of the exposure factors is used to demonstrate the zygomatic arches.

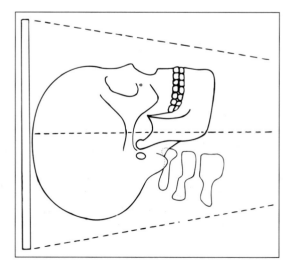

18   Submentovertex (base) view.

30° Fronto-occipital (Towne's view) skull radiograph (T)

This is shown in **19**. In this projection, the patient is positioned facing away from the film with both the radiographic baseline and the median sagittal plane at right angles to it. The X-ray tube is angled 30° caudally, so that the centre of the beam is directed to pass 5 cm above the glabella and emerge via the foramen magnum. To demonstrate the condylar necks of the mandible, the beam is angled 35° caudally and the patient's mouth is opened widely, as in the figure.

Transcranial radiograph of the temporomandibular joint (TMJ)

This is shown in **20**. This technique demonstrates oblique views of the glenoid fossa and mandibular condylar head. Several variations of this projection have been described, some of which compensate for the oblique orientation of the joints to the mid-sagittal plane. Typically, the patient's head is positioned with the interpupillary line at right angles to, and the mid-sagittal plane parallel to, the film. The X-ray tube is angled 25° caudally and 20° anteriorly on the contralateral side so that the centre of the beam passes through the joint adjacent to the film. Two exposures are made of each joint, one with the patient in centric occlusion and the other with the mouth wide open. An additional radiograph is sometimes taken with the jaws slightly parted in the rest position.

Temporomandibular joint arthrography (TMJA)

Whilst plain radiography and tomography demonstrate the osseous components of the temporomandibular joint, they provide little information about the soft tissue structures such as the position of the articular disc. In temporomandibular joint arthrography, a radio-opaque contrast medium is injected into one or both joint compartments. This dynamic study demonstrates joint function and in particular the position of the disc during the various phases of jaw opening. In addition, abnormalities such as disc perforation may be revealed. The procedure is usually performed under fluoroscopic control and the images may be stored on videotape.

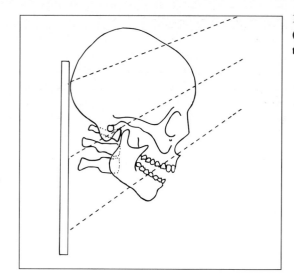

19 35° fronto-occipital (Towne's) view with the mouth open.

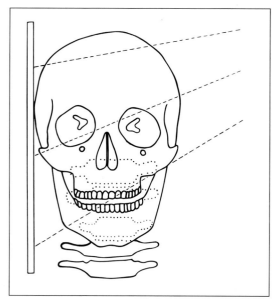

20 Transcranial view of the temporomandibular joint.

23

Tomography (TG)

This technique (**21**) demonstrates selected planes of part of the body by blurring out structures in other planes. This involves movement of the X-ray tube and film, which are connected so as to rotate about a pivot. They move in opposite directions about a stationary object so that there is a fixed plane at which there is no relative movement between them (the pivot point). This plane is referred to as the tomographic cut; Structures in adjacent planes are blurred due to movement and therefore not visualized. The thickness of the tomographic cut (or plane) is determined by the angle of travel taken by the X-ray tube, a small angle producing a thicker layer, a large angle a thinner. The position of the tomographic layer depends upon the relative movement of the tube and the film.

The simplest form of movement involves the X-ray tube and the film moving synchronously in straight lines in opposite directions. This is referred to as linear tomography. This may result in streaking of the radiograph due to false shadows from dense structures lying just outside the image layer which are not completely blurred out. The problem may be overcome by using more complex tube film movements such as circular, elliptical, spiral and hypocycloidial. By taking a series of adjacent tomograms in parallel planes, a composite image of a tissue or organ can be obtained. Tomography can also be performed by using a multiplanar cassette which contains several sets of intensifying screens of different speeds placed one upon the other.

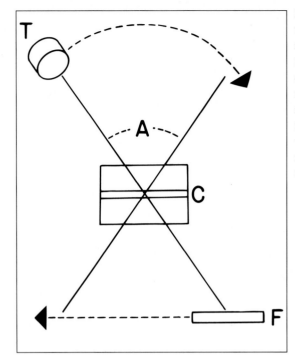

21 The principle of tomography. The X-ray tube (T) and film (F) rotate in opposite directions around a fixed plane (C) which remains in focus. The thickness of the plane visualized is determined by the angle of travel (A) of the tube.

Sialography

Sialography is a technique whereby a radio-opaque contrast medium is injected into the main parotid or submandibular salivary gland duct via a cannula, in order to demonstrate the anatomy of the duct system. Either water-soluble or oil-based media are used and may be introduced by a hand-held syringe, a hydrostatic pressure technique, or by means of a constant infusion pump. Radiographs are taken when the ducts are fully occluded by the contrast medium, with the cannula left *in situ* to prevent leakage. Initially only the duct system is delineated but with continued injection acinar filling is observed. The latter may assist in the detection of space occupying lesions. Following removal of the cannula, a post-evacuation radiograph may be taken to assess glandular emptying (clearance view).

Scintiscanning (SC)

Radioactive materials are used in a number of diagnostic imaging investigations when they are referred to as radiopharmaceuticals or radionuclides. One of the most commonly used radiopharmaceuticals is the metastable isomer technetium (^{99m}Tc). This radionuclide is obtained from a molybdenum–technetium generator as technetium pertechnetate. It has a short half-life of six hours and emits a gamma ray with an energy of 140 keV which falls within the energy range suitable for diagnostic imaging. As pertechnetate is metabolized by the the salivary and thyroid glands, it is suitable for imaging these organs. The selection of other radiolabelled compounds which are preferentially metabolized by other organs, allows them also to be imaged. For example, phosphate compounds (e.g. ^{99m}Tc methylene diphosphonate) which are concentrated in the skeleton, and sulphur colloid which is metabolized by the liver, facilitate the imaging of these structures. Functional information about an organ can be obtained if the change in the level of radioactivity of that organ is plotted against time in a time/activity curve.

Ultrasonography (US)

Diagnostic ultrasound imaging relies on high-frequency, mechanical vibrations which are transmitted through the tissues. These are produced by a transducer constructed of a piezoelectric material, such as lead zirconate titanate (PZT), which converts electrical signals into sound-waves which are transmitted into the tissues as a series of pulses. The transducer also receives those sound-waves which are reflected back from the tissues and reconverts them into electrical signals for processing into an image. The frequencies used for diagnostic ultrasound range from 1 to 20 megahertz (MHz), typically 3 to 7 MHz, well above the audible range. As sound travels through the tissues it loses energy by absorption, but a small proportion of the sound is reflected back from the boundaries of tissues which have different acoustic impedances (resistances), the remainder continuing deeper into the tissues. The reflected waves are received by the transducer and displayed on a monitor and recorded. Air and bone do not readily transmit ultrasound waves hence limiting the usefulness of ultrasound imaging in the maxillofacial region. It is, however, of value in the examination of space occupying lesions in the soft tissues, including for example the parotid gland.

No detectable, hazardous biological effects have as yet been demonstrated with ultrasound below a peak intensity of 100 mW cm^{-2} and the vast majority of such diagnostic apparatus operates below this threshold level. It is therefore a safe alternative to the use of ionizing radiation for the detection of tumours involving the soft tissues.

Computerized tomography (CT)

Computerized—or computed—tomography is an imaging system in which information received by a series of X-ray detectors is digitized and converted mathematically into a grey scale image. The X-ray-generating apparatus produces a number of tightly-collimated, highly-filtered X-ray beams which traverse the patient. The attenuated beams are then received by a series of detectors which convert this information into electrical impulses, each of which is proportional to the amount of radiation received. These data are fed into a computer which generates an image consisting of a matrix of pixels, each one representing the attenuation value of the radiation at a particular point.

Most examinations are performed with the patient in the supine position; a localizing view, or scanogram, is obtained from which the area to be recorded, and the number of slices required, is determined. Scans are recorded in the axial direction but direct coronal scans of the head and neck region can also be performed by extending the patients neck and tilting the gantry of the CT apparatus. Alternatively, scans in the coronal and sagittal planes may be obtained by reformatting contiguous axial scans, although this procedure results in some loss of detail. It is also possible to generate three-dimensional images which may be of value in the assessment of abnormalities of the facial skeleton arising during development or from trauma. CT, with or without the administration of intravenous contrast media, is helpful in the evaluation of soft tissue lesions.

Attenuation values, or Hounsfield numbers, have been allocated to different tissues according to their densities, that for air being -1000, for water 0 and for dense compact bone +1000. By setting the window level to the appropriate value and the window width to a range of values, it is possible to display both soft tissues and bone (or simply the bony tissues) on the same tomogram.

Artefacts can occur either from the apparatus itself as ring artefacts or emanate from the patient through movement or the presence of metallic or other high-density objects such as amalgam restorations.

Magnetic resonance imaging (MRI)

Magnetic resonance imaging is a technique which uses a combination of magnetic fields and radiofrequency waves to generate images of the body. As with CT, the images can be restricted to narrow planes and so multisectional views of the head and neck may be obtained.

Human tissues consist of molecules containing hydrogen nuclei (protons). Each proton has an axial spin and, because of its charge, behaves like a small magnet (22a). Normally the protons are randomly arranged (22b); however, when the patient is placed in a strong magnetic field (B), the direction of spin of the protons aligns with that of the field (22c). In addition, the protons precess or wobble with a frequency determined by the strength of the magnetic field, but out of phase with each other. The application of a pulsed, resonant, radiofrequency causes the protons to be deflected from their alignment and to precess in phase. With cessation of the radiofrequency, the protons realign with the applied magnetic field by transferring their acquired energy to their surroundings and revert to precessing out of phase. The rate at which the protons realign is referred to as the T_1 relaxation time; the T_2 relaxation time is the period in which protons remain in phase before returning to a random pattern. The energy released by the relaxation of the hydrogen nuclei is converted into a visual image. The introduction of paramagnetic contrast agents, which act by shortening the T_1 relaxation times, improves the detection of tumour masses.

25

Diagnostic MRI has the following advantages:
• It allows multiplanar imaging.
• There are no known harmful effects.
• It has better soft tissue contrast compared with CT.

However, it does have some limitations. Bone is not well displayed as it has a low signal intensity and it may be contraindicated in patients with ferromagnetic surgical clips and cardiac pacemakers.

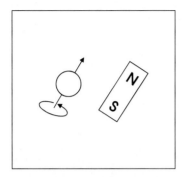

22a A diagrammatic representation of the influence of a powerful magnetic field on the tissue hydrogen nuclei in nuclear magnetic resonance (see text).

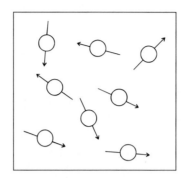

22b A diagrammatic representation of the influence of a powerful magnetic field on the tissue hydrogen nuclei in nuclear magnetic resonance (see text).

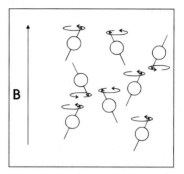

22c A diagrammatic representation of the influence of a powerful magnetic field on the tissue hydrogen nuclei in nuclear magnetic resonance (see text).

2

Normal radiographic anatomy

Introduction

Knowledge and understanding of the radiographic appearances of normal anatomical structures is essential for radiological interpretation. Whilst overall there is little fundamental difference between individuals in normal radiological anatomy, from time to time there are variations that can cause confusion in diagnosis and which may simulate pathological entities. On the other hand, variation in the projection geometry of the X-ray beam relative to the film, or unanticipated superimposition effects, may result in the failure to image a structure normally present on radiographs taken in the same anatomical location. Furthermore, some anatomical structures may alter with age, although the rate at which these changes occur varies from individual to individual. Outstanding examples are the developing dentition and the changes in bone density and remodelling of the alveolus that follow tooth extraction. Because there are some minor variations of detail between individuals, it is not practical to demonstrate the complete range of radiological appearances presented by normal anatomical structures. However, this chapter illustrates those most commonly seen, together with some variations from the normal. With many of the extra-oral techniques, it is now conventional clinical practice to use a collimated X-ray beam to expose only the fields of interest to irradiation. However, in many of the views illustrated, films taken before this practice was introduced have been chosen deliberately in order to illustrate the anatomical features more clearly.

The dentate jaws

Bitewing radiograph

23 A bitewing radiograph, BW. This demonstrates the lack of overlap of the contact points of contiguous teeth, the normal relationship between the alveolar crest and the amelocemental junctions of the adjacent teeth, and the arrangement of the trabeculae in the interdental septa, which are horizontal in the lower jaw. E: enamel; B: dentine; P: pulp chamber; L: periodontal ligament space; D: lamina dura; A: alveolar crest; R: root canal.

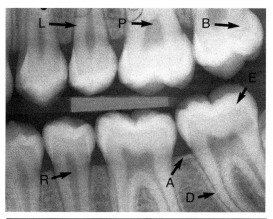

Periapical radiograph

<small>MAXILLARY TEETH – PARALLELING TECHNIQUE</small>
24 The pathway of the X-ray beam and the anatomical features that commonly appear on a maxillary incisor periapical radiograph taken by the paralleling technique. N: floor of the nose; A: anterior nasal spine; F: incisive foramen.

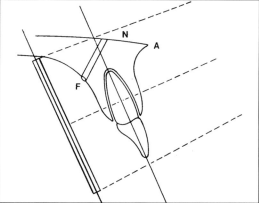

25 Periapical – P – ⌊123 region, paralleling technique. I: incisive canal; A: alveolar crest line.

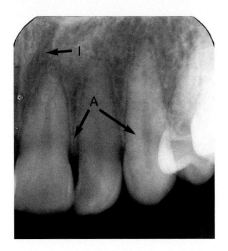

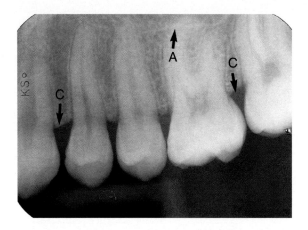

26 Periapical – P – ⌊456 region, paralleling technique. C: alveolar crest line; A: floor of the antrum.

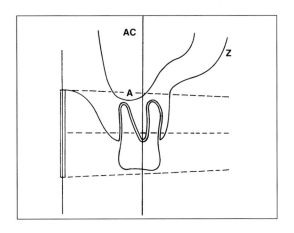

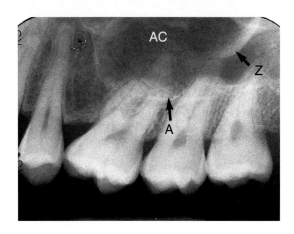

28 Periapical – P – ⌊678 region, paralleling technique. A: floor of the antrum; AC: antral cavity; Z: root of the zygoma.

27 The pathway of the X-ray beam and some of the anatomical features that commonly appear on a maxillary molar periapical film taken by the paralleling technique. The diagram demonstrates how the X-ray beam is directed below the root of the zygoma so that its image is not superimposed upon that of the roots of the adjacent molars. Further, there is minimal foreshortening of the image of the buccal roots of the molars compared with the bisecting angle technique. AC: antral cavity; A: floor of the antrum; Z: root of the zygoma.

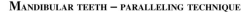

MANDIBULAR TEETH – PARALLELING TECHNIQUE

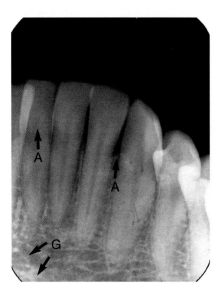

29 Periapical – P – ⌈123 region, paralleling technique. A: alveolar crest line; G: genial tubercles.

30 Periapical – P – 2345 region, paralleling technique. A: alveolar crest line; F: mental foramen; H: film holder.

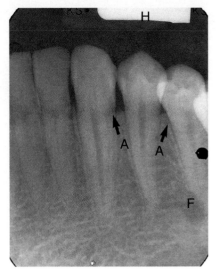

31 Periapical – P – 5 78 region, paralleling technique. O: oblique ridge; I: inferior cortical plate; C: inferior alveolar canal; F: mental foramen; A: alveolar crest line. Note that 6 is absent.

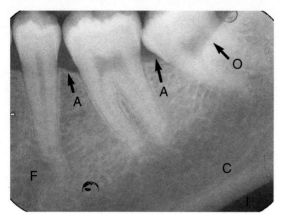

MAXILLARY TEETH – BISECTING ANGLE TECHNIQUE

32 The pathway of the X-ray beam and some of the anatomical features that commonly appear on a maxillary incisor periapical film taken by the bisecting angle technique. N: floor of the nose; A: anterior nasal spine; F: incisive foramen.

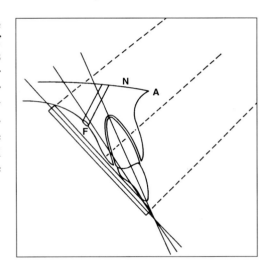

33 Periapical – P – 21|12 region. E: enamel; P: pulp chamber; R: root canal; A: root apex; D: lamina dura; L: periodontal ligament space; M: anterior midline suture; C: cingulum; I: incisal edge. The unlabelled arrowheads indicate the incisive foramen.

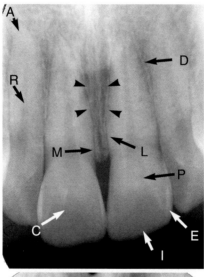

34 Periapical – P – 21|12 region, bisecting angle technique, demonstrating the trabecular pattern of the alveolar bone. N: lateral margin of the floor of the nose; S: nasal septum; NC: nasal cavity; T: inferior turbinates, covered with soft tissue; M: anterior midline suture.

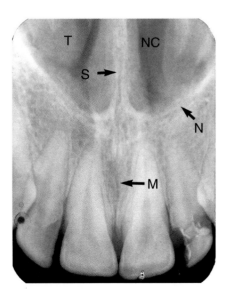

35 Periapical – P – 21|12 region, bisecting angle technique. N: lateral margin of the floor of the nose; S: nasal septum; NC: nasal cavity; F: incisive foramen; A: anterior nasal spine; M: anterior midline suture; T: soft tissue outline of the nose.

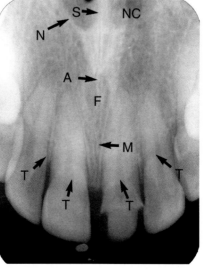

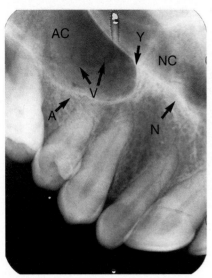

36 Periapical – P – 54321⌋ region, bisecting angle technique. A: floor of the antrum; AC: antral cavity; V: vascular canals in the antral wall; N: floor of the nose; NC: nasal cavity; Y: point of confluence of the structures making up the Y formation of Ennis, i.e. lateral margin of the floor of the nose and anterior part of the floor of the maxillary antrum.

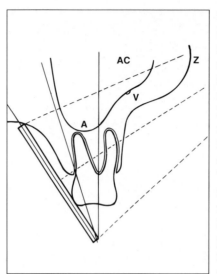

37 The pathway of the X-ray beam and some of the anatomical features that commonly appear on a maxillary molar periapical film taken by the bisecting angle technique. In this technique, the X-ray beam passes through the root of the zygoma so that its image is superimposed upon that of the roots of the adjacent molars. The image of the buccal roots of the posterior teeth tends to be foreshortened so that their apices lie at a lower level than that of the palatal roots. AC: antral cavity; A: floor of the antrum; V: vascular canal in the antral wall; Z: root of the zygoma.

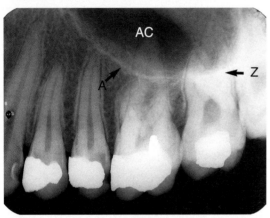

38 Periapical – P – ⌊345678 region, bisecting angle technique. A: floor of the antrum; AC: antral cavity; Z: root of the zygoma.

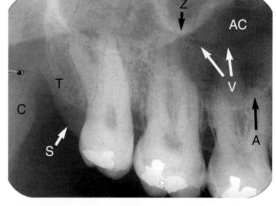

39 Periapical – P – 876⌋ region, bisecting angle technique. A: floor of the antrum; AC: antral cavity; Z: root of the zygoma; C: coronoid process of the mandible; T: maxillary tuberosity with mucosal covering; V: vascular canals in the antral wall; S: soft tissue outline of the tuberosity mucosa.

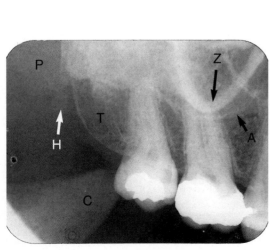

40 Periapical – P – 87⌋ region, bisecting angle technique. A: floor of the antrum; Z: root of the zygoma; T: maxillary tuberosity with mucosal covering; H: pterygoid hamulus; P: pterygoid plates; C: coronoid process of the mandible.

MANDIBULAR TEETH – BISECTING ANGLE TECHNIQUE

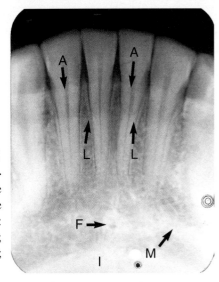

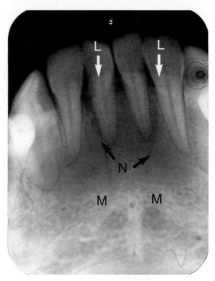

41 Periapical – P – 321̄|̄123 region, bisecting angle technique. This demonstrates the spiny interdental crests and the trabecular pattern of the bone. M: mental ridge; F: lingual foramen; L: lip line; A: alveolar crest line; I: inferior cortical plate.

42 Periapical – P – 321̄|̄123 region, bisecting angle technique. N: Hirschfield's nutrient (vascular) canals; L: lip line; M: mental ridge.

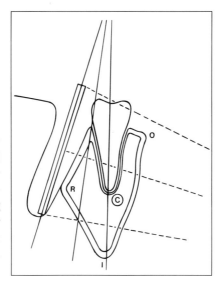

43 Periapical – P – |̄12345 region, bisecting angle technique. This demonstrates the trabecular pattern of the bone. A: alveolar crest line; I: inferior cortical plate.

44 The pathway of the X-ray beam and some of the anatomical features that commonly appear on a mandibular molar periapical film, taken by the bisecting angle technique. C: inferior alveolar canal; O: oblique ridge; R: mylohyoid ridge; I: inferior cortical plate.

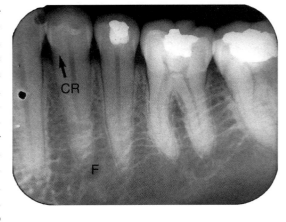

45 Periapical – P – |̄34567 region, bisecting angle technique. This demonstrates the plateau form of the interdental crests and the horizontal distribution of the trabeculae in the alveolar bone, both interdentally and interradicularly. F: mental foramen; CR: cervical radiolucency due to the relative contrast between – on the one hand – the enamel covered crown superiorly and the bone-invested part of the root inferiorly, and – on the other hand – the cervical part of the root, which is covered by neither.

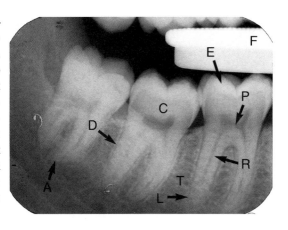

46 Periapical – P – 876| region, bisecting angle technique. E: enamel; P: pulp chamber; R: root canal; T: bony trabeculae in the interdental septum; L: periodontal ligament space; D: lamina dura; A: root apex; C: coronal dentine; F: film holder.

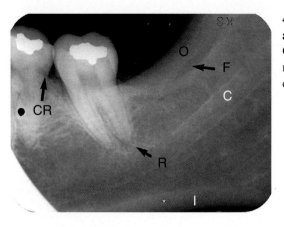

47 Periapical – P – ⌐78 region, bisecting angle technique. C: inferior alveolar canal; O: oblique ridge; R: mylohyoid ridge; F: retromolar fossa; I: inferior cortical plate; CR: cervical radiolucency.

Occlusal radiograph

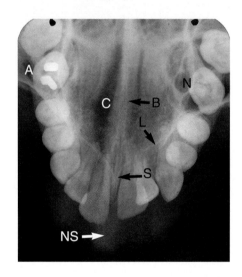

48 Upper standard (anterior) occlusal, USO. N: nasolacrimal canal; A: maxillary antrum; L: lateral margin of the floor of the nose; C: nasal cavity; S: anterior nasal spine; B: nasal septum; NS: soft tissue of the nose.

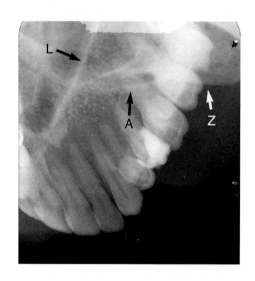

49 Upper oblique occlusal, UOO. L: lateral margin of the floor of the nose; Z: root of zygoma; A: floor of the maxillary antrum.

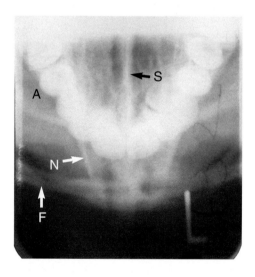

50 Upper vertex occlusal, VO. F: frontal bone; N: nasal bones; A: maxillary antrum; S: nasal septum.

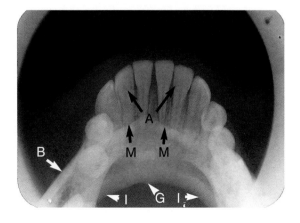

51 Lower anterior occlusal, LAO. M: mental ridge; G: genial tubercle; A: alveolar crest line; I: inferior cortical plate; B: buccal cortical plate.

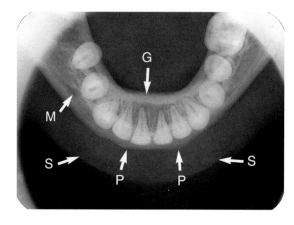

52 Lower true occlusal, LTO. M: mental foramen; S: outline of the soft tissues of the lip and chin; G: genial tubercle; P: mental protruberance.

Dental panoramic radiograph

53 Dental panoramic radiograph – DPR – of the jaws of an adult.

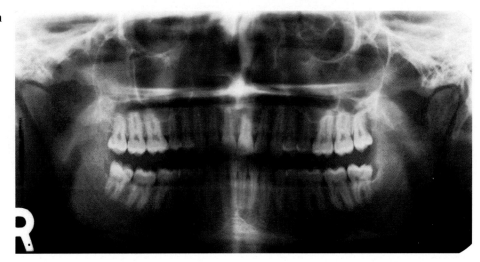

54 Line drawing of 53. 1: orbital cavity; 2: nasal cavity and turbinates; 3: nasal septum; 4: maxillary antrum; 5: root of the zygoma; 6: zygomatic arch; 7: styloid process; 8: glenoid fossa; 9: head of the mandibular condyle; 10: coronoid process of the mandible; 11: hard palate; 12: soft palate (dotted outline); 13: nasopharynx (dotted outline); 14: oropharynx (dotted outline); 15: pharyngeal air space (dotted outline); 16: pinna of the ear; 17: inferior alveolar canal; 18: mental foramen; 19: hyoid bone; 20: epiglottis (dotted outline).

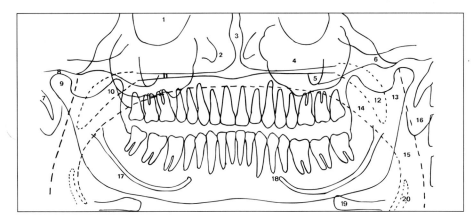

55 DPR of the jaws of a six-year-old. There is considerable variation between individuals in the pattern and chronology of tooth eruption but **55–59** illustrate a commonly occurring sequence. In this child, all the teeth of the primary dentition are erupted and present. All the first permanent molars are erupting into the oral cavity and the remainder of the permanent teeth, apart from the third molars, are unerupted and at various stages of development.

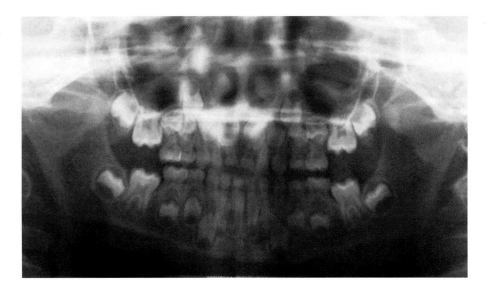

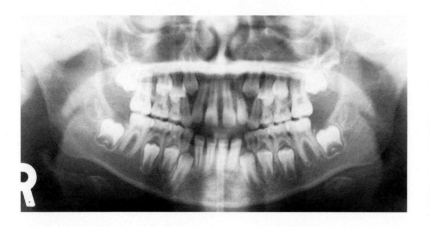

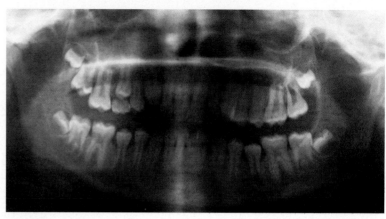

56 DPR of the jaws of a nine-year-old. All the permanent incisors and first molars are erupted, the primary incisors having been shed. The primary canines and molars are still present, their roots being at progressive stages of resorption owing to the development of the underlying permanent canines and premolars. Crown formation is complete in the second permanent molars and is just commencing in the third molars.

57 DPR of the jaws of a 12-year-old. All the permanent teeth, apart from the third molars and 5⌋, are erupted. Of the primary dentition, only E⌋ remains. Development of the roots of the canines, premolars and second molars and of the crowns of the third molars is still incomplete.

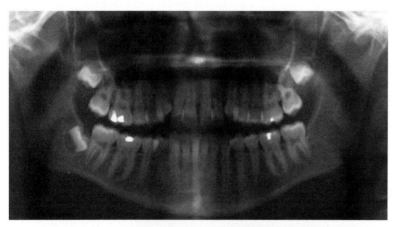

58 DPR of the jaws of a 15-year-old. The root development of most erupted teeth is now complete and is about to commence on the third molars. Note the absence of ⌊8 .

Oblique lateral mandible radiograph

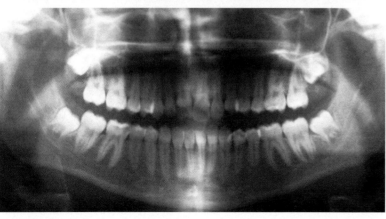

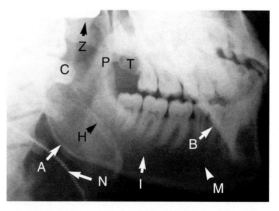

59 DPR of the jaws of an 18-year-old. Root development of all the erupted teeth is complete. The third molars, in which root formation is approximately half complete, are close to eruption into the oral cavity.

60 Oblique lateral mandible, OLM. M: mental foramen; I: inferior alveolar canal; H: hyoid bone; A: angle of the mandible; C: cervical vertebra obscuring the condylar process of the mandible; Z: zygomatic arch; P: coronoid process; T: maxillary tuberosity; B: inferior border of the opposite side of the mandible; N: metal necklace.

The edentulous jaws

Periapical radiograph

MAXILLA

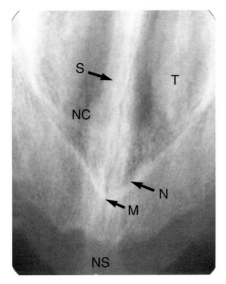

61 Periapical – P – anterior region of edentulous maxilla. N: floor of the nose; S: nasal septum (bony and cartilaginous portions); T: inferior turbinate bones covered with soft tissue; NC: nasal cavity; M: anterior midline suture; NS: soft tissue of the nose.

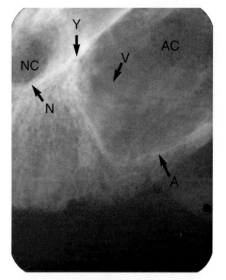

62 Periapical – P – left premolar region of edentulous maxilla. N: floor of the nose; NC: nasal cavity; A: floor of the antrum; AC: antral cavity; Y: Y formation of Ennis; V: vascular canals in the lateral wall of the antrum.

MANDIBLE

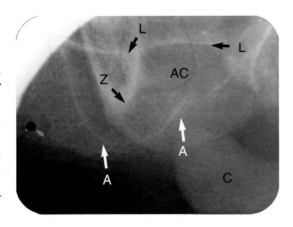

63 Periapical – P – left molar region of edentulous maxilla. A: floor of the antrum; AC: antral cavity; Z: root of the zygoma; C: coronoid process; L: lateral margin of the floor of the nose.

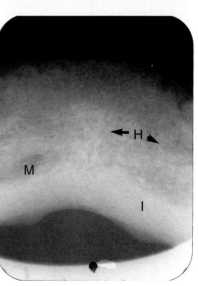

64 Periapical – P – incisor region of edentulous mandible. H: nutrient canals (Hirschfield's canals); I: inferior cortical plate of the mandible; M: mental ridge.

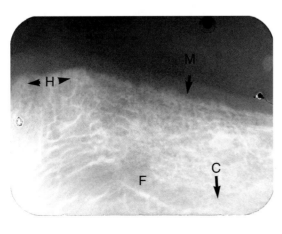

65 Periapical – P – left premolar region of edentulous mandible. H: nutrient canals (Hirschfield's canals); F: mental foramen; C: inferior alveolar canal; M: ridge mucosa.

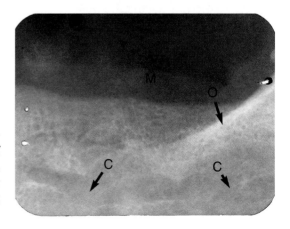

66 Periapical – P – left molar region of edentulous mandible. C: inferior alveolar canal; O: oblique ridge; M: ridge mucosa.

35

Occlusal radiograph

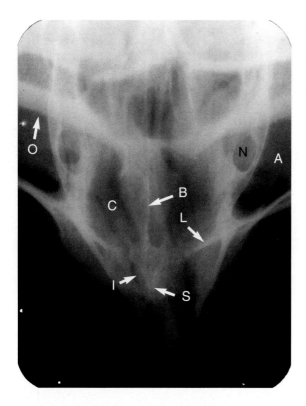

67 Upper true occlusal, UTO. N: naso-lacrimal canal; A: maxillary antrum; L: lateral margin of the floor of the nose; S: anterior nasal spine; I: incisive foramen; C: nasal cavity; B: nasal septum; O: infra-orbital margin.

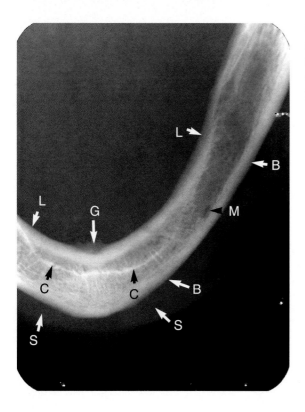

68 Lower true occlusal of one side of the mandible, LTO. M: mental foramen; G: genial tubercle; S: soft tissues of the lip and chin; C: crest of the alveolar ridge; B: buccal cortical plate; L: lingual cortical plate.

69 Dental panoramic radiograph – DPR – of the edentulous jaws. Following extraction of the teeth there has been resorption of much of the alveolar bone so that the antral floor and inferior alveolar canal on each side of the jaws become closer to the crest of the bony ridge. In addition, some soft tissue images – often obscured by the teeth – become more obvious. L: lip line; N: nasolabial fold.

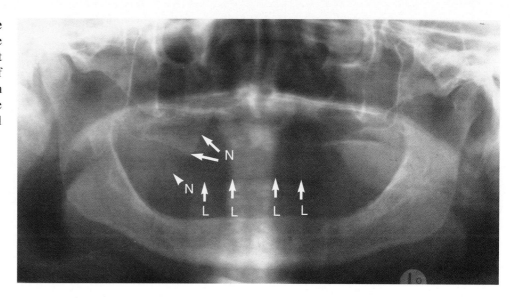

70 Oblique lateral mandible – OLM – of an edentulous jaw. C: condylar process; P: coronoid process; O: oblique ridge; F: mandibular foramen.

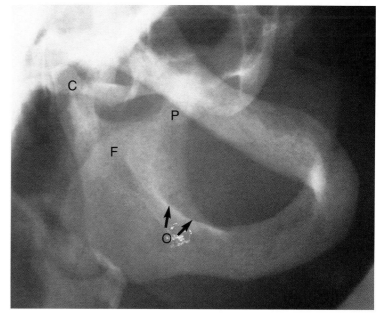

The skull

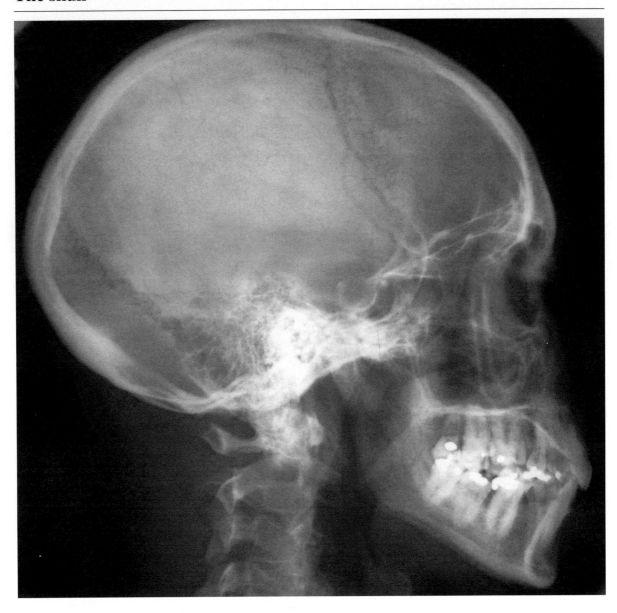

71 Lateral skull radiograph. L.

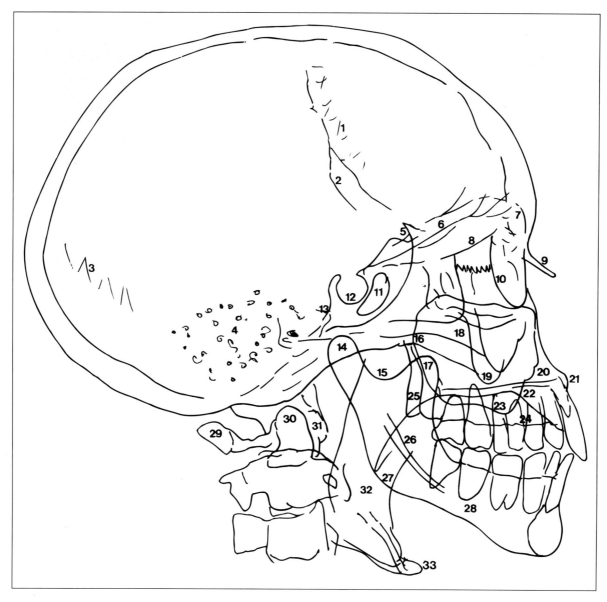

72 Line drawing of 71.

1. coronal suture	12. pituitary fossa (sella turcica)	23. floor of the maxillary antrum
2. meningeal grooves	13. clivus	24. alveolar ridge of the maxilla
3. lambdoid suture	14. head of the mandibular condyle	25. pterygoid plates
4. mastoid air cells	15. sigmoid notch	26. inferior alveolar canal
5. anterior wall of the middle cranial fossa	16. posterior wall of the maxillary antrum	27. angle of the mandible
6. floor of the anterior cranial fossa	17. coronoid process of the mandible	28. body of the mandible
7. frontal sinus	18. body of the zygoma	29. posterior arch of the atlas vertebra
8. cribriform plate	19. zygomatic process of the maxilla	30. odontoid process of the axis vertebra
9. nasal bones	20. anterior wall of the maxillary antrum	31. anterior arch of the atlas vertebra
10. anterior border of the lateral wall of the orbit	21. anterior nasal spine	32. pharyngeal air space
11. sphenoidal sinus	22. hard palate	33. hyoid bone

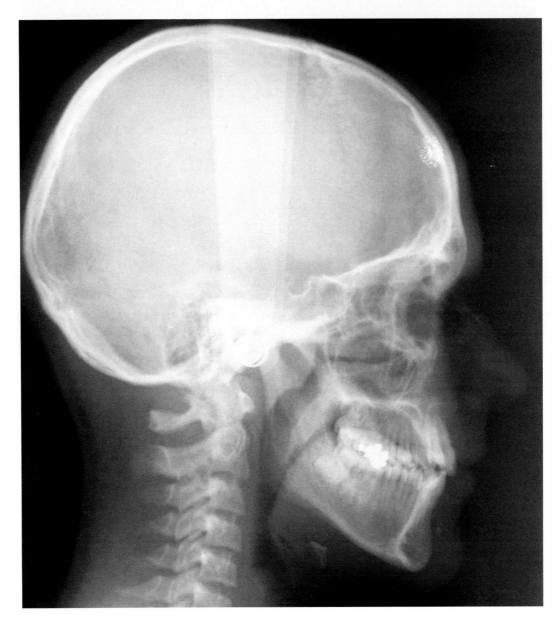

73 Lateral skull radiograph (cephalometric technique), LC. A cephalometric radiograph showing the relationship between the maxilla and the mandible in a patient with a Class I occlusion, and demonstrating the soft tissue profile of the face. Note the broad, radio-opaque band running vertically across the middle of the skull formed by part of the craniostat and also the circular ear-plugs.

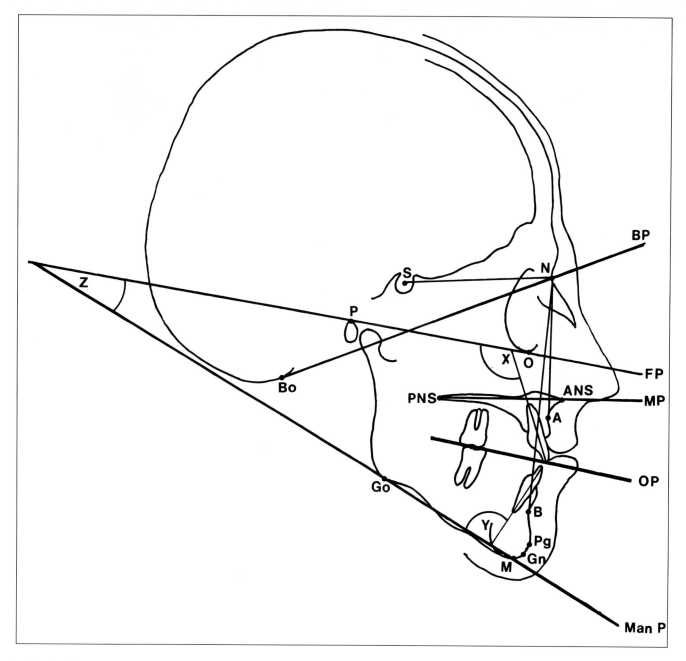

74 Line diagram of a cephalometric radiograph, LC. This illustrates some of the commonly-used anatomical landmarks, planes and angles in cephalometric analysis.

S	sella	Go	gonion	X	maxillary incisal angle
P	porion	N	nasion	Y	mandibular incisal angle
A	'A' point	O	orbitale	Z	Frankfort mandibular plane angle
B	'B' point	Bo	Bolton point	SNA	angle between the anterior part of
ANS	anterior nasal spine	BP	Bolton plane		the maxilla and the base of the
PNS	posterior nasal spine	FP	Frankfort plane		skull
Pg	pogonion	MP	maxillary plane	SNB	angle between the anterior part of
Gn	gnathion	OP	occlusal plane		the mandible and the base of the
M	menton	Man P	mandibular plane		skull

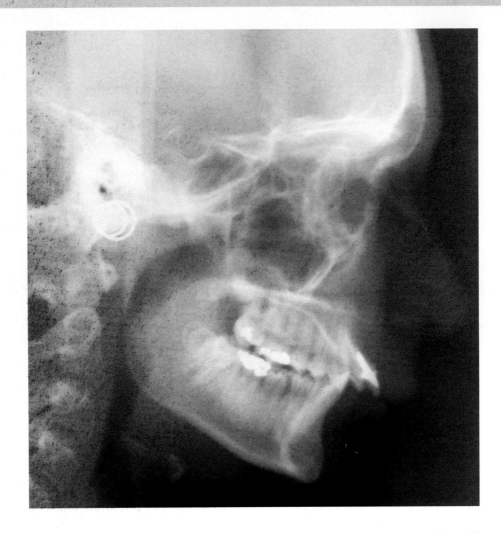

75 **A collimated cephalometric radiograph – LC – in a patient with a Class II occlusion.**

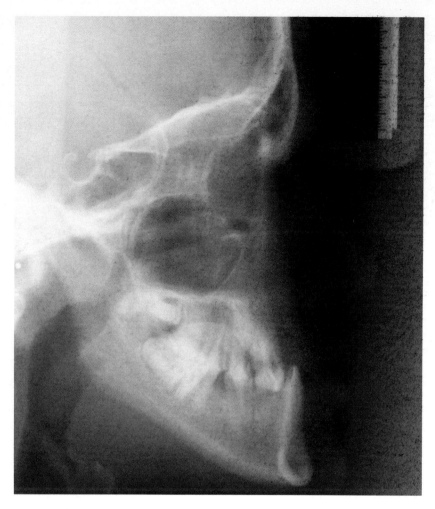

76 A collimated cephalometric radiograph – LC – in a patient with a Class III occlusion. Note the scale for assessing the magnification factor in cephalometric measurements.

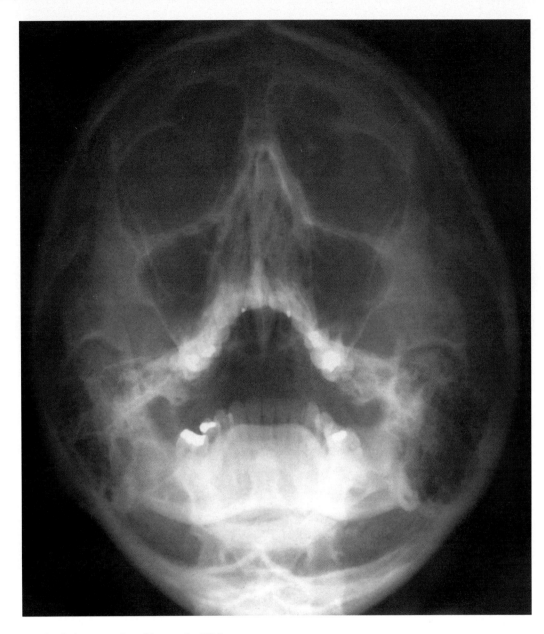

77 Occipitomental radiograph. OM.

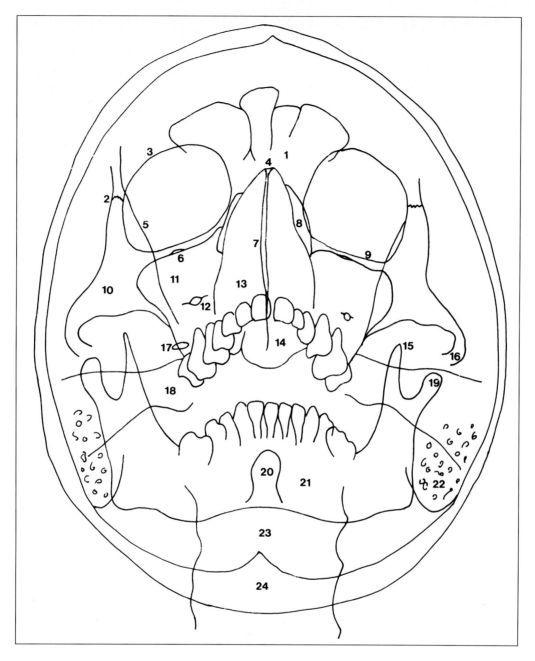

78 Line drawing of 77.

1. frontal sinuses	9. infra-orbital margin	17. foramen ovale
2. frontozygomatic suture	10. zygomatic bone	18. petrous part of the temporal bone
3. supra-orbital margin	11. maxillary antrum	19. condylar head of the mandible
4. nasal bones	12. foramen rotundum	20. odontoid process of the axis vertebra
5. linea innominata	13. nasal cavity and turbinate bones	21. body of the mandible
6. infra-orbital foramen	14. sphenoidal sinus	22. mastoid air cells
7. nasal septum	15. coronoid process of the mandible	23. cervical vertebrae
8. anterior ethmoidal sinuses	16. zygomatic arch	24. occipital bone

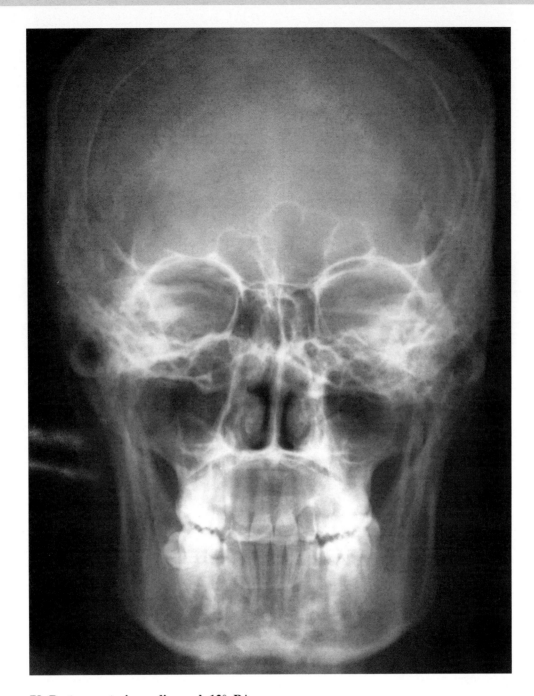

79 Postero-anterior radiograph 12°. PA.

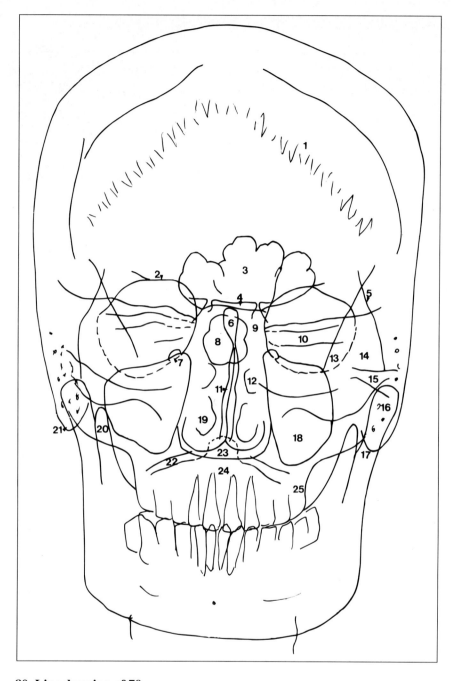

80 Line drawing of 79.

1. lambdoid suture	8. sphenoidal sinus	15. external auditory canal	22. intervertebral space between the atlas and the axis vertebrae
2. supra-orbital margin	9. ethmoidal sinuses	16. head of the mandibular condyle	23. odontoid process of the axis vertebra
3. frontal sinuses	10. internal auditory canal	17. neck of the mandibular condyle	24. hard palate
4. dorsum sellae	11. nasal septum	18. maxillary antrum	25. alveolar process of the maxilla
5. zygomatic process of the frontal bone	12. middle turbinate bone	19. inferior turbinate bone	
6. crista galli	13. linea innominata	20. coronoid process of the mandible	
7. foramen rotundum	14. frontal process of the zygomatic bone	21. mastoid process	

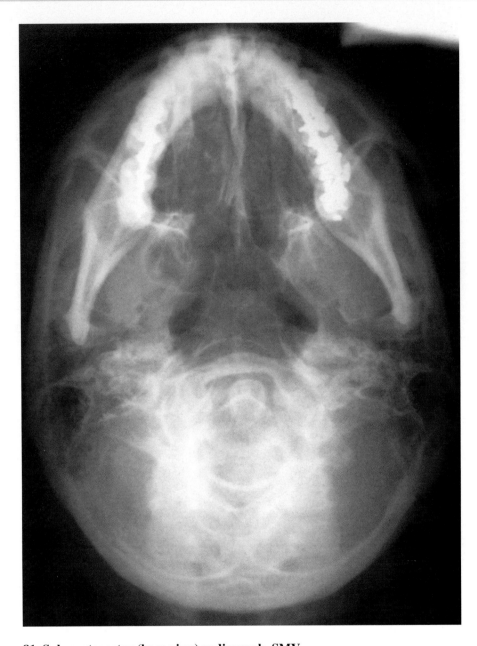

81 Submentovertex (base view) radiograph. SMV.

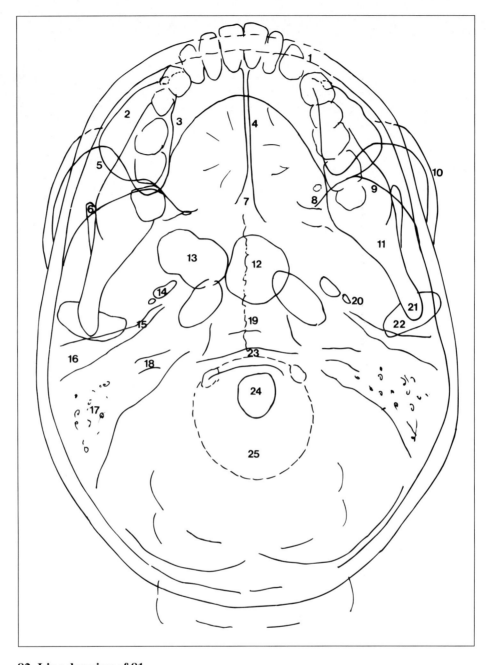

82 Line drawing of 81.

1. frontal bone	10. zygomatic arch	18. internal auditory canal
2. maxillary antrum	11. ramus of the mandible	19. clivus
3. medial wall of the maxillary antrum	12. sphenoidal sinus	20. foramen spinosum
4. nasal septum	13. ethmoidal sinus	21. ramus of the mandible
5. lateral wall of the orbit	14. foramen ovale	22. mandibular condyle
6. coronoid process of the mandible	15. pharyngotympanic (Eustachian) tube	23. anterior arch of the atlas vertebra
7. posterior border of the vomer	16. external auditory canal	24. odontoid process of the axis vertebra
8. greater palatine foramen	17. mastoid air cells	25. foramen magnum
9. anterior wall of the middle cranial fossa		

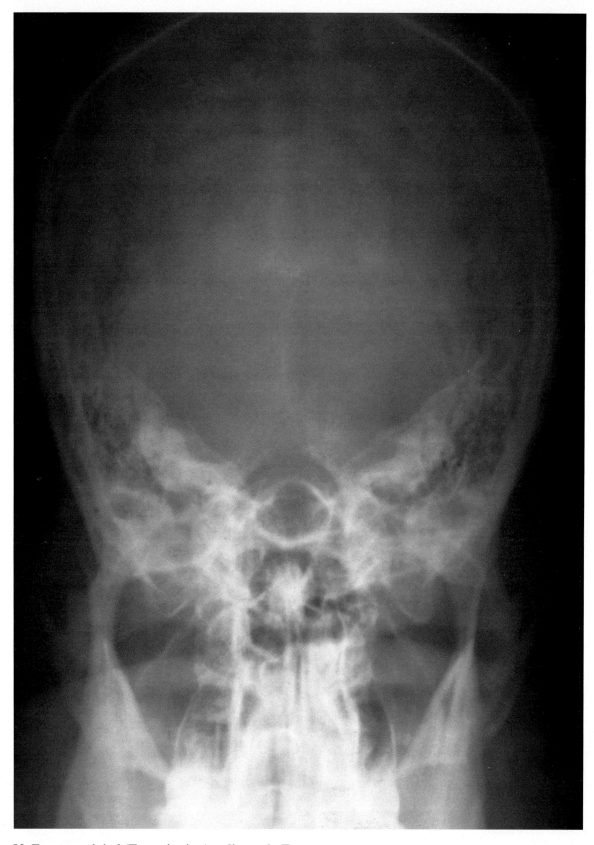

83 Fronto-occipital (Towne's view) radiograph. T.

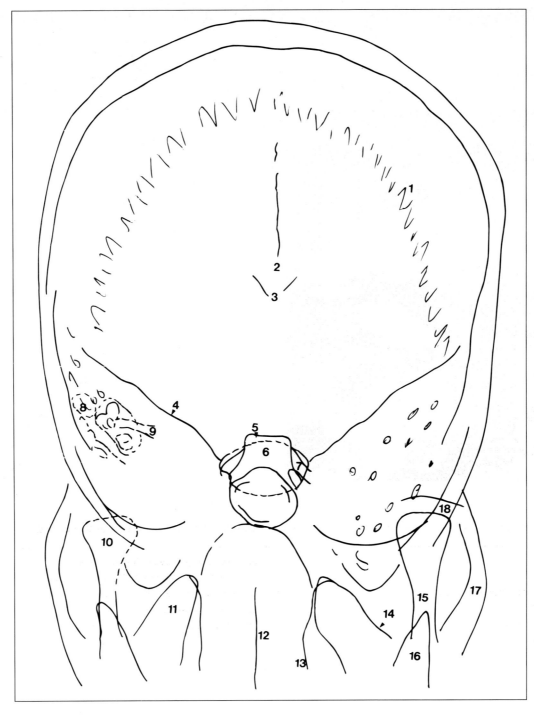

84 Line drawing of 83.

1. lambdoid suture	6. dorsum sellae	11. maxillary antrum	15. neck of the mandibular condyle
2. internal occipital crest	7. foramen magnum	12. nasal septum	16. coronoid process of the mandible
3. occiput	8. mastoid air cells	13. mesial wall of the maxillary antrum	17. zygomatic arch
4. petrous ridge of the temporal bone	9. internal auditory canal	14. roof and wall of the maxillary antrum	18. temporomandibular joint space
5. posterior clinoid process	10. head of the mandibular condyle		

The temporomandibular joint

Transcranial radiograph

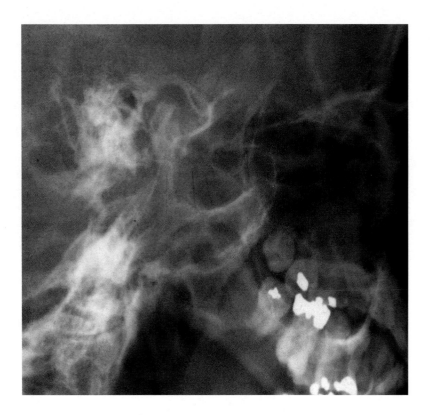 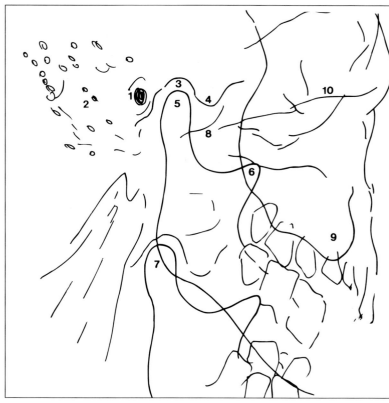

85, 86 Transcranial radiograph of the temporomandibular joint – TMJ – and line drawing with the mouth closed.

1. external auditory meatus	6. coronoid process of the mandible
2. mastoid air cells	7. mandibular condyle of the opposite side
3. articular fossa of the temporomandibular joint	8. medial rim of the articular fossa
4. articular eminence	9. maxillary antrum
5. head of the mandibular condyle	10. floor of the anterior cranial fossa

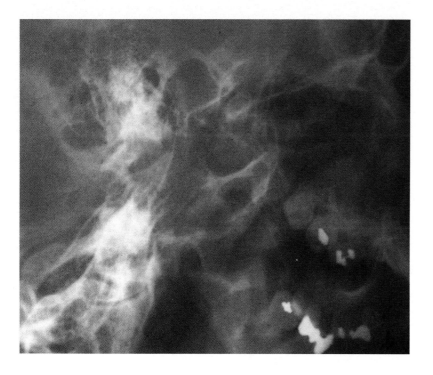

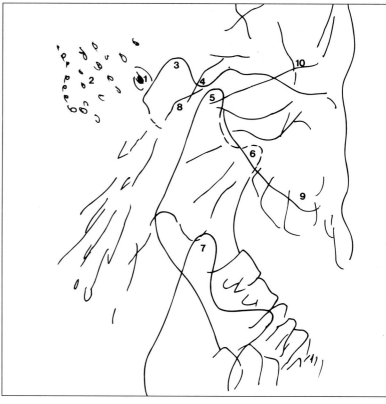

87, 88 Transcranial radiograph of the temporomandibular joint – TMJ – and line drawing with the mouth fully open.

1.	external auditory meatus	6.	coronoid process of the mandible
2.	mastoid air cells	7.	mandibular condyle of the opposite side
3.	articular fossa of the temporomandibular joint	8.	medial rim of the articular fossa
4.	articular eminence	9.	maxillary antrum
5.	head of the mandibular condyle	10.	floor of the anterior cranial fossa

Arthrogram

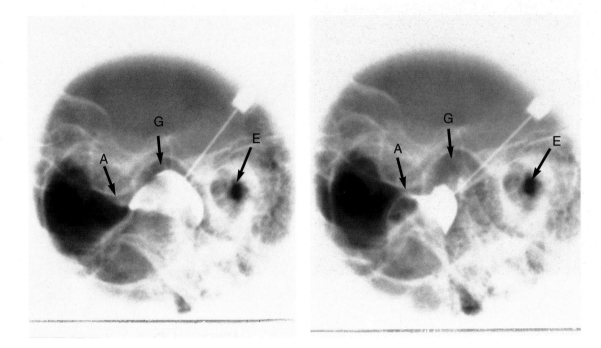

89, 90 An arthrogram – A – of a normal temporomandibular joint with the mouth in the closed and open positions. The radio-opaque medium has been injected into the inferior joint space and forms a cap overlying the head of the condyle. In the closed position (**89**) the majority of the medium occupies the posterior compartment of the space, extending well down the neck of the condyle to the posterior attachment of the capsule and the disc. Rather less medium occupies the smaller anterior compartment. As the mouth is opened (**90**) the head of the condyle and the overlying articular disc move forward over the articular eminence so tensing the anterior part of the joint capsule and squeezing the medium almost entirely into the posterior compartment, which now assumes a dome shape. E: external auditory meatus; A: articular eminence; G: glenoid fossa.

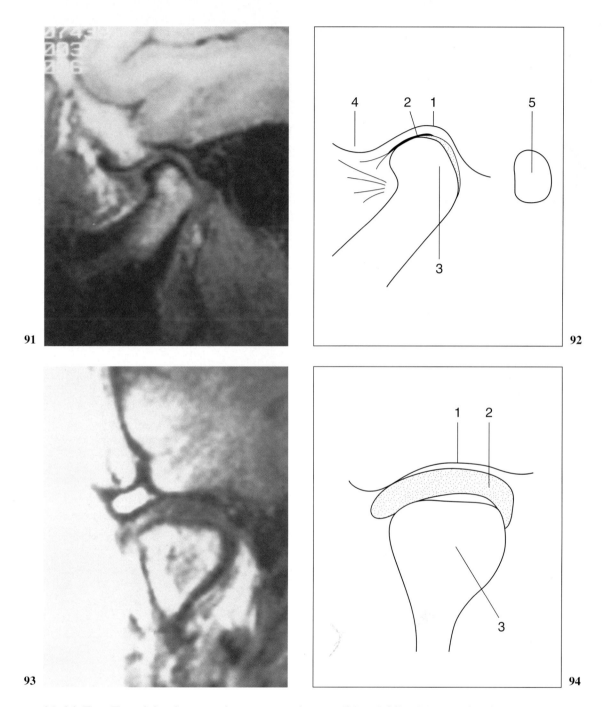

91

92

93

94

91–94 Two T₁-weighted magnetic resonance images (91 and 93) – MRI – with line drawings (92 and 94) of the temporomandibular joint. With this technique, cortical bone appears black – having a low signal – whereas cancellous bone appears much whiter because its fat content provides a higher signal. The articular disc has an intermediate grey appearance. In **91** and **92**, the joint is viewed in the sagittal plane; in **93** and **94** it is viewed in the coronal plane. 1: superior bone margin of the glenoid fossa; 2: articular disc; 3: head of the mandibular condyle; 4: articular eminence; 5: external auditory meatus.

The salivary glands

Parotid sialogram

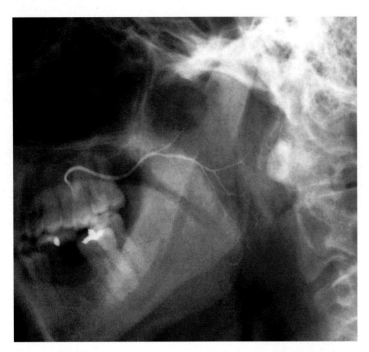

95 A sialogram – SL(L) – of a normal parotid gland in which the outline of the duct system is highlighted by the radio-opaque contrast medium. The main duct runs posteriorly from opposite the maxillary first molar into the body of the parotid gland, the image of which overlies that of the ramus of the mandible. The duct outline is continuous and approximately 1 mm in width; where it penetrates the buccinator muscle anteriorly it exhibits a typical hook shape. The first branch of the duct superiorly is that from the accessory lobe of the parotid gland. Thereafter, at each bifurcation, there is a reduction in the width of the ducts, which ultimately form a fine, complex, branching pattern.

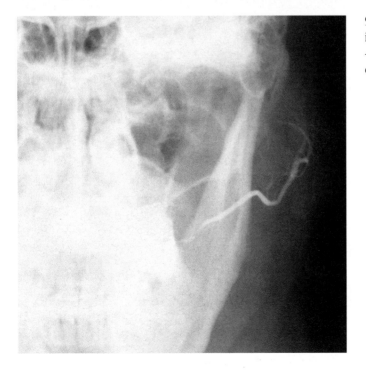

96 A sialogram of a normal parotid gland in which the outline of the duct system is highlighted by the radio-opaque contrast medium. Postero-anterior view – SL(PA) – in which the superficial position of the duct relative to that of the body of the gland is clearly displayed.

97 A sialogram – SL(L) – of a normal, right submandibular salivary gland taken immediately after injection of the contrast medium. The main duct, which is of normal and regular width, passes obliquely backwards from its outlet in the anterior part of the floor of the mouth, to a point, superimposed upon the inferior border of the mandible, where it curves sharply forwards. This point represents the posterior border of the mylohyoid muscle, above which lies the deep part and below which lies the superficial part of the gland. In both parts, there are several smaller branches from which the terminal ramifications of the duct system derive, forming a typical branching pattern. Note the smooth, regular, radio-opaque arc formed by the medium in the cannula, which lies on the patient's skin and the excess medium which has pooled in the floor of the mouth.

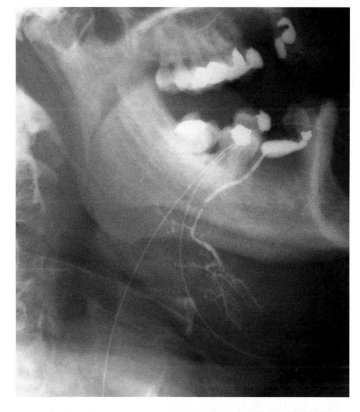

98 In submandibular sialography, radio-opaque medium does not usually gain access to the multiple small ducts of the sublingual salivary gland. Occasionally, when there is a substantial single duct from the latter, medium enters it and so, in addition to the duct system of the submandibular gland, that of the sublingual gland is also displayed more anteriorly. Again there is pooling of excess medium in the floor of the mouth.

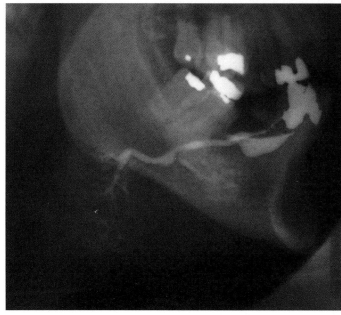

Scintigram (time/activity uptake curve)

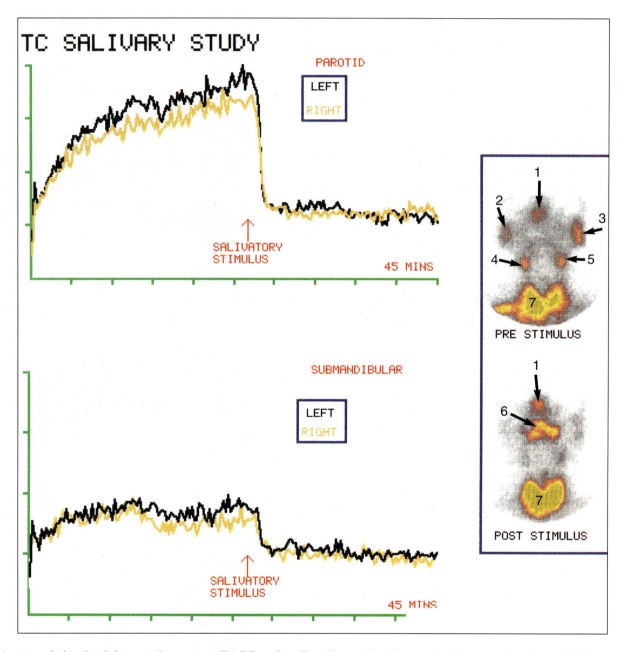

99 A normal time/activity uptake curve – TASC – of radioactive technetium pertechnetate showing a similar rate of uptake in both parotid salivary glands and in both submandibular salivary glands. Following administration of a sialogogue, there is rapid and almost complete excretion of the radioactive material from all four glands. The scintigrams to the right of the illustration demonstrate, at the top, the accumulated radioactivity in the four major salivary glands immediately prior to the administration of the sialogogue and, at the bottom, shortly afterwards when the glands are 'cold'. Also illustrated in the upper scintigram is the accumulation in the nasal glands prior to stimulation. Following excretion, the radioactive material accumulates in the oral cavity, as shown in the lower scintigram. The activity in the thyroid gland remains essentially unaltered by the sialogogue. 1: nasal glands; 2: right parotid gland; 3: left parotid gland; 4: right submandibular gland; 5: left submandibular gland; 6: activity in the oral cavity; 7: thyroid gland.

Computerized tomogram

100, 101 Computerized tomogram – CT – and line drawing at the level of the first cervical vertebra.

A   maxillary alveolar ridge
B   tongue
C   pterygoid hamulus
D   mandibular foramen
E   retromandibular vein
F   external carotid artery
G   styloid process
H   oropharynx
I   atlas vertebra
J   odontoid process of the axis vertebra
K   sternocleidomastoid muscle
L   parotid gland
M   medial pterygoid muscle
N   masseter muscle
O   buccal pad of fat

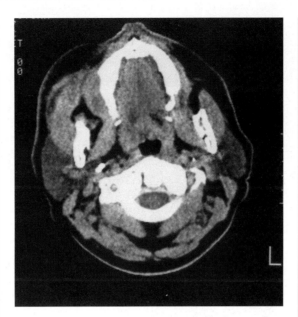
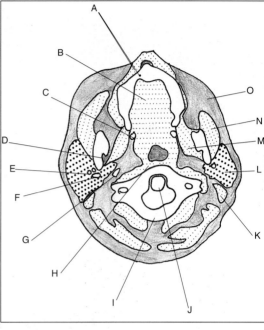

Some variations on normal radiographic anatomy

102 The incisive canal. Usually the incisive canal is not well displayed on intra-oral radiographs (apart from its palatal end, the incisive foramen). However, under the circumstances when it is not obscured by superimposition of the roots of the teeth, and when the angulation of the X-ray beam permits, the whole length of the canal may be visible. In this example, in an edentulous maxilla, the palatal and nasal foramina (arrows) at each end of the canal are clearly displayed, with the incisive canal bounded by a thin, corticated lamina. UOO.

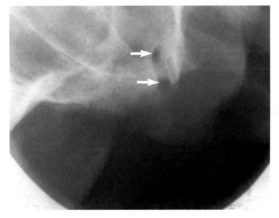

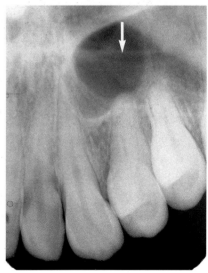

103 Antral locule. This shows an unusually prominent radiolucent locule of the left maxillary antrum, overlying the apex |4 , simulating a radicular cyst. The presence of the nutrient canal (arrow) running transversely indicates that this is part of the normal bony wall of the antrum. In such cases, a second radiograph, taken with the X-ray beam at a different angle, helps to confirm that this appearance is a normal variation of antral anatomy. P.

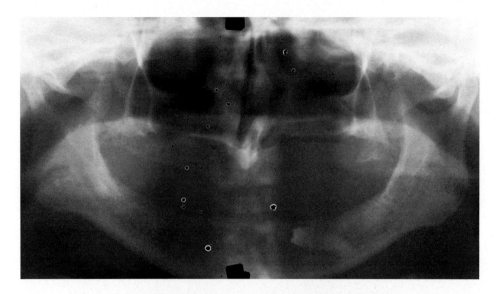

104 Nasal soft tissues. Occasionally, if the patient is positioned a little posteriorly in the dental panoramic machine, the cartilagnious part of the nasal septum and the nasal soft tissues may form a prominent image in the midline of the upper jaw. At first sight, this image may appear similar to that of an unerupted tooth and lead to confusion in diagnosis. If the anterior teeth are missing, and/or the septum is deviated from the midline, the image may be more obvious as in this example. Careful comparison with the unerupted |5 , which is conveniently present in this otherwise edentulous jaw, confirms the distinction from a tooth structure. This radiograph also shows a cystic lesion in the left maxilla. DPR.

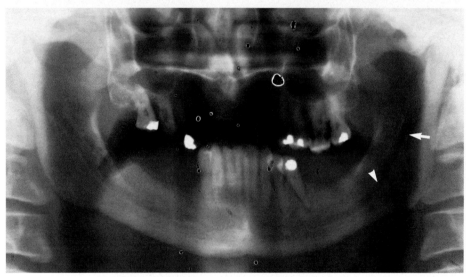

105 (left), 106 (below) Branched inferior alveolar canal. In the example in the left side of the mandible (**105**) there are two minor branches of the main canal, one at the level of the mandibular foramen (arrow) and one in the third molar region (arrowhead). The latter shows a second dichotomy in the second molar region. The second example (**106**) shows a branched canal arising from the left mandibular foramen. The smaller branch loops inferiorly from the main canal and unites with it at the level of the single molar tooth. In addition, the incisive branch (arrows) running anteriorly from the mental foramen (arrowhead) is clearly shown on both sides of the mandible. DPR.

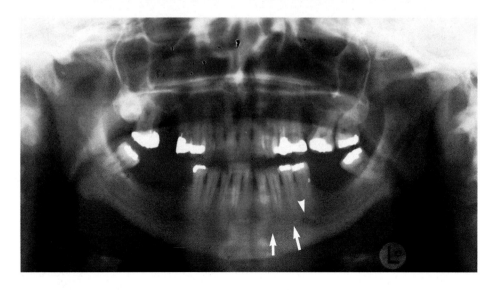

107 Simulated pathological lesions. The superimposition of the image of one structure upon another may lead to artefactual appearances simulating pathological lesions. Here, the combined effects of the superimposition of the radiolucent air shadow of the pharynx and the radio-opaque, spinous processes of two vertebrae, have formed a circumscribed radiolucency in the base of the ramus of the mandible, simulating a cystic defect (arrowheads). A view of the same area with a different beam orientation would confirm that this appearance is an artefact. OLM.

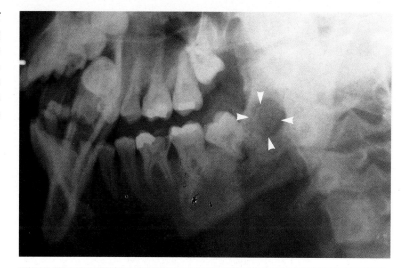

108 Mineralized ligaments. Ligaments are prone to undergo mineralization, usually as part of the ageing process; occasionally this may become very pronounced and even occur in younger patients, as in this case, affecting both stylohyoid ligaments. The ligament on the left is discontinuous and is deviated anteriorly at its lower end. DPR(J).

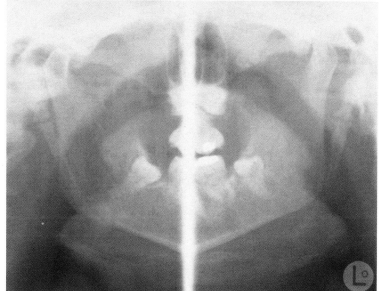

109 The frontal air sinuses. There is great variation among individuals in the configuration of the frontal air sinuses, to such an extent that use is made of this in the forensic identification of skulls. In this example, the frontal sinus is present only on the right side and is heart-shaped in outline (compare with **77** and **79**). OM.

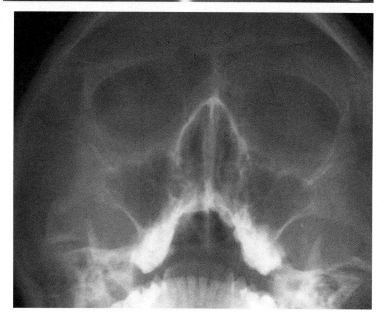

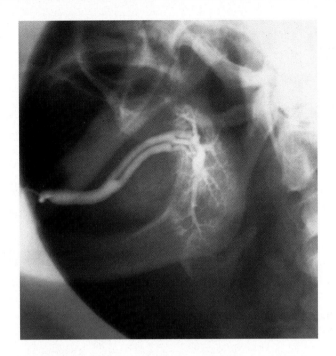

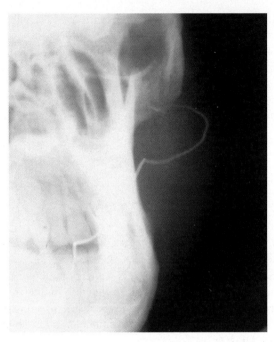

110 Submandibular sialogram. In this submandibular sialogram, the gland has been displayed on an oblique lateral mandible projection rather than on a true lateral mandible radiograph. For practical reasons, the sialogram was performed on the right gland with the X-ray tube positioned to expose the left side of the mandible. This has demonstrated particularly clearly a not uncommon variation in the structure of the submandibular duct, which is bifid in its distal portion. This appearance is exaggerated because the duct is dilated. OLM.

111 Masseteric hypertrophy. This is not uncommon in patients with parafunctional habits, such as bruxism and is usually bilateral. Occasionally, an enlarged masseteric muscle may be confused with a parotid gland swelling. If a parotid sialogram is undertaken in such a patient, the curve of the duct of the gland is deflected more laterally than normal by the increased muscle mass. This illustration shows how the deflection affects mostly the anterior, extraglandular part of the duct. SL(RPA).

3

Some technical errors and artefacts

Introduction

Whilst a knowledge and understanding of normal anatomical radiographic features is fundamental to radiological diagnosis, it is likewise important to be aware of the technical errors that can affect the final radiographic image. Some of the more common errors and artefacts are illustrated in this chapter. In general, faults may arise at any stage of the recording of the image or subsequently during the processing of the film. For convenience of presentation, they have been grouped in relation to intra-oral radiographic techniques, extra-oral radiographic techniques, processing of films and other radiographic and imaging techniques. With regard to intra-oral techniques, some of the errors described (particularly those relating to the positioning of the X-ray tube and bending of the film) are more likely to occur in the bisecting angle technique than in the paralleling technique. Some extra-oral techniques, in particular panoramic

radiography, require relatively long exposure times and so patient movement is more likely to occur during the process. Thus there are some patients for whom the technique is not suitable, including the very young and those with various neurological or neuromuscular disorders, which may prevent them from keeping still. As in any technical procedure, the processing of films requires a consistent standard of care and attention to detail. Films should always be processed according to the manufacturer's instructions and failure to do so may lead to faults. The avoidance of the human factor by the use of automatic processing machines makes the occurrence of errors in film development and fixation less likely. Many of the more modern radiographic and imaging techniques are very sophisticated and require highly trained personnel to perform them.

Errors associated with intra-oral radiographic techniques

Incorrect angulation of the X-ray tube

As described in Chapter 2, the taking of intra-oral radiographs requires the X-ray beam and film to be appropriately aligned relative to each other to avoid distortion of the resulting image. A common error, when using the bisecting angle technique, is the failure to direct the X-ray beam at right angles to the bisector. Insufficient vertical angulation will result in elongation of the image (**112**) whereas excessive vertical angulation will produce foreshortening (**113**).

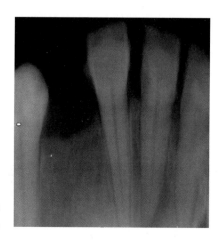

112 Incorrect tube angulation (elongation). P.

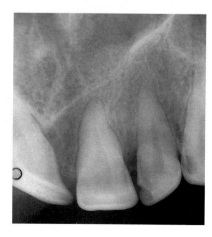

113 Incorrect tube angulation (foreshortening). P.

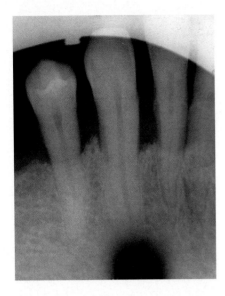

114 Incorrect centring of cone. P.

Incorrect centring of the X-ray cone (coning)

Collimation of the X-ray beam is an important feature in radiation protection. However, failure to correctly centre the X-ray cone to the film may result in only part of the film being exposed. The unexposed portion of the film appears clear as in **114** where the limit of the radiation field is illustrated. In addition, light has reached the film prior to exposure, causing fogging in the apical region 3|, simulating an apical radiolucency. This type of film fogging results in an area of profound radiolucency often with a diffuse periphery. It is usually a consequence of damage to the film packet; the use of plastic, rather than paper, packaging makes this error less likely.

BENDING AND FOLDING OF THE FILM

Bending of the film during exposure may lead to distortion of the resulting image. If the film becomes excessively bent whilst being held in place by the patient, part of it will be incorrectly aligned in relation to the X-ray beam. Consequently, there may be distortion of part of the image. In **115**, 54| are projected normally, but the roots of 321| are markedly elongated. If a film has been folded prior to exposure, the emulsion may be damaged and react abnormally resulting in a dark line on the film (**116**).

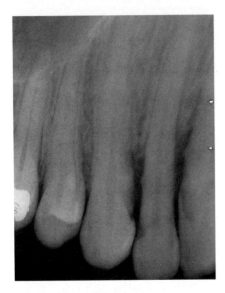

115 Bent film. P.

Positioning the film the wrong way round

A film placed back to front will be underexposed due to interposition of the lead foil backing between the emulsion and the X-ray source (**117**). In addition, as shown in this example, the herring bone pattern of the foil may be superimposed upon the image.

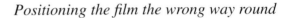

117 Film placed back to front. P.

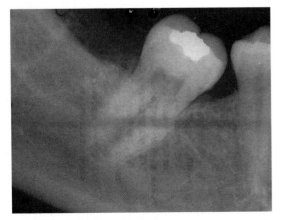

116 Folded film. P.

Patient movement

Movement of the patient or film during exposure, may result in blurring or superimposition of several images of the same structure (**118**).

Foreign body in the X-ray cone

Rarely, a metallic foreign body may be present in the X-ray cone, producing an unexplained radio-opaque image (**119**) as seen overlying 2|.

Incorrect film exposure

Overexposure of a film produces overall darkening (**120**) whereas underexposure results in a film which lacks density (**121**). Although incorrect exposure is a common cause of such faults, there are other factors that can produce similar appearances: a dark film may also arise from overdevelopment or from fogging by light while a pale film may be the result of inadequate development. Double exposure of a film may produce a confusion of images (**122**).

120 Overexposure of film. P.

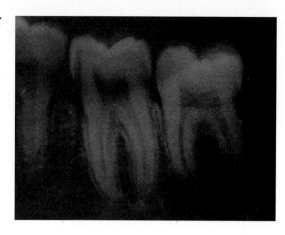

118 Patient movement. P.

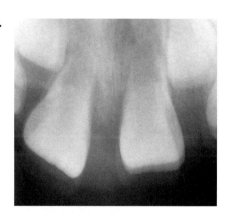

119 Metallic body in X-ray cone. P.

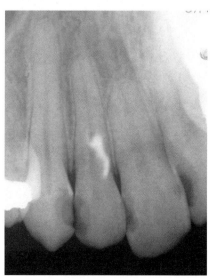

121 Underexposure of film. P.

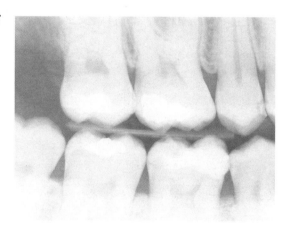

122 Double exposure of film. P.

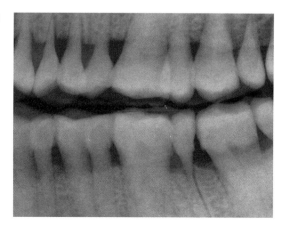

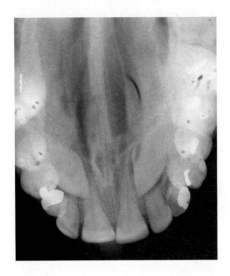

123 Bitemarks on film. USO.

Bitemarks on the film

In techniques where the film is placed between the opposing teeth during exposure, such as occlusal views, defects may arise when the emulsion is damaged by the patient biting too firmly on the film. In **123** there are a number of punctate radiolucent marks overlying the cusps of the premolar and molar teeth. In addition, there is a radiolucent arcuate line overlying the radiolucency of the left nasal cavity due to film damage produced either by a finger nail indentation or crimping during its removal from the packet.

Errors associated with extra-oral radiographic techniques

Incorrect patient preparation

In panoramic radiographs, the images of extra-oral objects (commonly ear-rings) may be superimposed upon the facial structures. In the patient (**124**) wearing stud ear-rings, the image of each ear-ring is clearly displayed on its own side; in addition a second image is projected on to the opposite side of the jaw at a higher level due to the upward angulation of the X-ray tube. These images are enlarged and blurred and are superimposed upon the maxillary antra. Another patient (**125**) has annular ear-rings, the projected images being superimposed mostly over the body of the mandible on the opposite side. Again they are enlarged, blurred and at a slightly higher level than the image on the side where they are positioned. In addition, this patient is also wearing a metallic hair-clip on the left side, but only a small part of the second image (arrow) – projected over the antrum on the right side – is apparent. Note that this is also at a higher level. The projected image of annular ear-rings may be misinterpreted as a cyst ('ear-ring cyst') if it is superimposed over the appropriate part of the maxilla. In **126** there is an 'ear-ring cyst' (arrowhead) overlying the left antrum and, in addition,

124 Patient wearing stud ear-rings. DPR.

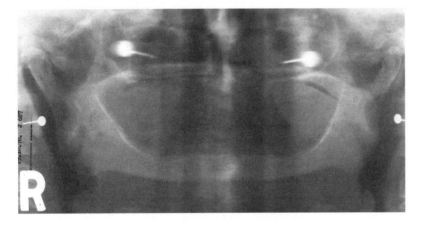

125 Patient wearing annular ear-rings. DPR.

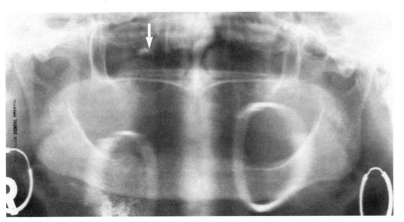

126 Patient wearing annular ear-rings. DPR.

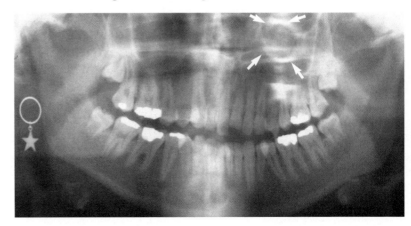

there is an opacity overlying the apices |456 due to projection of the image of the star pendant of the ear-ring. Such examples emphasize the importance of removing all such radio-opaque artefacts prior to the taking of radiographs. These include dentures (**127**), spectacles (**128**), hair-clips (**129**) and nasal studs, necklaces and bib chains.

Incorrect patient positioning

Whereas patient positioning is important in all techniques, it is particularly relevant in dental panoramic radiography because of the finite constraints of the focal trough. There are many errors of positioning that can lead to different faults in the resulting film.

If the patient has been positioned too far forward (anteriorly) in relation to the focal trough, a loss of definition and apparent narrowing of the anterior teeth results. In **130** all the teeth mesial to the molars are affected. Conversely, positioning of the patient too far posteriorly (relative to the focal trough) results in loss of definition and magnification of the anterior teeth, particularly in a mesial/distal

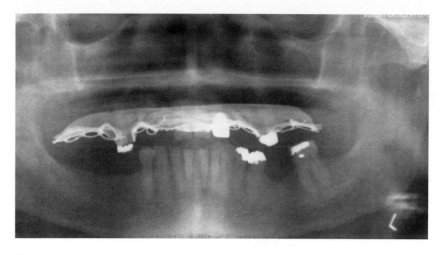

127 Patient wearing chrome–cobalt denture. DPR.

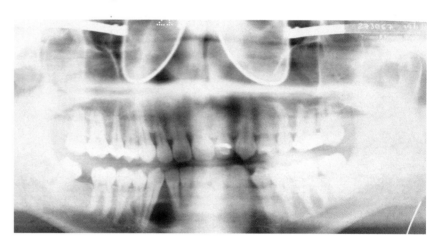

128 Patient wearing spectacles. DPR.

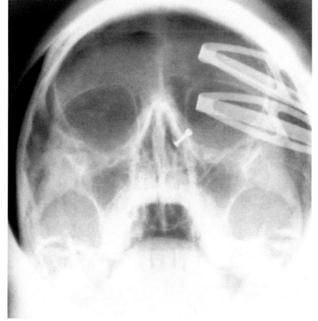

129 Patient wearing hair-clip. OM.

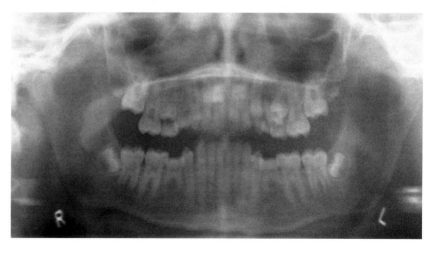

130 Patient positioned too far forward. DPR.

direction (**131**). The different sizes of the images of the teeth are a consequence of the teeth not being correctly located within the focal trough, being placed too near or too far from the film. Moving out of the focal trough also results in a reduction in definition. For similar reasons, rotation of the head in the vertical plane results in magnification of the images on one side and reduction on the other. Those teeth which lie further from the film (the side to which the head has been turned) will appear magnified and less sharp, whereas those lying closer to the film will appear narrower and less distinct. In **132** the patient's head was rotated towards the left side so that the incisors, canines, premolars and first molars on that side are magnified and blurred, and the premolars on the right side appear narrowed. With correct positioning, the patient's Frankfort plane

should be horizontal so that the occlusal plane runs obliquely downwards in a postero-anterior direction, making a small angle with the horizontal plane. If the patient is positioned with the chin up, the slope of the occlusal plane is reversed so that the roots of the upper anterior teeth lie palatal to the focal trough and may not be recorded (**133**). In addition, the image of the hard palate may be projected over those of the upper anterior teeth, so obscuring them and the rami of the mandible may be projected posteriorly to, or beyond, the posterior limits of the film. Conversely, over-tilting in a downward position (chin down) results in the apical parts of the lower anterior teeth being positioned out of the focal trough so that they are poorly imaged (**134**). This 'chin down' position may be a consequence of failure to position the patient sufficiently upright in the machine, so that

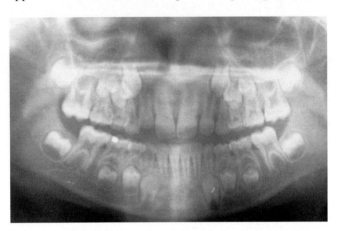

131 Patient positioned too far back. DPR.

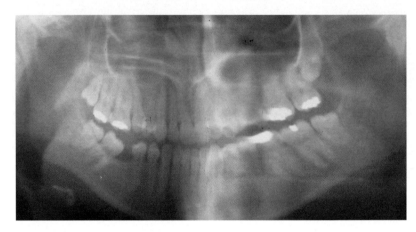

132 Patient's head rotated. DPR.

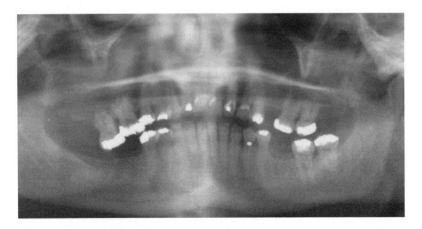

133 Patient positioned with chin up. DPR.

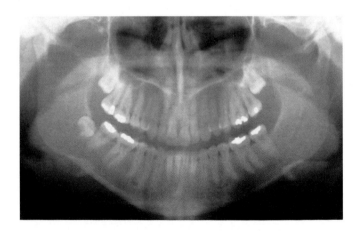

134 Patient positioned with chin down. DPR.

the cervical spine is flexed, or sometimes because of physical incapacity. If the film is exposed in this position, there is greater attenuation of the X-ray beam by the spine, which may result in a centrally-positioned, radio-opaque band obscuring the anterior teeth (**135**). Positioning of the patient's head either too low or too high relative to the film will result in the loss of part of the images of the lower or upper jaws respectively.

In addition to the patient's head being positioned relatively too high (**136**) other errors are present on this film. The relatively high position has resulted in the inclusion of the horizontal, densely radio-opaque metallic bars of the chin support. Failure to remove a necklace has produced a half-elliptical radio-opacity in the midline which overlies most of the anterior teeth. In addition, the film drum was incorrectly aligned so that it had completed its path of rotation prior to the completion of the X-ray exposure. As a consequence the image of the left ramus of the mandible is absent and in its place there is a vertical band of dense radiolucency. On the right side there is some alternating, radiolucent and radio-opaque banding, due to mechanical wear of the apparatus causing uneven film exposure.

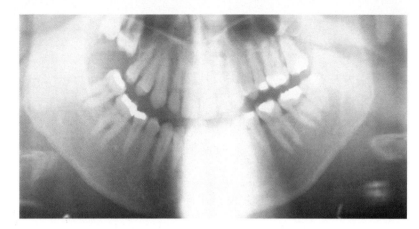

135 Patient slumped forward. DPR.

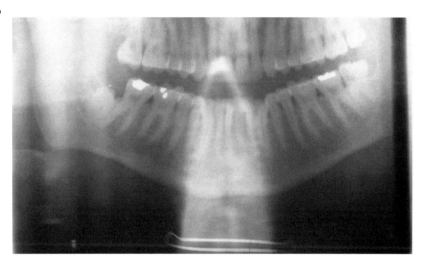

136 Patient too high. DPR.

Patient movement

Because of the relatively long exposure time of dental panoramic radiographic films, patient movement may occur leading to distortion and/or blurring of the image. When this involves the mandible alone, only the image of that jaw is affected. If the movement involves the whole head then the distortion will affect both jaws. In **137** the patient's head moved briefly with the result that there is only a small part of the film in the upper

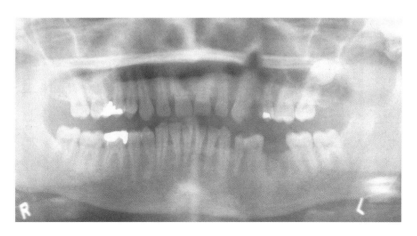

137 Patient movement. DPR.

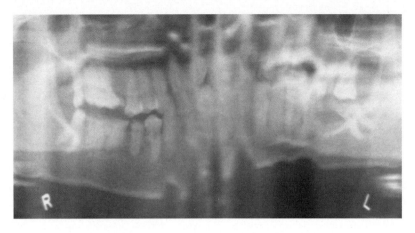

138 Patient movement. DPR.

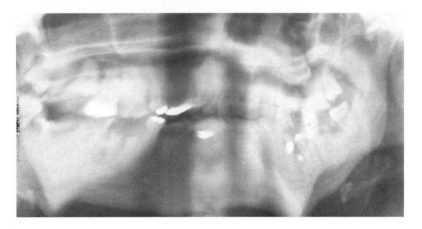

139 Patient movement. DPR.

and lower left premolar region, which is blurred. In the next illustration (**138**) the head movement occurred during the middle of the exposure period, so the images of the more anterior parts are distorted and blurred but those of the posterior part of the jaws on both sides are reasonably sharp. When the movement is prolonged (**139**) nearly all the image is markedly distorted and blurred.

Incorrect cassette handling

Cassettes containing extra-oral films need to be correctly prepared and positioned before exposure. If a focused grid is placed in front of the cassette the wrong way round (**140**), the central part of the film remains exposed but the more peripheral parts are obscured due to incorrect angulation of the oblique lead slats in this part of the grid (see **10**), forming a series of linear radio-opacities across the film. Sometimes the cassette may not be closed tightly, either due to distortion or worn clips – under these circumstances the two sides may not be closely apposed to the film over its whole area. This results in an image which is sharp in part but becomes progressively blurred towards that part which is contiguous with the loosely apposed sides of the cassette. In **141** the image is blurred on the right side but sharp on the left. If the cassette is positioned the wrong way round during exposure, images of the extraneous structures on the outside of the back of the cassette will appear on the film. Various vertical and oblique radio-opaque lines are present (**142**) as a result of this incorrect positioning of the cassette. In dental panoramic radiographs, positioning of the cassette the wrong way round results in an underexposed film except where there is a rectangular plastic window on the back of the cassette (**143**).

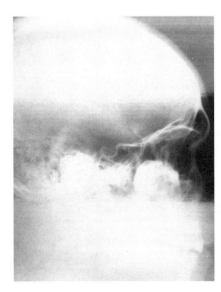

140 Incorrectly inserted grid in cassette. L.

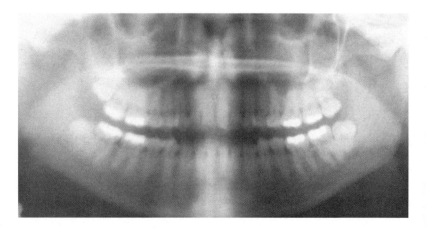

141 Incorrectly closed cassette. DPR.

142 Incorrectly positioned cassette. TMJ.

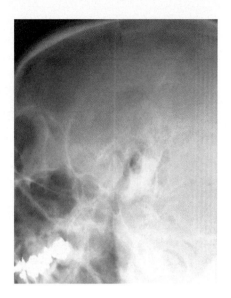

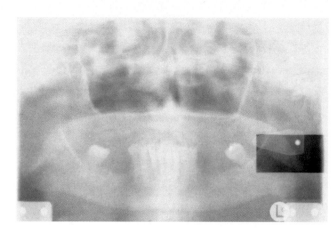

143 Incorrectly positioned cassette. DPR.

Errors arising during processing of films

Electrostatic discharge

Electrostatic discharge during the handling of films may take two forms. During sudden movements over the film surface, electrostatic discharge may occur without any light formation, causing a series of irregular, branched, dark tracks (**144**) which have been variously described as 'naked tree' or 'forked lightening' in appearance. This type of discharge may occur when the film is withdrawn from its packet or cassette and arises from friction between the film and the packaging. It is more likely to occur in a warm, dry environment.

The other form of electrostatic discharge probably results from sparks and follows a path induced by dust or other irregularities on the surface of the film. It produces numerous, rounded ill-defined dark spots of varying size over those parts of the film affected by the discharge. In **145** the top and bottom of the film are affected. The wearing of rubber gloves during processing of the film increases the incidence of this artefact.

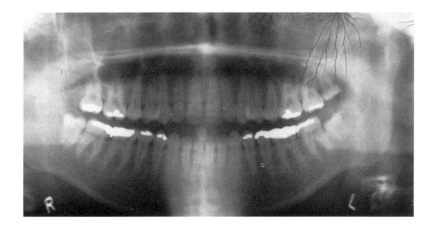

144 Electrostatic discharge. DPR.

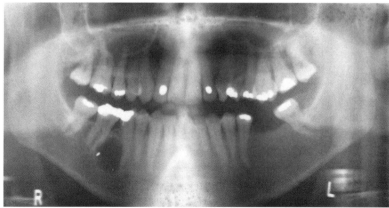

145 Electrostatic discharge. DPR.

Incorrect development and fixation

It has already been stated that overexposure (see **120**) and underexposure (see **121**) result in poor quality films. Inadequate development (**146**) may also result in poor quality films if the developer solution is insufficiently agitated. Furthermore, if the film is incompletely immersed in the developer, that part of the film which remains exposed to the air appears clear. This fault is particularly well demonstrated if there are air bubbles on the surface of the developing fluid (**147**). Premature contact of the film with either developer solution or fixative will also cause film abnormalities.

The example (**148**) was contaminated by developer prior to processing, both from the operator's thumb, producing a dark thumb print overlying much of the film, and from droplets splashed upon it. In **149**, fixative has been splashed on to the film prior to development, resulting in clear areas. This film has also been partly coned off. Similarly, prolonged overfixation may result in the loss of some of the metallic silver grains decreasing the film density (**150**).

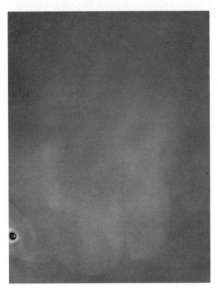

146 Inadequately agitated developer solution. P.

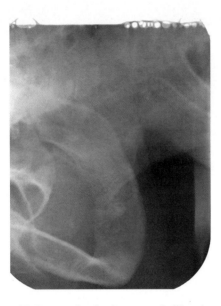

147 Incompletely immersed film in developer solution. OLM.

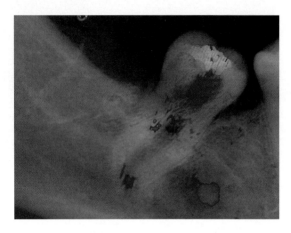

148 Premature contamination of film by developer. P.

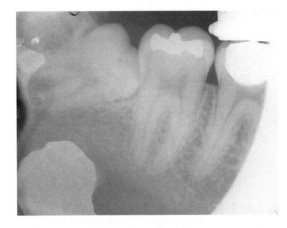

149 Premature contamination of film by fixative. P.

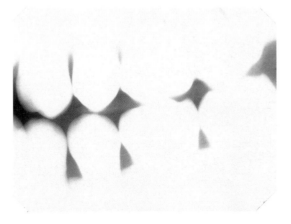

150 Overfixation of film. P.

Scratching of film

Scratching of the film emulsion, which is most likely to occur after it has been processed but is still wet, results in clear defects as seen anterior to the molar tooth in **151**. Small defects may be caused by the clip used to suspend the film in the processing fluids and such defects can be seen on most hand-processed films, as in the middle of the right-hand margin of the example.

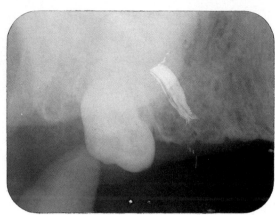

151 Scratching of film. P.

Errors and artefacts arising with other radiographic and imaging techniques

Faulty sialographic technique

Sialography requires considerable practical skill, without which errors may be introduced. For example, if too much pressure or volume of contrast medium is used, the ducts may be damaged, with medium escaping into the periductular tissues. As a consequence, the duct architecture may become obscured (**152**) and the gland appears as a more uniformly radio-opaque structure. When an oil-based medium is used, as in this example, it may take many weeks to be fully resorbed and to disappear completely. Due to the narrowness of the orifices of the salivary gland ducts, particularly that of the submandibular gland, cannulation can present difficulties and occasionally perforation of the duct ensues. Radio-opaque medium may then be inadvertently introduced into the soft tissues in the floor of the mouth (**153**). In this example, a water-based medium was used and a second film (**154**), taken 30 minutes later, demonstrates that much of it has already dispersed.

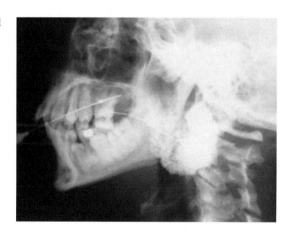

152 Overfilled parotid gland. L.

153 Perforated sub-mandibular duct. OLM.

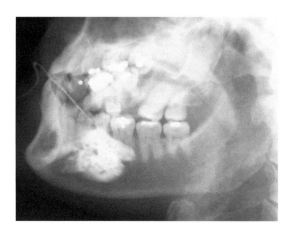

154 Perforated sub-mandibular duct. OLM.

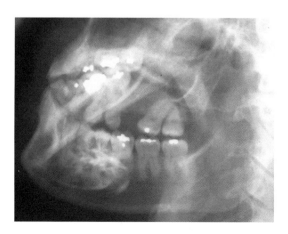

73

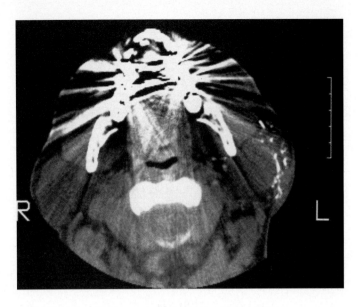

155 'Star bursts' around metallic restorations. CT.

Artefact in computerized tomography

A common form of artefact arising during CT of the face and jaws is the presence of 'star bursts' of radially-arranged, alternating bands of radiolucency and radio-opacity. These artefacts arise when structures of low and high attenuation are close together, causing a hardening of the X-ray beam. Therefore they are particularly likely to occur when metallic objects are present within the tissues, for example, metallic dental restorations. When numerous restorations are present (**155**) the detail of the surrounding tissues can be totally obscured.

4

The teeth

Introduction

The radiographic examination of the teeth and their supporting tissues is commonly performed in dental practice to confirm a diagnosis or in the assessment of a disorder or abnormality. Intra-oral radiographs are preferred where detailed information is required, as, for example, in the detection of early dental caries or apical bone loss, or where a limited area of the jaw is being investigated. DPRs, on the other hand, are useful for general screening of the dentition, in the assessment of unerupted teeth and for the demonstration of extensive or multiple lesions associated with the teeth. Although they may lack the fine definition of intra-oral radiographs, DPRs demonstrate a number of conditions well, due to their inherent high contrast. The anatomical arrangement of the teeth in an arch form allows them to be imaged in a buccolingual plane or as a plan view but not in a mesiodistal direction. However, this limitation does not present a major problem in clinical practice.

The long-term review of patients with diseases of the teeth may require repeated radiographs of the jaws over a number of years. Although the irradiation from each dental radiograph is relatively small, it is essential that the clinician is satisfied with the justification for every exposure, in order to minimize the accumulated dose.

Developmental conditions

Unerupted teeth

It is not unusual for one or more teeth of the permanent dentition to fail to erupt, the most common cause being insufficient space. Although any tooth of the permanent dentition may be affected, it most commonly involves those teeth that naturally erupt late in the formation of the dentition, i.e third molars and canines. Failure to erupt is often accompanied by the impaction of the unerupted tooth against an adjacent one. To assess an impacted tooth fully it is necessary to obtain information about the shape and state of its crown, the shape, size and number of its roots, its relation to adjacent structures, e.g. the inferior alveolar canal, and the nature and level of the enveloping bone. As a consequence, radiographs giving the most detailed information, intra-oral films, are particularly helpful. Since unerupted teeth, especially third molars, are often multiple, DPRs have the advantage of showing all the teeth on the same film and also the full depth of the supporting bone. To determine the spatial relationship of the unerupted tooth to adjacent structures in the plane of the X-ray beam, it is often necessary to take two radiographs employing the principles of parallax or to use radiographs taken at right angles to each other.

MANDIBULAR MOLARS

In the permanent dentition, mandibular third molar teeth commonly become impacted and so fail to erupt fully. If partially erupted, the overlying soft tissues are prone to recurrent episodes of infection (pericoronitis) and the impacted teeth may become carious, whereas when deeply embedded they are often symptomless. Impacted mandibular third molars are classified according to the position in which they lie relative to the longitudinal axis of the second molars into vertical, mesio-angular, disto-angular, horizontal and transverse impactions.

In the vertically impacted ⎡8̅ (**156**), the distal aspect of the crown is encased in bone and is surrounded by a normal, radiolucent follicular space and a thin, radio-opaque, cortical lamina. Its occlusal surface is slightly below that of ⎡6̅7̅ . The impacted tooth has two mesial roots, the apices of

which are curved distally. Note the dense, radio-opaque shadow of the film holder above ⎡6̅ , which is also present in a number of subsequent radiographs. Another vertically impacted ⎡8̅ (**157**) has fused roots and the crown is covered in bone disto-occlusally. The radiolucent follicular space is of normal width around much of the crown, the mesial part of which slightly overlaps ⎡7̅ cervically. The inferior alveolar canal runs obliquely across the apices of the roots but shows no evidence of narrowing and hence possible grooving of the roots (see **172–175**).

Mandibular third molars are commonly impacted in a mesio-angular direction. The slightly mesio-angularly impacted ⎡8̅ (**158**) is partially erupted and has at least four separate root apices. The number of roots is better demonstrated (**159**) where the tube angulation has been altered

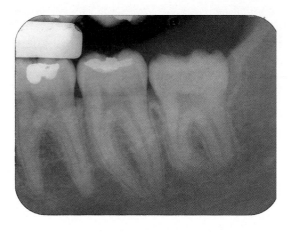

156 Vertically impacted mandibular third molar. P.

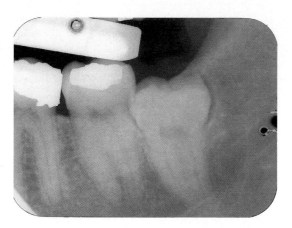

157 Vertically impacted mandibular third molar. P.

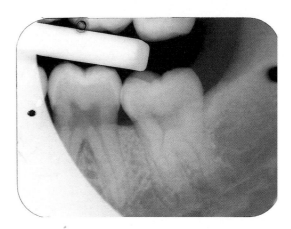

158 Mesio-angularly impacted mandibular third molar. P.

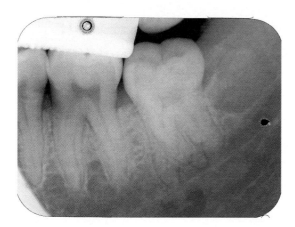

159 Mesio angularly-impacted mandibular third molar. P.

upwards in a vertical direction. In the more markedly mesio-angularly impacted 8̲| (**160**), the distal part of the crown is partially erupted. The tooth has two stout roots, whereas 7̲| has a single, conical root. When partially erupted, an impacted third molar provides an area of stagnation that may predispose to dental caries and/or localized periodontal disease. The next example of a mesio-angularly impacted |8̄ (**161**) has a large occlusal carious lesion. There is also bone loss interdentally |78 where the alveolar crest is radiolucent, which is further evidence of stagnation around the impacted tooth. The roots of |78 are both conical, and the inferior alveolar canal – the cortical lamina of which remains intact – runs obliquely across the apex |8̄. In addition to the impacted tooth, the adjacent tooth is also prone to dental caries, as in the example (**162**) of a mesio-angularly impacted |8̄ with a grossly carious crown impacted into a cavity on the distal aspect |7̄. |8̄ has two roots, both of which exhibit marked mesial curvature apically. The surrounding bone is densely radio-opaque with increased trabeculations (osteosclerosis), probably in response to local irritation from the focus of stagnation where the teeth are impacting.

Impacted teeth are frequently diagnosed about the time of their expected eruption, when their root formation is incomplete, as in the mesio-angularly positioned 8̲| (**163**). Its crown is surrounded by a normal,

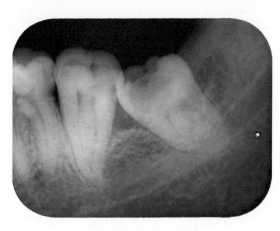

161 Mesio-angularly impacted mandibular third molar. P.

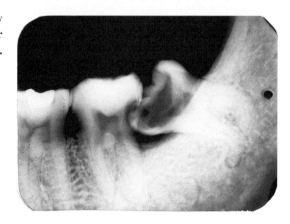

162 Mesio-angularly impacted mandibular third molar. P.

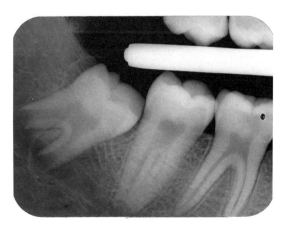

163 Mesio-angularly impacted mandibular third molar. P.

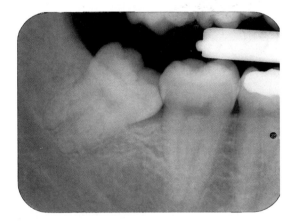

160 Mesio-angularly impacted mandibular third molar. P.

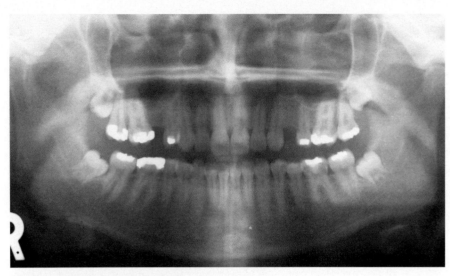

164 Unerupted third molars. DPR.

radiolucent follicular space and a thin radio-opaque, cortical lamina. In **164** there are four unerupted third molars, all with incompletely formed roots. $\overline{8|8}$ are mesially inclined and $\underline{8|8}$ distally inclined, $|8$ being higher than $8|$.

With disto-angularly impacted mandibular third molars, the impaction is into the thick cortical bone of the anterior margin of the ascending ramus of the mandible, rather than into an adjacent tooth. Around the crown of the disto-angularly impacted $\overline{8|}$ (**165**), there is a well-defined, radiolucent follicular space and a thin, radio-opaque cortical lamina. The tooth has two roots and the apical part of the mesial root is curved distally.

In horizontal impactions, the third molar is usually impacted against the tooth in front, commonly the second molar and, as with other types of impaction, its position in the vertical plane may vary. In **166**, the distal part of the crown $\overline{8|}$ lies at the same occlusal level as the adjacent second molar and $\overline{8|}$ has two roots, the apex of the distal root being slightly hooked. Horizontal impactions may also predispose to stagnation, although much less commonly than in mesio-angular impactions, as illustrated by the $\overline{|8}$ (**167**), impacted against $\overline{|7}$, which has a large carious cavity distally. $\overline{|8}$ is two-rooted, but the apices are not visible on this radiograph. There is a large, cervical overhang from the disto-occlusal amalgam restoration $\overline{|6}$, which has a periapical radiolucency with loss of lamina dura on the distal root. The interdental crest $\overline{|67}$ is irregularly radiolucent, indicating the early bone loss of chronic periodontitis.

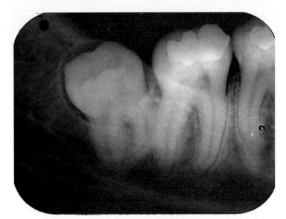

165 Disto-angularly impacted mandibular third molar. P.

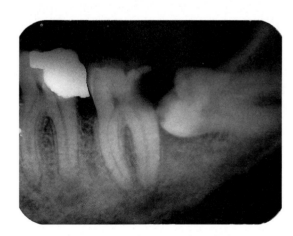

167 Horizontally impacted mandibular third molar. P.

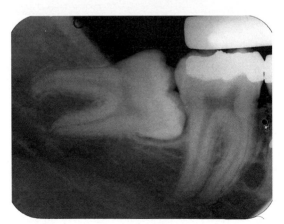

166 Horizontally impacted mandibular third molar. P.

Impactions of third molars usually relate to abnormal positioning of the tooth in the anteroposterior plane. Much less commonly the impaction may relate to an abnormal position in the transverse plane, as in the $\overline{8|}$ (**168**) lying distally to a grossly carious $\overline{7|}$. It is not possible to be certain from this radiograph whether the crown of $\overline{8|}$ lies on the buccal or lingual side of the alveolus, but since the crown is more clearly defined than the roots, it is probable that it lies closer to the film, i.e. lingually. To confirm this, a lower true occlusal view is required. An occlusal radiograph from another patient (**169**) shows the position of the crown (arrow) of the transversely impacted $\overline{8|}$ to be lying lingually. Occasionally, third molars develop in an atypical position and remain unerupted, as in the unusually positioned unerupted $\overline{8|}$ (**170**) with the crown distally angled, lying high up in the ramus of the mandible. The root is fully formed and there is an enlarged, radiolucent follicular space around the crown. Another unusual form of mandibular third molar impaction is shown on the left side of the mandible (**171**), where the $\overline{|8}$ is impacted into the crown of the disto-angularly unerupted $\overline{|7}$. The two teeth share a common radiolucent follicular space. There is also a disto-angularly impacted $\overline{8|}$ and a mesio-angularly impacted $\underline{8|}$.

Unerupted mandibular third molars may lie close to the inferior alveolar canal or indeed their roots may be grooved or even penetrated by the neurovascular bundle. Surgical removal of mandibular third molars may therefore result in damage to the inferior alveolar nerve leading to various degrees of sensory disturbance of the dependent tissues. The pre-operative assessment of the spatial relationship of the inferior alveolar neurovascular bundle to the roots of an impacted tooth is therefore critical. It is possible for the roots of any lower posterior tooth to be close to the inferior alveolar canal. However, because impacted teeth are often more deeply positioned in the alveolar bone than normal, some part of their roots may be at the same horizontal level as that of the inferior alveolar canal and so their images may be superimposed upon each other. This superimposition will occur despite the fact that the two structures are not contiguous and that some bone is present between them. Under these circumstances, the outline of the cortical boundaries of the inferior alveolar canal will remain continuous as it runs across the image of the tooth roots (see **157**) and there will be no narrowing.

169 Transversely impacted mandibular third molar. LTO.

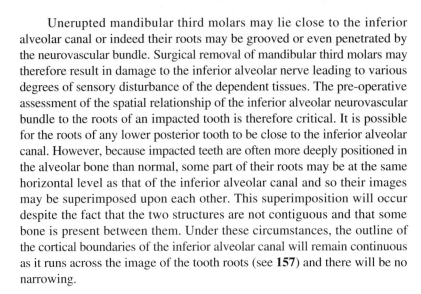

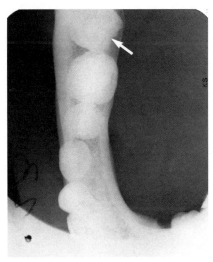

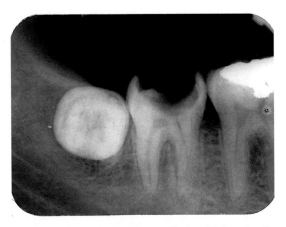

168 Transversely impacted mandibular third molar. P.

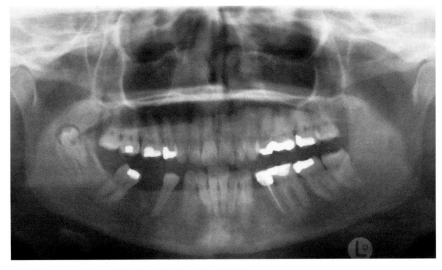

170 Unerupted mandibular third molar. DPR.

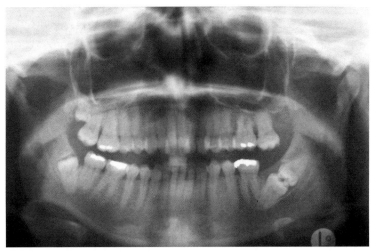

171 Unerupted mandibular third molars. DPR.

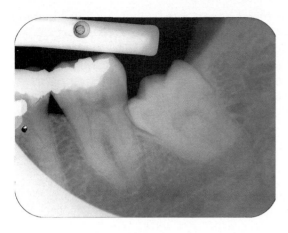

172 Mesio-angularly impacted mandibular third molar involving the inferior alveolar canal. P.

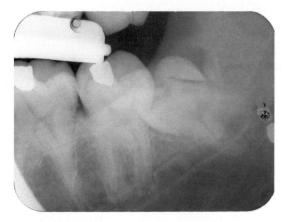

173 Mesio-angularly impacted mandibular third molar involving the inferior alveolar canal. P.

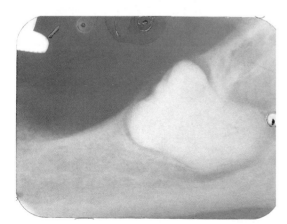

174 Mesio-angularly impacted mandibular third molar involving the inferior alveolar canal. P.

The main radiological features of a tooth root that is grooved or perforated by the inferior alveolar neurovascular bundle are one or more of the following:

- Increased radiolucency of the root where it is traversed by the canal.
- A change in the direction of the canal as it crosses the root.
- Loss of one or both cortical margins of the canal.
- Apparent narrowing of the canal as it crosses the root.

The extent of these changes will depend upon the degree of notching of the tooth root by the neurovascular bundle, or if the root is actually penetrated by the bundle, which is a rare event.

In the mesio-angularly impacted $\overline{8}$ (**172**) with a conical root, the inferior alveolar canal runs transversely over its apical part. The radio-opaque laminae demarcating the bony walls of the canal are continuous across the root and exhibit slight narrowing. In addition, the root is less radio-opaque in this region, suggesting that its surface is indented by the canal. Another example of a mesio-angularly impacted $\overline{8}$ (**173**) shows more marked narrowing of the laminae of the walls of the inferior alveolar canal as it crosses both roots. Again, there is a marked reduction in the radiodensity of the roots in this region, suggesting that they are deeply grooved. There is a large, radiolucent follicular space with a radio-opaque lamina on the distal aspect of the crown. The dark line running obliquely across the distal part of the crown $\overline{8}$ is a finger nail indentation (see **123**). In **174** and **175**, the fused roots of a deeply-placed, mesio-angularly positioned unerupted $\overline{8}$ in an otherwise edentulous jaw, have caused narrowing and deviation of the inferior alveolar canal.

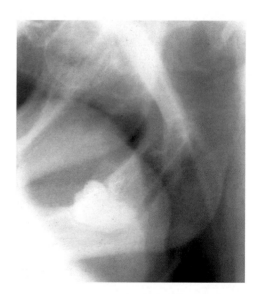

175 Mesio-angularly impacted mandibular third molar involving the inferior alveolar canal. OLM.

Maxillary molars

As in the mandible, with the maxilla it is the third molars that most commonly remain unerupted. They may be vertically or disto-angularly positioned, often with a slight buccal inclination. The tooth also may be mesio-angularly impacted into the second molar, or more rarely inverted. Although the root morphology demonstrates some variation, most tend to be conically shaped. When multirooted the individual roots are often fine or hooked. The crown of the almost fully formed, unerupted |8 (176) is surrounded by a radiolucent follicular space and a thin, radio-opaque layer of cortical bone. The root of the zygoma lies above |6 and running posteriorly from it is the zygomatic arch, its inferior border crossing |8 cervically. Note the coronoid process of the mandible and the pterygoid plate distal to the tuberosity. The distally inclined 8| (177) is inverted and lying in close proximity to the floor of the maxillary antrum. Its root is incompletely formed and the tooth is totally enclosed in bone. The soft-tissue shadow of the mucosa overlying the tuberosity is shown clearly and a root fragment 6| is also present.

Maxillary canines

It is unusual for the maxillary canine to be absent congenitally, therefore if it fails to appear at its expected time of eruption it is probably unerupted, indeed, after third molars, maxillary canines are the next most common teeth not to erupt. As a result the primary predecessor is often retained long after its expected time of shedding. One of both canines may fail to erupt, most often adopting a palatal position relative to the incisor roots, nevertheless radiological confirmation of their position is necessary. This may be performed by employing the parallax method (see 9) or by vertex occlusal (VO) radiography. In addition to determining the buccopalatal location, the angulation and depth in bone of the unerupted canine should be assessed. Other features to note include the stage of root development, root length, root curvature and the size of the follicular space. The unerupted maxillary canine may displace the root of the adjacent maxillary incisor or occasionally induce root resorption.

The two parallax views of the mesially inclined, unerupted |3 (178, 179) demonstrate that its crown lies palatally. In the first radiograph (178) the tip of the crown of the unerupted tooth overlies the apical part of the root |1 . The X-ray tube has been positioned more distally in the second radiograph (179) and the crown of the unerupted tooth has moved in the same relative direction and now overlies the apical part of the root |2 . Another example of the use

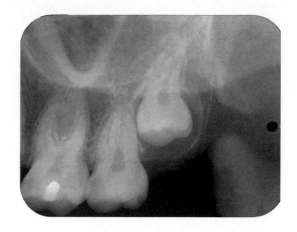

176 Unerupted maxillary third molar. P.

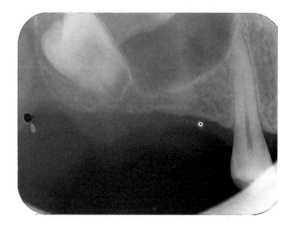

177 Unerupted maxillary third molar. P.

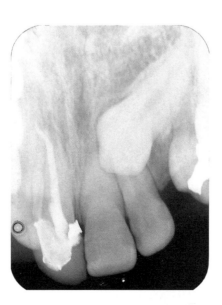

178 Unerupted maxillary canine. P.

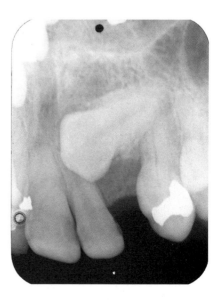

179 Unerupted maxillary canine. P.

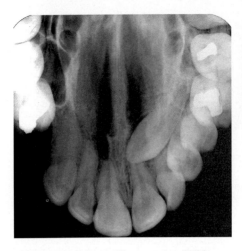

180 Unerupted maxillary canine. USO.

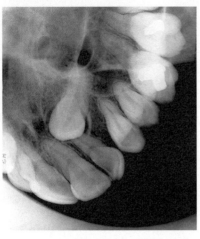

181 Unerupted maxillary canine. UOO.

of parallax demonstrates that the mesially inclined, unerupted ⌐3 (**180**, **181**) lies palatally to the incisor teeth. In the first illustration (**180**), the tube was centred over the midline, as demonstrated by the clear contact 1⌐1 mesially, and in the other (**181**) between ⌐24 . Again, the crown of the unerupted tooth has moved in the same direction as the tube. Both nasolacrimal canals are clearly demonstrated, one of them being superimposed upon the periapical region of the unerupted tooth in the oblique occlusal view. In the example (**182**) of a VO radiograph, the crown 3⌐ is displayed palatally to 4C2⌐ and, although little other information can be obtained, note that 1⌐ is missing.

The decision on how to treat a patient with unerupted maxillary canines usually involves a full orthodontic assessment. The next four radiographs (**183–186**) are, collectively, an example of such an orthodontic assessment and treatment in a 12-year-old patient. The first two (**183**, **184**) show

$$
\begin{array}{cccc|cccc}
8 & 7 & & 3 & 3 & & 7 & 8 \\
\hline
8 & 7 & 5 & & & & & 8
\end{array}
$$

to be unerupted, and C⌐ and E⌐ retained. ⌐3 is in a favourable position to erupt but there is insufficient space in the arch. On the other hand, 3⌐ is less favourably positioned, being mesially inclined, with an enlarged, radiolucent, follicular space around its crown. When an unerupted maxillary canine appears relatively large on a DPR, it is usually indicative of its palatal position. Its apex lies above 5⌐ , close to the floor of the nose, as demonstrated in the lateral radiograph (**184**) in which the two unerupted canines are superimposed.

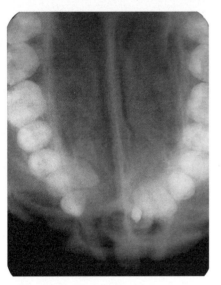

182 Unerupted maxillary canine. VO.

183 (below) Unerupted maxillary canines. DPR.

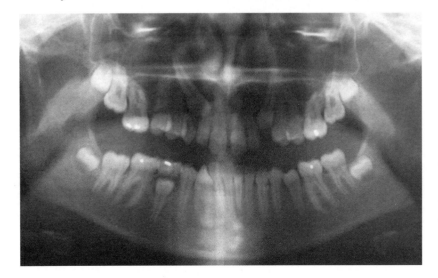

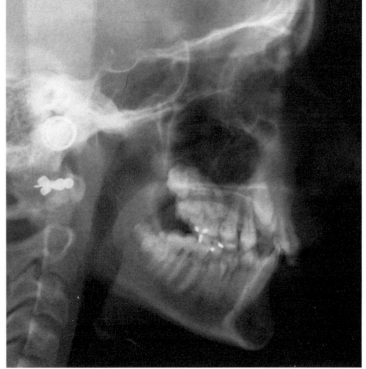

184 Unerupted maxillary canines. LC.

In the next two illustrations taken with the X-ray tube at different angles (**185, 186**), treatment has started with the patient wearing a fixed orthodontic appliance, |3 has erupted and 3| is still unerupted in a palatal position (parallax). Note that stud ear-rings (**183**) have caused linear opacities bilaterally at the lower border of the orbits (see **124**).

Although the crowns of unerupted canines usually lie palatally to the roots of the erupted teeth (as in the examples already given), less commonly they may be buccally placed. The two parallax views (**187, 188**) of an unerupted 3|, taken with the X-ray tube more mesially placed in the second radiograph, demonstrate that the crown lies buccally to the adjacent teeth. In the first radiograph the crown of the unerupted tooth obscures much of the width of the apical part 2| and appears to lie close to 1|, whereas in the second, more of the root 2| is visible as the 3| has moved distally relative to the incisors. C| is retained with a large, carious cavity distally and there is advanced resorption of the root. Although root resorption of the retained deciduous predecessor tooth is to be anticipated, the rate at which this occurs varies greatly.

Resorption of the roots of other adjacent permanent teeth by an unerupted canine is sometimes an undesirable complication. The unerupted, impacted 3| (**189**) has caused apical resorption 2| in a 14-year-old. The apex of the resorbed tooth is irregularly blunted and lacks a distinct periodontal ligament space and lamina dura, so that the follicular radiolucency around the crown 3| abuts directly onto the root, suggesting that the resorptive process is active. On the other hand, the root of the retained C|, although irregularly shortened, is surrounded by a periodontal ligament space and lamina dura indicating that any resorption is proceeding slowly. Note the dilaceration 1| apically, indicated by the curvature of its root canal, and that |3 is also unerupted. Root resorption is an intermittent process, periods of resorption often being followed by periods of temporary repair. Resorption caused by unerupted teeth usually slows down and eventually ceases when the normal age of full eruption of the impacted tooth has been reached. In the example (**190**) in an adult, the unerupted 3| has caused apical resorption of the roots 21|, which are shortened and flattened. Both roots are surrounded by a distinct radiolucent periodontal ligament space and a radio-opaque lamina dura, the crown 3| by a normal, follicular radiolucency, suggesting that the resorptive process is no longer active.

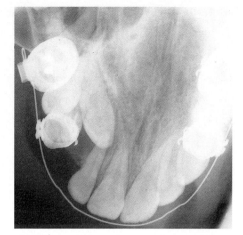

185 Unerupted maxillary canines. UOO.

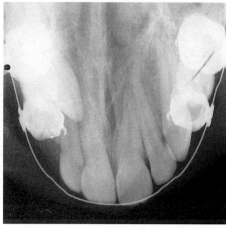

186 Unerupted maxillary canines. USO.

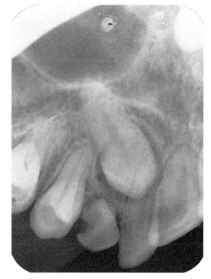

187 Unerupted maxillary canine. P.

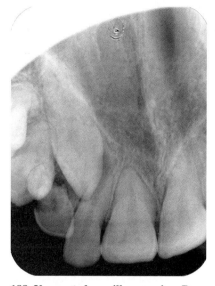

188 Unerupted maxillary canine. P.

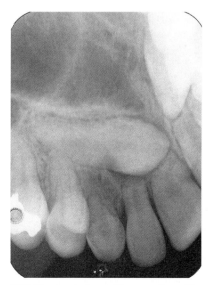

189 Unerupted maxillary canines. P.

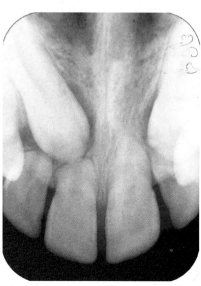

190 Unerupted maxillary canine. P.

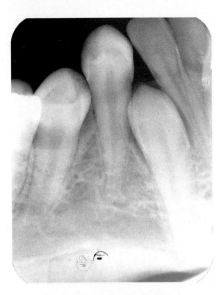

191 Unerupted mandibular canine. P.

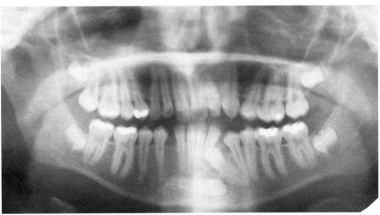

192 Unerupted mandiubular canines. DPR.

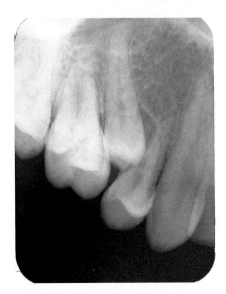

193 Unerupted maxillary premolar. P.

MANDIBULAR CANINES

Mandibular canines remain unerupted less frequently than maxillary canines and are usually unilateral, although bilateral impactions do occur. The unerupted $\overline{3|}$ (191) in a 12-year-old is vertically impacted between $\overline{4|}$ and $\overline{2|}$, which have drifted mesially and distally respectively. There is a normal follicular radiolucency around the crown $\overline{3|}$; the slightly hooked apex lies close to the inferior border of the mandible. The unerupted teeth may assume a position deep within the bone of the body of the mandible, as in 192 showing bilateral, unerupted impacted canines with resultant diastemas in a 15-year-old. $\overline{3|}$ lies horizontally beneath the incisors and $\overline{|3}$ is mesio-angularly impacted against $\overline{|2}$, the crown of which is tilted distally. The follicular space around the crown $\overline{3|}$ is enlarged and is contiguous superiorly with that surrounding $\overline{|3}$.

MAXILLARY PREMOLARS

Second premolars, more commonly than first premolars, may fail to erupt fully, particularly when there is insufficient space to accommodate both teeth in the arch. They are most commonly displaced palatally. The unerupted, mesio-angularly impacted $5|$ (193) lies between $6|$ and $4|$, which are tilted mesially and distally respectively. A normal follicular space surrounds the crown $5|$ and there is a slight curvature of the root apex. In the second example (194) – a 13-year-old patient – the image of the unerupted $5|$ is markedly foreshortened due to its palatal inclination, so that its long axis lies roughly in the same plane as that of the X-rays. The root is dilacerated and has an open apex. $6|$ is mesially tilted, the root formation $7|$ is incomplete and $8|$ is only partially formed and unerupted.

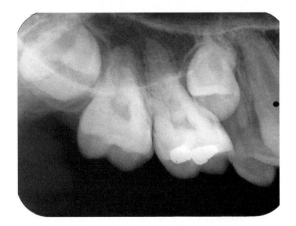

194 Unerupted maxillary premolar. P.

MANDIBULAR PREMOLARS

As with maxillary premolars, it is the mandibular second premolar that is more likely to remain unerupted and they are most commonly inclined lingually. Sometimes, when they are more deeply embedded, they are positioned horizontally and are often not discovered until later life when the patient may be edentulous.

The unerupted, mesio-angularly inclined $\overline{5|}$ (**195**) lies between $\overline{6|}$ and $\overline{4|}$, which are tilted mesially and distally respectively. There is a follicular radiolucency around the crown and a slight distal curvature of the root. It is difficult to be certain on periapical radiographs whether the crown of such an unerupted tooth lies lingually or buccally. However, the greater definition of the crown compared with that of the root suggests that the crown is closer to the film, i.e. lingually. Its position is confirmed (arrow) on the occlusal radiograph (**196**). In the further example (**197**) of a mesio-angularly impacted $\overline{5|}$ in a 13-year-old, $\overline{4|}$ is tilted distally and has an incompletely formed root, which exhibits apical bifurcation of the root canal suggestive of taurodontism. Both roots $\overline{6|}$ are retained and are carious. There is a normal follicular space around the crown $\overline{5|}$ mesio-inferiorly, but distosuperiorly there is an enlarged, poorly defined, radiolucent area that is confluent with a periapical radiolucency around $\overline{6|}$ roots. A cortical lamina is continuous from the distal aspect of the distal root $\overline{6|}$ to the distal cervical region of the $\overline{5|}$. The roots $\overline{7|}$ and $\overline{5|}$ are not completely formed.

With deeply embedded teeth in older patients, the alveolar bone may have been resorbed and remodelled following extraction of the erupted teeth and hence the unerupted tooth becomes closer to the surface and may even become exposed in the oral cavity. In **198**, the unerupted $\overline{5|}$ lies horizontally in an edentulous mandible. The definition of the crown is better than that of the root, suggesting that the former is lingually positioned. The tooth appears to be lying anteroposteriorly in the jaw but its oblique position is indicated in the occlusal view (**199**). The lingual position of the crown, which has perforated the cortical plate and become carious, is

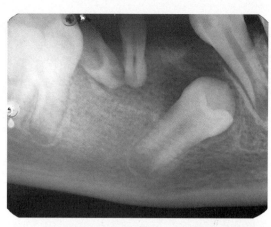

197 Unerupted mandibular premolar. P.

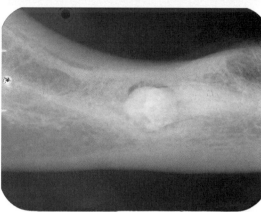

198 Unerupted mandibular premolar. P.

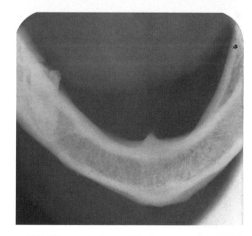

199 Unerupted mandibular premolar. LTO.

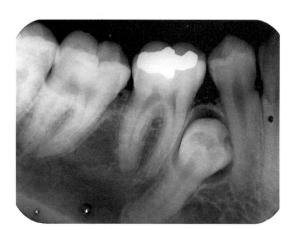

195 Unerupted mandibular premolar. P.

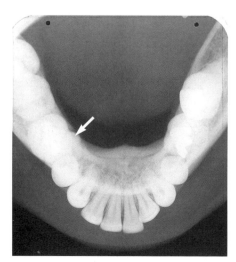

196 Unerupted mandibular premolar. LTO.

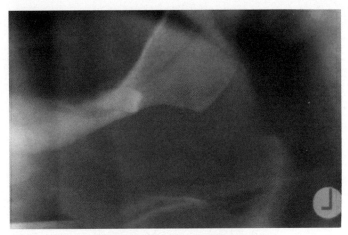

200 Unerupted mandibular premolar. DPR.

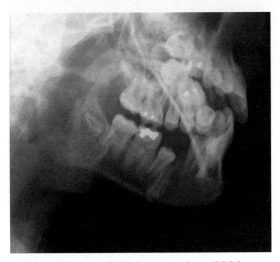

201 Unerupted mandibular premolars. OLM.

confirmed. Another example (**200**) shows an unerupted 5̲ which is disto-inferiorly displaced with the crown perforating the lower border of the mandible and the apex projecting through the edentulous ridge. Following exposure to the oral environment, the root apex has become carious, as demonstrated by the irregularly shaped radiolucent defect. The inferior alveolar canal deviates inferiorly beneath the tooth before looping upwards anteriorly to reach the superior aspect of the mandibular ridge, indicating a close relationship between the canal and the unerupted tooth. Another example (**201**) shows an unusual unerupted premolar in a 13-year-old, this time a 4̲, which is inverted. The crown has perforated the inferior border of the mandible and 5̲ is also unerupted.

MAXILLARY INCISORS

Occasionally maxillary incisors fail to erupt; when this occurs it is almost always due to some abnormality of the tooth or the adjacent tissues, rather than lack of space. Common causes include the presence of a supernumerary tooth (see **221**, **213**), an odontome (see **233**, **234**) or, when the erupting tooth is dilacerated, sometimes as a consequence of trauma. The unerupted 1̲ (**202**, **203**) has a dilacerated root following traumatic displacement at an early stage of root development by the intrusion of the overlying A̲. On the periapical radiographs the tooth is grossly foreshortened because it is lying transversely in the alveolar bone. Parallax views (**202**, **203**) indicate that the crown lies buccally. Its position is confirmed on a true lateral view of the anterior maxilla (arrow), which demonstrates the spatial relationships of the tooth more clearly (**204**). These radiographs were taken when the patient was nine years old and the root formation of 2̲1̲|2̲ is still incomplete, |3̲ is unerupted and 2̲| is already tilted mesially with some loss of space. Another unerupted and dilacerated 1̲ (**205**) is shown in an older patient. 1̲ is foreshortened and rotated, and 2̲| is markedly tilted in a mesial direction so that it now contacts |1̲ with almost complete loss of the space.

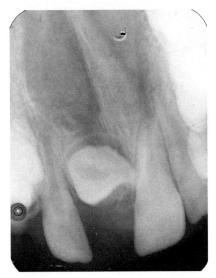

202 Unerupted maxillary central incisor. P.

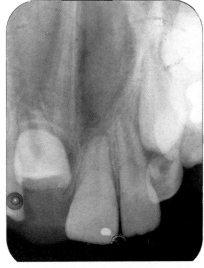

203 Unerupted maxillary central incisor. P.

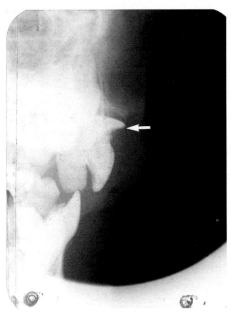

204 Unerupted maxillary central incisor. TLM.

Tooth transposition

Tooth transposition is uncommon but is most likely to affect the maxillary permanent canine which has a long path of eruption and normally erupts after the adjacent premolar teeth. In **206**, |34 are transposed and |3 is rotated and impacted between |45 . In addition, this patient has hypodontia, |2 , 5| and 5̄| are missing, and 2| is smaller than usual. 3| is unerupted, lying above the retained C| , and |5̄ is impacted. All four third molars are at an early stage of development.

Supernumerary teeth

Supernumerary teeth are not uncommon, occurring in approximately 0.5% of the population. They are most commonly found in the anterior part of the maxilla, where they may exist in one of two forms: conical or tuberculate. The conical form, or mesiodens, tends to occur either side of the midline. Its chronological development is between the formation of the primary and secondary dentitions, so that it may erupt before the permanent teeth. The mesiodens (**207**) which has erupted in the midline of the maxilla in a five-year-old, has a conical crown and the root formation is complete. In contrast, root formation in the unerupted 21|12 , the images of which are superimposed, has only just commenced. A| is missing and root resorption |A is advanced. Another example (**208**) of an erupted mesiodens, this time in an adult, shows the small conical crown lying between 1|1 . Conical supernumerary teeth often remain unerupted as in the mesiodens (**209**), the crown of which is inclined disto-occlusally, in the midline of the maxilla of a nine-year-old.

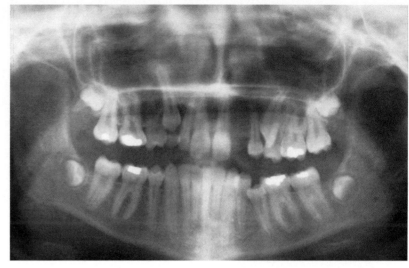

206 Transposed maxillary canine. DPR.

207 Mesiodens. P.

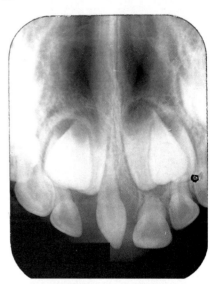

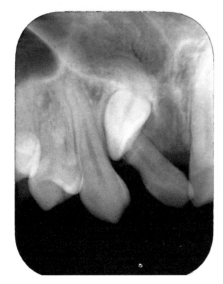

205 Unerupted maxillary central incisor. P.

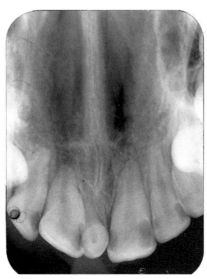

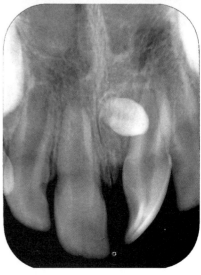

208 Mesiodens. P.   **209 Mesiodens. P.**

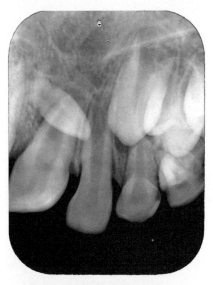

210 Mesiodens. P.

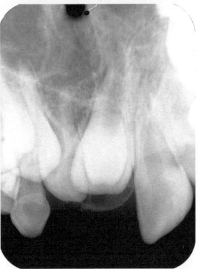

211 Tuberculate super-numerary tooth. P.

The root is dilacerated (**210**) with the apex pointing occlusally. These two films show by parallax that the crown lies palatally and the root lies buccally to ⌞1 , which is rotated.

The tuberculate form of supernumerary teeth develops slightly later than the permanent incisors so they are usually found to be at a less advanced stage of development than the adjacent permanent teeth. As a consequence, they are less likely to erupt and often impede the eruption of the permanent incisors. The unerupted tuberculate, supernumerary tooth (**211**) in the anterior maxilla, has caused delayed eruption 1⌟ in a nine-year-old. The outline of the supernumerary tooth overlies 1⌟ , the root of which is more fully formed than that of the supernumerary tooth. Note the unerupted 32⌟ and erupted C⌟ .

Both forms of supernumerary tooth may occur singly or in pairs and in the case of the latter the two teeth are usually of the same form. In **212** there are two unerupted, distally inclined, inverted supernumerary teeth with conical crowns lying above the apices of the maxillary incisors. The apex of the right tooth is hooked. It is not uncommon for supernumerary teeth in the anterior maxilla to be inverted. Two unerupted supernumerary teeth (**213**) are shown inhibiting the eruption of ⌞1 in a ten-year-old. The more apically placed one is inverted, conically shaped and has a complete root. The more occlusally placed one is tuberculate, incompletely formed and probably the cause of the delayed eruption ⌞1 . It is unusual to find both types in the same patient. Root formation ⌞1 is nearly complete and the space between 1⌟ and ⌞2 is partially closed. Note the unerupted ⌞345 .

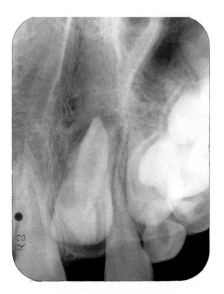

213 Supernumerary teeth. P.

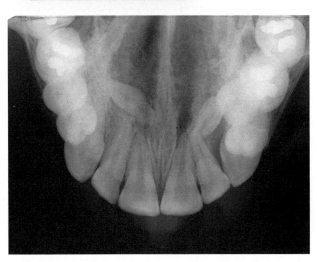

212 Supernumerary teeth. USO.

Supplemental teeth

In contrast to supernumerary teeth, supplemental teeth are morphologically similar to those of the normal dentition but, as in the tuberculate form, they commence their development after the adjacent permanent teeth. In this respect, they are regarded as representing a third and even sometimes a fourth dentition. In **214** there is an incompletely formed, unerupted, supplemental, left mandibular premolar. The developing tooth is surrounded by a radiolucent follicular space and a thin, radio-opaque lamina. The next example (**215**) shows two unerupted, impacted, supplemental, right mandibular premolars. Note that $\overline{5|5}$ are rotated. Extra mandibular molars are less frequent than premolars. The horizontally impacted, supplemental molar (**216**) is lying occlusally to an unerupted third molar (paramolar), which is also horizontally impacted. Supplemental maxillary molar teeth are, however, not uncommon and in the radiograph of a 14-year-old (**217**), there are two supplemental maxillary molars on each side in addition to the developing upper third molars (arrows). The lower arch has a normal complement of molar teeth.

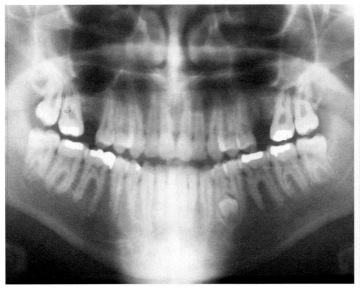

214 Supplemental mandibular premolar. DPR.

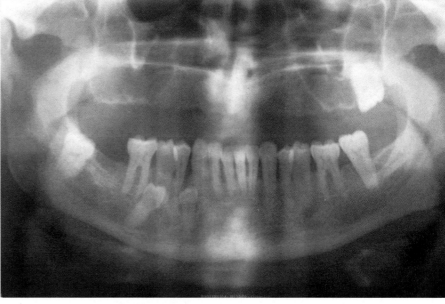

215 Supplemental mandibular premolars. DPR.

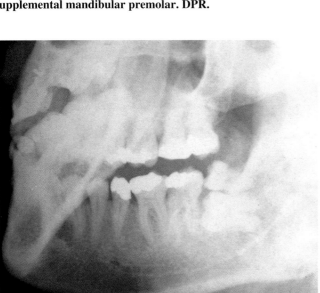

216 Supplemental mandibular molar. OLM.

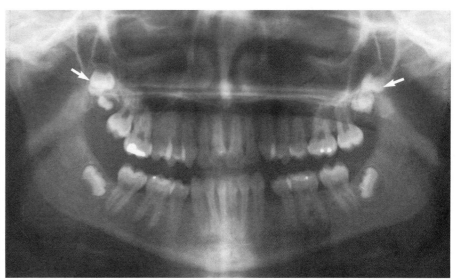

217 Supplemental maxillary molars. DPR.

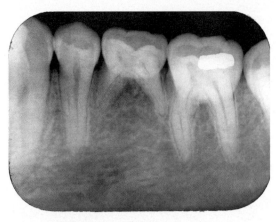

218 Retained primary second molar. P.

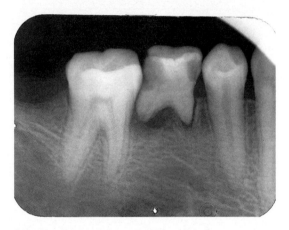

219 Retained primary second molar. P.

Hypodontia (partial anodontia)

Missing teeth, or hypodontia (partial anodontia), is usually a familial condition observed in both the primary and the permanent dentitions. In the former it most commonly affects a maxillary incisor tooth, but in the latter the teeth, which are most often absent, include third molars, mandibular second premolars, maxillary lateral incisors and mandibular central incisors. The condition may be mild, when one or a few teeth are affected, or more severe when numerous teeth fail to develop. Absence of a permanent tooth may result in retention of its primary predecessor for a longer period than normal. This commonly occurs with second premolars and, as a consequence, the primary second molar is retained. Their roots may remain relatively normal (**218**) or show evidence of past resorption (**219**). In the latter there are two large radiolucent carious lesions, one mesially and one distally in the retained second primary molar, with periapical radiolucencies on both roots. The outline of the radiolucent areas is indistinct.

Less commonly, the process of root resorption, which is intermittent with alternate periods of repair, may lead to ankylosis between the tooth root and the surrounding bone. Under these circumstances, the primary tooth becomes fused to the bone and, as the permanent teeth on each side continue their normal pattern of eruption, it appears at a relatively lower occlusal level as a submerged primary molar. In **220** there has been complete resorption of the roots |E and only the crown remains. The boundary between the tooth and the surrounding bone is indistinct and no lamina dura is present, indicative of bony ankylosis. The occlusal level of the crown |E is apically positioned relative to that of |4 and |6 , which are distally and mesially inclined respectively. In the case of missing maxillary permanent lateral incisors, the canine frequently erupts into their site. In **221** and **222**, |3 has erupted into the position normally occupied by |2 ; |C has been retained.

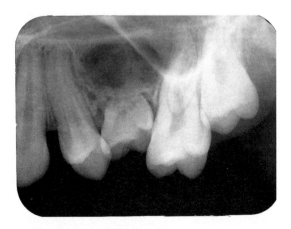

220 Submerged primary molar. P.

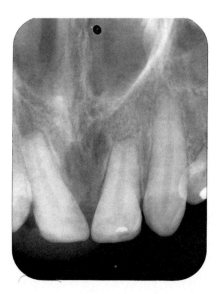

221 Hypodontia (partial anodontia). P.

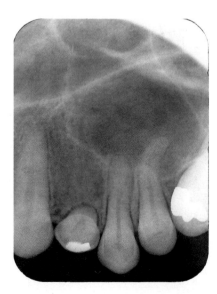

222 Hypodontia (partial anodontia). P.

In more severe cases several teeth may be absent. In **223** – a 15-year-old – the only permanent teeth to have developed are

$$\frac{7\,6 \quad\quad 1\,|\,1 \quad\quad 6}{7\,6 \quad 3\,2\,1\,| \quad\quad 6}.$$

In the intervening spaces the following primary teeth are retained:

$$\frac{E\,D\,C \quad\quad B\,C\,D\,E}{E\,D \quad\quad A\,B\,C\,D\,E}.$$

$\frac{|6}{|6}$ both have a single conical root and root canal, which is a further manifestation of the condition.

Ectodermal dysplasia

A severe variety of partial anodontia may occasionally be associated with the more generalized, genetically determined disorder of ectodermal dysplasia in which the adnexal structures of ectodermal origin may be abnormal or absent and the teeth may be affected to a varying extent. In this five-and-a-half-year-old with severe involvement of the dentition (**224**), many teeth are absent and those that have developed exhibit pronounced conical form and bulbosity of their crowns. The only teeth present are

$$\frac{6\,E \quad C\,B \quad |\,1\,B\,C \quad E\,6}{6 \quad\quad | \quad\quad 6},$$

none of the permanent teeth having yet erupted. The absence of teeth has resulted in failure of the alveolar bone to develop and the jaws exhibit less vertical height than normal.

Odontomes

Odontomes are developmental malformations (hamartomata) of the mineralized dental tissues, which may (invaginated odontome; geminated odontome; enameloma) or may not (compound odontome; complex odontome) resemble a normal tooth in structure. The former usually erupt into the mouth, whereas the compound and complex odontomes tend to remain embedded in bone. Odontomes develop at the same time as the normal dentition and so if they remain unerupted they may impede the eruption of the adjacent teeth.

INVAGINATED ODONTOME
This condition – invagination of the odontogenic epithelium into the dental papilla prior to the secretion of the mineralized matrix – produces the appearance of a tooth within a tooth (dens in dente). It most commonly affects maxillary lateral incisors and is often bilateral.

In **225**, the crown $\underline{2}$ is conical in outline and contains an invaginated mass, which is lined by a densely radio-opaque layer of enamel. The root is of normal structure. Pulpal necrosis commonly occurs in this condition due to direct bacterial penetration of the invagination and consequently

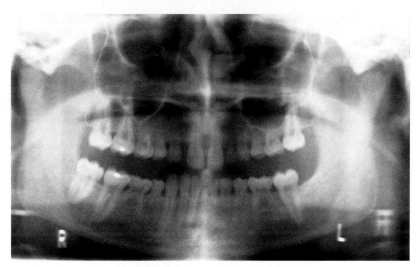

223 Hypodontia (partial anodontia). DPR.

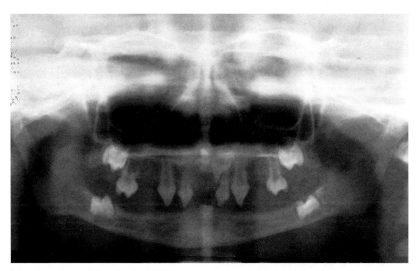

224 Ectodermal dysplasia. DPR.

225 Invaginated odontome. P.

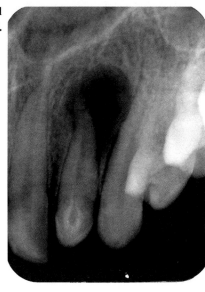

periapical lesions may be seen. In this example there is a large, clearly defined, periapical radiolucency, with absence of the apical lamina dura.

If the epithelial invagination occurs in the radicular part of the developing tooth, a dilated form of odontome arises (**226**) where the crown 2| is conical and the cervical part of the root is widened by a radiolucent dilatation lined by a thin, radio-opaque layer of enamel. The invagination has displaced the pulp chamber into the apical half of the root. Such invaginations may weaken the tooth and, in this example, a thin, radiolucent fracture line is present, running obliquely across the widest part of the invagination.

Another example (**227**) is shown, in which the crown of |4 is enlarged and contains a convoluted mass of dental tissues projecting mesially into the coronal part of the pulp chamber. The root is also enlarged with a widened root canal. As a sequel to pulpal necrosis, there is a periapical radiolucency, which extends along the entire mesial aspect of the root up to the alveolar crest, with loss of the lamina dura.

GEMINATED ODONTOME

In geminated odontomes, the affected structure usually has two crowns, which are separated to a variable extent, and a single root. These structures may arise from fusion of two separate tooth germs or from twinning of a single tooth germ. In the odontome (**228**) replacing B| in an eight-year-old, there are two distinct crowns, each with its own pulp chamber and a common root with two separate root canals. There is slight resorption of the root, with irregularity of part of the surface. 2| is missing and the unerupted 43| have drifted mesially, 3| lying beneath the odontome.

Another lesion in the lower incisor region (**229**) has probably arisen from the fusion of the tooth germs of |1 and |2 . In their place there is a single tooth structure with a large incisiform crown (megadontia) and a single, large root canal and pulp chamber with two elongated pulp horns.

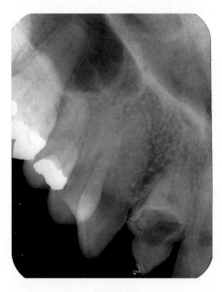

226 Invaginated odontome. P.

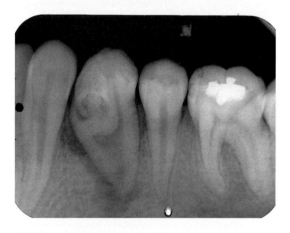

227 Invaginated odontome. P.

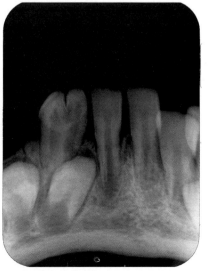

228 Geminated odontome. P.

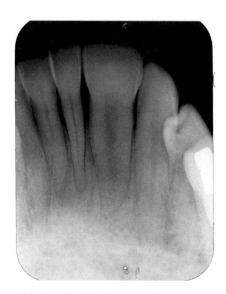

229 Geminated odontome. P.

In **230**, in the maxillary incisor region, |1 has a large crown partially separated by a centrally placed, vertical cleft. There is a large pulp chamber with two prominent pulp horns and a single wide root canal in the greatly enlarged root. The cingulum is composed of several small tubercles. 1| is also larger than normal and may be a mild expression of the same condition. Note the pronounced horizontal cervical radiolucency overlying the odontome, caused by the contrast of the relatively radiodense crown incisally and the crest of the alveolar bone apically.

A fourth example (**231**) shows 4|, which has two separate crowns, each with its own pulp chamber, joined approximately half way along their roots. At this level, the two separate root canals unite, forming a single, common root canal in the apical half. The disto-occlusal part of the crown is densely radio-opaque due to the convoluted pattern of the surface enamel. 5| has been displaced buccally by the odontome and its crown appears at a lower occlusal level than that of the adjacent teeth.

ENAMELOMA

An enameloma (enamel pearl) is a small nodule composed predominantly of enamel, located at or close to the level of the furcation of the roots and therefore appears as a dense radio-opacity at this site. It is more common in maxillary molars between the distobuccal and palatal roots. In **232**, there is a small, irregularly ovoid, densely radio-opaque mass on the mesiocervical aspect of the root |6 . Note the overhanging restoration and recurrent caries mesially |7 .

COMPOUND ODONTOME

These odontomes probably arise from aberrant proliferation of the dental lamina with the formation of multiple tooth germs, resulting in circumscribed collections of tooth-like structures (denticles). They are more common in the anterior regions of the jaws and are usually mature when discovered.

The lesion (**233**), which has prevented the eruption of 1| in a ten-year-old, is circumscribed by a clearly-defined, capsular radiolucency and a thin radio-opaque lamina, and contains numerous small radio-opaque denticles. The mass overlies the crown 1|, which appears wider and less clearly defined than that of |1 , suggesting that it is more buccally placed.

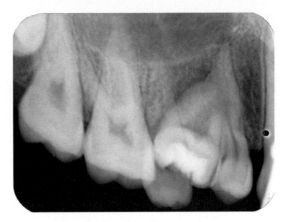

231 Geminated odontome. P.

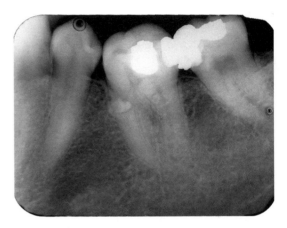

232 Enameloma. P.

230 Geminated odontome. P.

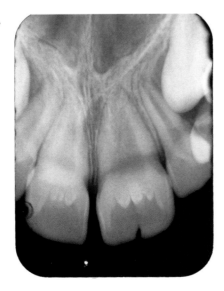

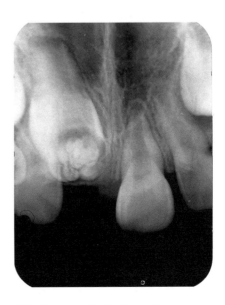

233 Compound odontome. P.

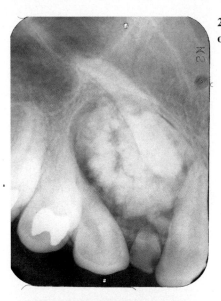

234 Compound odontome. P.

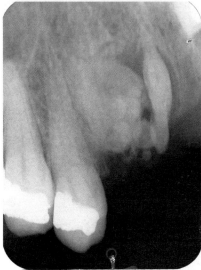

235 Compound odontome. P.

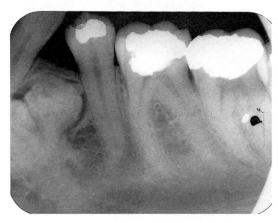

236 Complex odontome. P.

A larger lesion (**234**) has prevented the eruption of 2|, which is displaced superiorly. It is surrounded by a capsular radiolucency and a thin, radio-opaque lamina and is composed of numerous denticles superimposed upon each other, forming a mass of variable radio-opacity. The root 3| is displaced distally and the retained B| exhibits advanced root resorption.

A further lesion (**235**) is shown in the edentulous part of the premaxilla. The mass consists of a number of denticles of varying size, several of them exhibiting a root canal, enamel and dentine. It is clearly defined anteriorly where there is a radiolucent capsular space and a radio-opaque lamina, but less so superiorly and posteriorly, possibly as a consequence of infection. The occlusal surface of the mass lies in the soft tissues.

COMPLEX ODONTOME

In complex odontomes, the aberrant proliferation of the epithelium of a single tooth germ forms a complex structure in which the disordered mass of mineralized dental tissues bears no morphological resemblance to a tooth. They occur most commonly in the posterior part of the jaws.

The small lesion (**236**), which has displaced and prevented the eruption of |4, is variably radio-opaque and clearly defined, being surrounded by a radiolucent capsular space and a thin radio-opaque lamina. The roots |35 are displaced mesially and distally respectively.

A larger lesion (**237**) in the right body of the mandible has displaced 8| anteriorly and inferiorly. The mass is variably radio-opaque and oval in outline and surrounded by a clearly defined radiolucent capsule and a radio-opaque lamina of bone. The degree of radio-opacity of the lesion varies, containing some areas of similar density to those of the enamel and dentine of the adjacent displaced tooth. The follicular space around the crown 8| is clearly shown indicating that it is separate from the overlying lesion. Note the diffuse radio-opacity with parallel linear radiolucencies in the molar region and base of the left ramus of the mandible, formed by the ghost image of the odontome. Note also the root-filled 6|4 , both of which show excess radio-opaque root-filling material extruded into the periapical tissues.

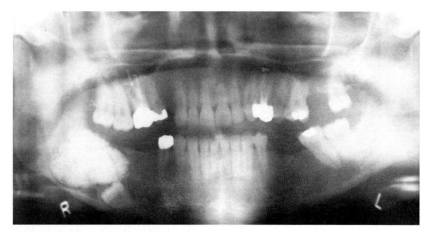

237 Complex odontome. DPR.

Periapical cemental dysplasia

This hamartomatous condition may affect one, or more commonly, multiple teeth and is more common in females, particularly those of negroid origin.

In **238** there are approximately circular, clearly defined, periapical radiolucencies at the apices of $\overline{2|12}$. The central aspect of each area is relatively radio-opaque due to the deposition of cementum. As a rule, the early lesion is radiolucent and is similar in appearance to a periapical inflammatory lesion. However, in periapical cemental dysplasia, the teeth retain their vitality. As the lesion matures, more mineralized cementum is formed and it becomes increasingly radio-opaque.

In **239** there are two well displayed lesions associated with the apices $\overline{6|}$ and $\overline{3|}$, each at different stages of development. Whereas the lesion $\overline{3|}$ is at an early stage, with a well defined, approximately circular, radiolucent area surrounded by a thin radio-opaque margin, that associated with $\overline{6|}$ is more mature and, although circular in appearance, contains a central area of radio-opacity. Its density is similar to that of the adjacent roots of the teeth. There are also other lesions, less well displayed, associated with the lower anterior teeth. Their presence was confirmed on periapical radiographs (**240**).

Gigantiform cementoma

This tumour of cementum also affects negresses more commonly and lesions may be found in all four quadrants of the jaws. Although believed to be a hamartomatous type of abnormality, the masses may not be diagnosed until later life, often when the jaws are edentulous and may reach a large size. The example (**241**) shows radiodense masses of cementum present in the alveolar part of the jaws, each of which are surrounded by a radiolucent capsule and thin radiodense lamina of cortical bone. Such lesions may become infected, particularly if they become exposed in the mouth as a consequence of bone remodelling after tooth extraction, as has occurred in the mass in the right mandibular premolar region.

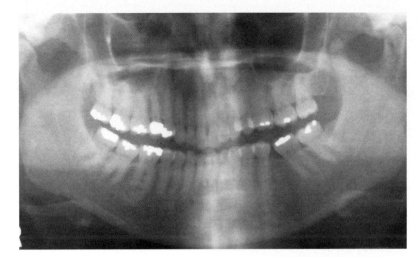

239 Periapical cemental dysplasia. DPR.

240 Periapical cemental dysplasia. P.

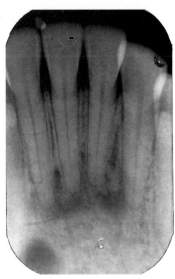

238 (left) Periapical cemental dysplasia. P.

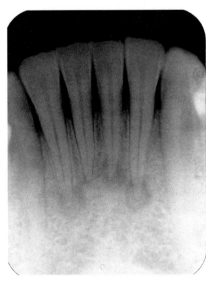

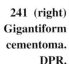

241 (right) Gigantiform cementoma. DPR.

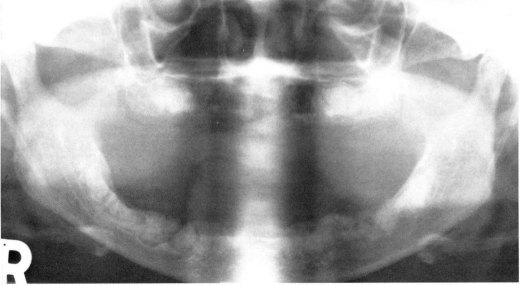

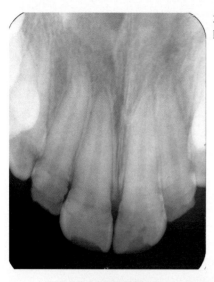

242 Enamel hypoplasia. P.

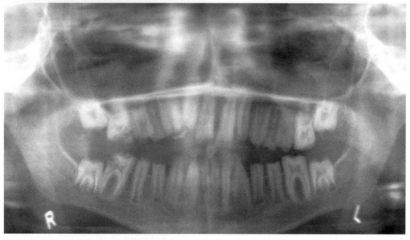

243 Amelogenesis imperfecta. DPR.

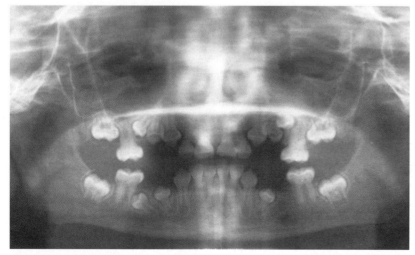

244 Dentinogenesis imperfecta. DPR.

Enamel hypoplasia

Abnormalities of tooth structure arise during the period of development of a tooth and may affect all the mineralized tissues. However, because the cementum is normally only a thin layer covering the root of the tooth and not clearly shown on radiographs, such abnormalities will be demonstrated only in the enamel and dentine. There is either a deficiency in the quantity (hypoplasia) or the quality (hypomineralization) of the tooth tissue, occurring either independently or together. These abnormalities occur either as a consequence of disturbances in the tissue environment of the developing tooth, or they are genetically determined. The environmental causes may be local (e.g. inflammation) or systemic (e.g. acute gastroenteritis; fluorosis) and result in horizontally placed, ring-like defects of the enamel, either single or multiple, according to the aetiology. Depending upon the age of the patient and the duration of the disturbance, a varying number of teeth are affected.

In the example of systemically caused hypoplasia (**242**) there are several bands of radiolucency running horizontally across the crowns of all the teeth, particularly in their cervical portions. These multiple rings of hypoplastic enamel are caused by repeated episodes of illness during the period when the teeth were forming. The enamel is generally thinner and less radio-opaque than normal and is virtually absent from the incisal edges of the lateral incisors, which are malformed. Attrition of the central incisors has resulted in the formation of concave incisal edges.

Amelogenesis imperfecta

This genetically transmitted disorder of the enamel affects the permanent and often the primary dentition. Usually the entire dentition is affected, although more localized forms do occur. In **243** a generalized form is shown in a ten-year-old in which all the permanent teeth are affected. There is no radiological evidence overall of the presence of enamel, except for a thin layer of dense radio-opacity on the occlusal surfaces of some of the teeth. Due to the enamel deficiency and the consequent rapid wear of the occlusal surfaces, the teeth have a more square outline, with an absence of cusps. There are clear gaps between the crowns of adjacent teeth.

Dentinogenesis imperfecta

This is a genetically transmitted disorder that mostly affects Caucasians. It may be associated with osteogenesis imperfecta, or affect only the teeth without systemic involvement. Dentinogenesis imperfecta is primarily a disorder of dentine, but the enamel may be thinner than normal and be weakly attached to the dentine. As in amelogenesis imperfecta, the entire permanent dentition is usually involved although the primary teeth may also be affected. Clinically, the teeth appear discoloured and are prone to attrition. Radiographically the teeth have bulbous crowns, constricted at the amelocemental junction and the roots appear short and blunted, with partial or complete obliteration of the pulp chambers and root canals.

In the nine-year-old shown in **244** many of the teeth are incompletely formed but the characteristic features of the disorder are clearly displayed. The crowns of all the teeth are markedly bulbous, and the pulp chambers and root canals of those teeth approaching the completion of development are becoming narrowed and obliterated.

The obliteration of the pulp chambers and the root canals due to excessive formation of abnormal dentine is seen more clearly in the second example (245, 246). The permanent incisors show almost total obliteration of the pulp chambers and root canals due to excessive formation of abnormal dentine. There is marked attrition of the incisal edges with only a thin layer of enamel interstitially. The roots are characteristically shortened and the teeth are separated by narrow diastemas. Note the small, irregular radio-opacity between the apices $\overline{111}$ due to the superimposition of the dense cortical bone of the genial tubercles.

Hereditary hypophosphataemia (Vitamin D-resistant rickets)

In this inherited disorder, the teeth of both dentitions may be involved; males are more severely affected than females. The pulp chambers are larger than normal and characteristically have prominent cuspal pulp horns extending close to, or up to, the amelodentinal junction.

In the example (247, 248) affecting the primary dentition, the changes in $\underline{C|}$ and $\overline{DC|}$ are particularly apparent. In the further example (249, 250) affecting the permanent dentition, all the teeth are involved to a greater or lesser extent. As a consequence of the pulpal extensions, pulpal infection and necrosis are not uncommon in teeth

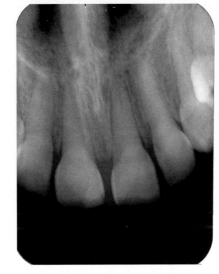

245 Dentinogenesis imperfecta. P.

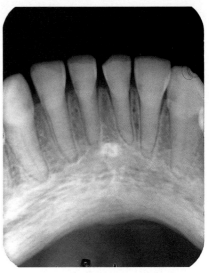

246 Dentinogenesis imperfecta. P.

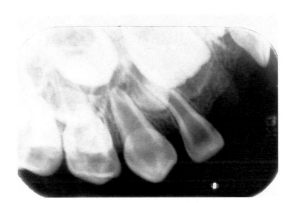

247 Hereditary hypophosphataemia. P.

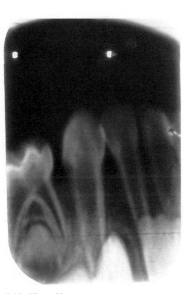

248 Hereditary hypophosphataemia. P.

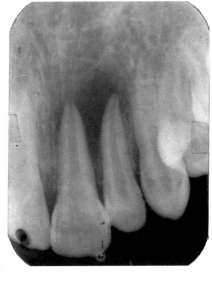

249 Hereditary hypophos-phataemia. P.

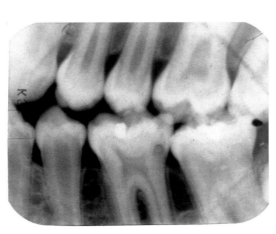

250 Hereditary hypophos-phataemia. BW.

that appear sound externally. Periapical lesions may ensue, as in **249** in which a periapical radiolucency affects the apices ⌊12 . In some patients there may also be generalized osteoporosis and the lamina dura around the teeth may be less clearly defined. In **249** and **250**, the trabeculations in the alveolar bone are sparse, particularly interdentally in the molar region.

Odontodysplasia

This condition (of uncertain pathogenesis) can affect any number of contiguous teeth and sometimes involves teeth on each side of the midline. The enamel and dentine of the affected teeth are markedly hypoplastic, so that the pulp chambers are large and the root canals wide. Thus they appear only a shadow of their normal selves, an appearance often referred to as 'ghost teeth'.

In **251**, in a ten-year-old, $\overline{32|}$ are unerupted and affected. There is no evidence of enamel on the crowns, the roots have only a thin outline of dentine and are shortened with wide pulp chambers. The radiolucent follicular space around the crowns of these teeth is widened due to the proliferation of odontogenic tissues, which is a feature of the condition.

251 Odontodysplasia. P.

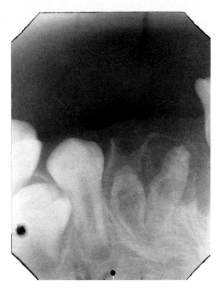

Concrescence

This is the fusion of the roots of adjacent teeth by cemental hyperplasia; it usually occurs as a consequence of chronic inflammation. It most commonly involves maxillary molars, as in **252**, where there is concrescence of the roots of 87| . 7| is tilted mesially with its root contiguous to that of 8| . There is no periodontal ligament space between the roots of these two teeth, although one is present around their roots mesially and distally. 8| contains an excess of temporary dressing material, which is overhanging the crown.

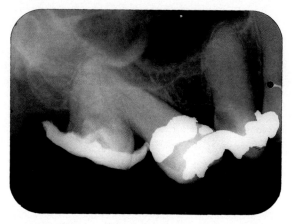

252 Concrescence. P.

Microbial conditions and their sequelae

Dental caries

Dental caries is a widespread disease and most commonly affects the occlusal and proximal surfaces of the teeth on which dental plaque readily forms. The interproximal surfaces, however, are not always readily accessible to direct clinical examination, so intra-oral radiographs are useful in the diagnosis of dental caries at this site. The use of bitewing radiographs in the posterior sextants of the mouth is the technique of choice as it provides a non-distorted image of the teeth, and, by including the crowns of both the maxillary and mandibular teeth on the same film, reduces the number of radiographs required and thus the amount of radiation exposure to the patient. Since enamel is highly mineralized, there is often a considerable loss of mineral before any radiographic changes are detected and the lesion is clinically more extensive than is shown on the radiograph. Lesions occurring on other surfaces of the teeth (e.g. buccally, cervically, or

adjacent to restorations as in recurrent caries) are not so clearly shown, particularly when small, because of superimposition effects.

The process of dental caries is accompanied by acid demineralization of the teeth. The initial carious lesion, when confined to the enamel, thus appears as a small and relatively well defined radiolucency. When the lesion spreads to involve the dentine, it extends pulpally and laterally along the amelodentinal junction and the margin is less well defined. Frequently, a zone of dentinal sclerosis is present between the carious lesion and the underlying pulp. This sclerotic dentine is a reaction of the healthy tissues to the toxic environment within the lesion. Eventually the enamel becomes unsupported and fragments, resulting in cavitation with a change in the outline of the crown. Ultimately the pulp becomes exposed although the exact time at which this occurs cannot be determined radiographically.

FISSURE CARIES

In fissure caries there is little radiological change until the lesion involves the underlying dentine. When this occurs it spreads along the amelodentinal junction before extending as a diffuse radiolucency towards the pulp chamber. Example **253** shows a slight widening of the central fissure 7| , beneath which the lesion has extended along the amelodentinal junction as a radiolucent band. There is a layer of radio-opaque dentinal sclerosis between the roof of the pulp chamber and the lesion. In |7 the caries is more advanced and appears as a larger, cone-shaped radiolucency in the dentine. In |6 and 6| the lesions are extensive, having spread further along the amelodentinal junction and more deeply into the dentine, although the enamel remains intact. Both teeth contain an occlusal amalgam restoration indicating that the caries is either recurrent or was incompletely removed prior to the placement of the restorations.

As the caries spreads, more of the tooth tissue is destroyed so that the overlying unsupported enamel fractures and is progressively lost, producing a cavity of increasing size. In the advanced lesion 7| (**254**) there is destruction of most of the crown and exposure of the pulp chamber involving both root canals. There is also a small interstitial lesion, distally |7 .

INTERSTITIAL CARIES

Caries starting at the contact points of adjacent teeth may affect one or both of the contacting tooth surfaces in the first instance. If both are involved, the two lesions may be of different sizes. Whilst confined to the enamel, caries appears as a triangular radiolucency at or just below the contact point. As in a fissure lesion, once the process has reached the dentine it spreads both pulpally and laterally along the amelodentinal junction. In **255** there are early interstitial carious lesions – distally 4| , mesially 5| , distally |5 and mesially 6| – resulting in triangular radiolucencies in the enamel just below the contact point, with the apex of the triangle towards the amelodentinal junction. More advanced caries – distally 5| , involving the enamel and the dentine – appears as a mushroom-shaped radiolucency with the stalk towards the outer enamel surface. The next example (**256**) shows a larger lesion distally 6| and a smaller one mesially 7| . In 6| , there is a small, radiolucent breach in the enamel surface distally, just below the

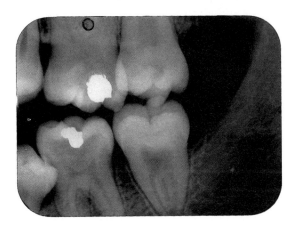

253 Fissure caries. BW.

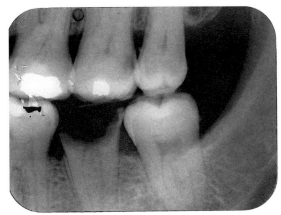

254 Fissure caries. BW.

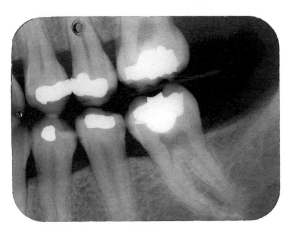

255 Interstitial caries. BW.

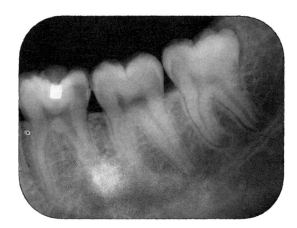

256 Interstitial caries. P.

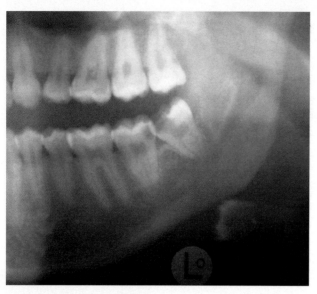

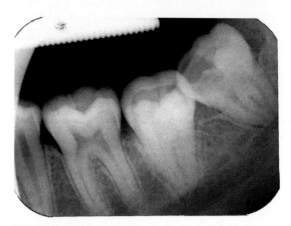

258 Interstitial caries. P.

257 Interstitial caries. DPR.

contact point, leading to a larger, more ill defined area of radiolucency in the dentine. A small amalgam restoration is present occlusally. Early caries mesially $\overline{7|}$ is restricted to the enamel.

More advanced carious cavities, $\overline{7|}$ distally and $\overline{|8}$ mesio-occlusally, are demonstrated clearly on the dental panoramic radiograph 257. There is loss of enamel and cavitation mesially $\overline{|8}$. The distal lesion $\overline{7|}$ is difficult to see on the intra-oral radiograph 258, although the degree of overlap of the crowns of the teeth is similar in the two views. This difference can be attributed largely to the incorrect vertical angulation of the X-ray beam in the latter view, resulting in the superimposition of bone and mineralized tooth tissues over the carious lesion, thus obscuring it.

The rate of progress of carious lesions varies not only from patient to patient, but also, as previously mentioned, from tooth surface to tooth surface in the same patient. The three radiographs (259, 260, 261) of the same patient, taken at yearly intervals, illustrate in particular the progressive development of cavities $\underline{5|}$ distally, $\overline{6|}$ mesially and $\overline{5|}$ distally. In the first radiograph (259), the distal lesions in the two premolars are not yet apparent. In the last radiograph (261), an amalgam restoration has been inserted $\underline{5|}$ disto-occlusally, although caries still remains cervically. There is also an occlusal cavity $\overline{7|}$ (259), which has been restored in the later radiographs.

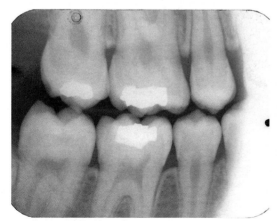

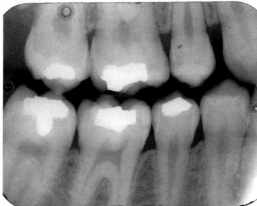

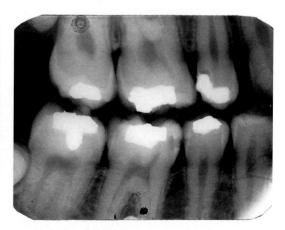

259 Interstitial caries. BW.

260 Interstitial caries. BW.

261 Interstitial caries. BW.

In anterior teeth, large interstitial lesions have a typically craterform outline as shown in the cavities (**262**) mesially ⌊2 and ⌊3 . There is also a lesion distally ⌊2 , which has been restored but from which the filling has been subsequently lost. The more clearly defined boundary of the radiolucency is due to the previous cavity preparation and contrasts with the less well-defined boundaries in the other two lesions. In addition there is lateral spread towards the incisal edge through the outermost layers of the dentine. More advanced caries is shown (**263**), which has resulted in the loss of most of the crowns ⌊2 and ⌊3 . A clearly defined, periapical radiolucency is present ⌊2 , and in ⌊3 and ⌊4 there are prominent radio-opaque zones of reactive dentinal sclerosis around the lesions.

CERVICAL CARIES

Cervical lesions occur typically on the labial, buccal, lingual and palatal aspects of the teeth and are less common in most communities than fissure or interstitial lesions. The margin of the cavity tends to be more clearly defined because the X-ray beam is parallel to the walls of the cavity, as in ⌐3 labially (**264**). Another example (**265**) shows a clearly defined, radiolucent defect 7⌐ partly superimposed upon the pulp chamber. A similar appearance will be produced whether the lesion lies buccally or lingually. However, with cervical lesions, it is not always possible to determine the relationship between the advancing edge of the lesion and the pulp chamber, as their images are superimposed and in the same plane as the X-ray beam.

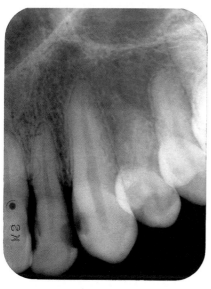

262 Interstitial caries. P.

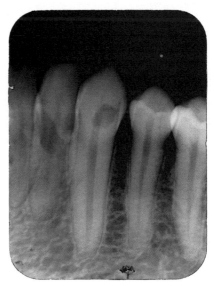

264 Cervical caries. P.

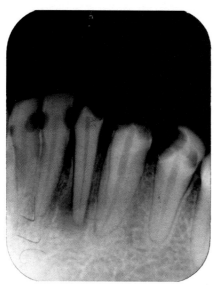

263 Interstitial caries. P.

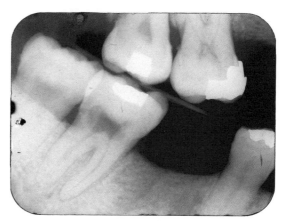

265 Cervical caries. BW.

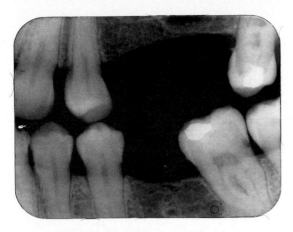

266 Cemental caries. BW.

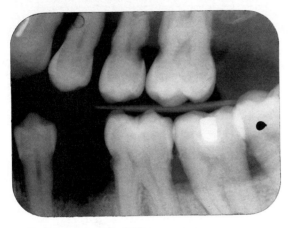

267 Cemental caries BW.

CEMENTAL CARIES

Cemental caries may occur when the cervical part of a tooth root becomes exposed to the oral environment, so permitting the accumulation of cariogenic dental plaque on the exposed surface. This is most commonly due to apical migration of the periodontal tissues along the root surface following destruction of alveolar bone in chronic periodontal disease. Cemental caries is therefore increasingly frequent in older patients. The lesions are most common on the labial and buccal aspects of the roots, but may also occur lingually, palatally and interstitially, usually when the periodontal disease is more advanced. As cementum is only a thin layer, the dentine becomes involved at an early stage and the lesions have many features of dentine caries. Radiographically, the cavity is typically saucer-shaped and although in early caries it is well defined, in larger lesions it is often ill defined.

The cemental caries distally 7| (**266**) is an early lesion that has extended into the dentine forming a small, punched-out radiolucency in the region of the amelocemental junction; compare this appearance with that of the normal cervical radiolucency 8| mesially. A further example (**267**) shows interstitial cervical lesions, which started in the cementum |56 and 6| . The early caries, 6| mesially, forms a punched-out radiolucency, whereas the more advanced cavities, |6 mesially and |5 distally, form saucer-shaped radiolucencies with poorly defined margins, partly undermining the cervical enamel. There is moderate loss of interdental bone and the presence of subgingival calculus indicative of chronic periodontitis.

Note the basic differences in shape between these cemental cavities and lesions in the enamel (**260**, **261**).

RAMPANT CARIES

In some individuals, often for poorly understood reasons, the teeth are particularly susceptible to rapid carious destruction and most, if not all, of the teeth are affected. In the 20-year-old (**268**), numerous carious lesions are present, many of them advanced, particularly 6| . |6 and 6| have already been extracted because of advanced disease.

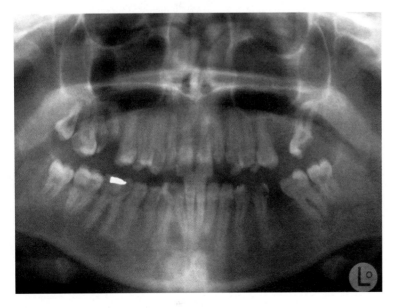

268 Rampant caries. DPR.

RECURRENT CARIES

Caries may be recurrent at the periphery of a restoration if the initial lesion has not been completely eradicated or if a defect develops between the restoration and the cavity wall. In **269** there is an extensive recurrent lesion 6| distally beneath an inadequate amalgam restoration. Other recurrent

lesions are present beneath the restorations 65|. Early interstitial cavities are also present at several contact points.

Acute periapical abscess

The consequences of untreated or unsuccessfully treated dental caries are, in the first instance, pulpitis and pulpal necrosis. Radiographic examination of the teeth is of no direct help in the diagnosis of these conditions. Extension of the inflammatory process into the periapical tissues results in the progressive loss of the adjacent bone. In early acute inflammation there is usually little evidence of bone destruction as it takes at least ten days before sufficient bone has been resorbed to become evident radiographically. On the other hand, in acute exacerbations of previously chronic inflammatory lesions, the bone loss associated with the chronic lesion will be apparent.

In **270**, however, the acute periapical inflammation has resulted in the displacement of |5 from its socket in an occlusal direction, with widening of the periodontal ligament space apically, although there is no evidence of previous periapical bone destruction due to chronic disease. The displacement is accompanied by the projection of the cusps of the tooth beyond the occlusal plane. There are large amalgam restorations in |4567 .

The acute abscess in the second example (**271**) has arisen in a pre-existing chronic inflammatory lesion 2|, the latter having caused the poorly-defined periapical radiolucency.

Periapical granuloma

Periapical granulomas are a common sequel of pulpal necrosis. These chronic inflammatory lesions are usually symptomless, their presence being suspected from the clinical signs and investigation of the associated tooth. The earliest radiographic change is thinning of the lamina dura apically, which subsequently becomes completely resorbed, together with progressive resorption of the adjacent bone trabeculae. In teeth with lateral root canals, granulomas may arise in relation to the lateral foramen. With multirooted teeth, granuloma formation may occur on each root. Although periapical granulomas are usually slow-growing, they may or may not be well defined. They rarely exceed 1.5–2.0 cm in diameter, but when smaller than this radiological differentiation from radicular cysts may not be possible. In addition to the lesion itself, there is usually evidence in the associated teeth of the pre-existing disease, such as dental caries or trauma, which has lead to the formation of the granuloma.

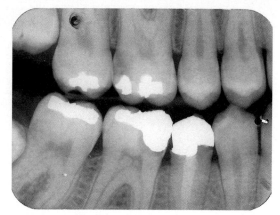

269 Recurrent caries. BW.

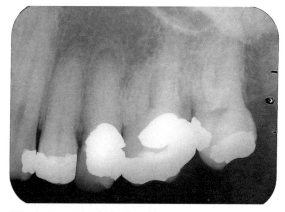

270 Acute periapical abscess. P.

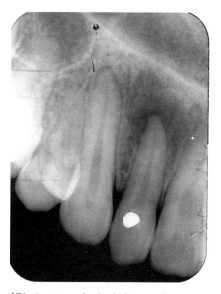

271 Acute periapical abscess. P.

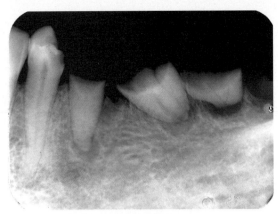

272 Periapical granulomas. P.

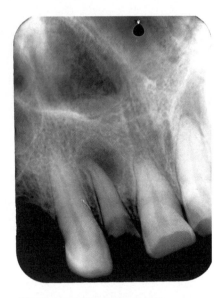

273 Periapical granuloma. P.

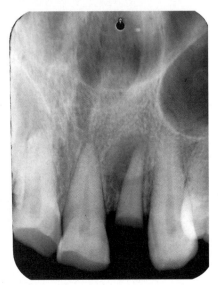

274 Periapical granuloma. P.

In **272**, advanced caries $\overline{5\ 78}$ has resulted in the destruction of the crowns; only portions of the roots remain. On each root there is a clearly defined periapical radiolucency, surrounded by a radio-opaque lamina, but the lamina dura is absent apically. The relatively superficial position of the root fragments $\overline{78}$ indicates that they are being exfoliated. There is a periodontal infrabony pocket distally $\overline{5}$.

Another example is shown (**273**, **274**, both in the same patient) of advanced carious destruction $\underline{2|2}$ and formation of periapical granulomas. Whereas the periapical radiolucency $\underline{2|}$ is clearly defined and surrounded by a thin, radio-opaque lamina, that associated with $|\underline{2}$, although of similar size, is less well defined. Within the radiolucent areas is a finer, less distinct, trabecular pattern due to the superimposition of the remaining overlying cortical and cancellous bone. The lesion $\underline{2|}$ is probably quiescent and that associated with $|\underline{2}$ is actively enlarging. There is advanced attrition of the incisal edges $\underline{1|1}$. These two examples illustrate the variable radiological appearances that such lesions may give.

In the next illustration (**275**) there are two radiolucent areas associated with the root $\overline{5}$, the larger being periapical with an indistinct outline. The smaller is on the distal aspect of the root. The lamina dura in relation to both lesions is absent. There is a large amalgam filling with recurrent caries mesiocervically. The large lesion is a periapical granuloma and the smaller one either an oblique extension of the lesion along the surface of the root or a separate granuloma arising from a lateral root canal.

The next example (**276**) shows two small, clearly defined, radiolucent areas (arrows) situated mesially $\overline{5|}$ and distally $\overline{4|}$, due to granulomas developing on lateral root canals in these inadequately root filled teeth with necrotic pulps. Both areas are surrounded by a thin, radio-opaque lamina and there is loss of lamina dura. Note that the periapical tissues are normal.

In maxillary posterior teeth a granuloma may cause a nodular elevation of the floor of the antrum, as in the example on a carious $\underline{5|}$ root (**277**). To each side of the radiolucent granuloma, the thin cortical lamina of the antral floor is clearly displayed and is continuous with the more diffuse, radio-opaque cortical thickening surrounding the antral surface of the lesion. This diffuse radio-opacity is a consequence of reactive osteosclerosis. There is absence of the lamina dura distally and apically $\underline{5|}$, with irregular destruction of the alveolar bone distally.

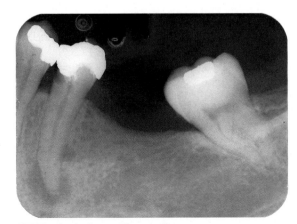

275 Periapical granulomas. P.

The outline of a periapical radiolucency associated with the lower anterior teeth may appear to be associated with the apices of more than one tooth, although only one is actually implicated. In **278** there is a triangular radiolucency associated with the roots of the lower incisors. The lesion originated on ⌐1, which has a large distal cavity filled with radio-opaque dressing material, and has spread to involve 1⌐ and 2⌐. The lamina dura is missing ⌐1 and indistinct 1⌐ apically, and the outline of the lesion is not clearly defined inferiorly. The finer, trabecular pattern of the overlying cortical and cancellous bone is clearly shown.

The illustration (**279**) shows small periapical granulomas on both roots ⌐6 having a large disto-occlusal carious cavity. The appearance of small periapical granulomas may be confused with that of the normal, apically-placed papillary tissue in an incompletely formed tooth root. The radiolucent lesions ⌐6 are surrounded by a thin, cortical lamina, which is continuous with the lamina dura mesially and distally on both roots. Compare this with the similar appearance on both roots ⌐7 apically, which is due to the persistence of papillary tissue in these incompletely formed roots. The apical foramina ⌐7 are still widely open.

When a periapical granuloma develops on a tooth in which the pulp has undergone necrosis due to trauma, abnormalities of the outline of the pulp chamber may be present, due to disturbances in dentinogenesis. A radiolucent periapical granuloma is shown in **280** in association with the apices 21⌐, where there is no lamina dura. The periphery is not well defined and the finer trabecular pattern of the overlying cortical and cancellous bone is clearly displayed. The lesion developed after trauma, and, following pulpal necrosis 1⌐, there has been premature cessation of dentinogenesis in the root, which has a relatively wide canal. Disturbance of odontogenesis 2⌐ has led to the formation of a flattened apex and progressive mineralization of the root canal, which is totally obliterated.

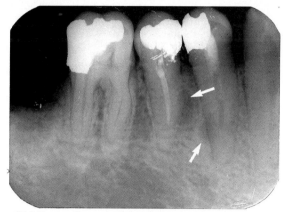

276 Laterally-positioned granulomas. P.

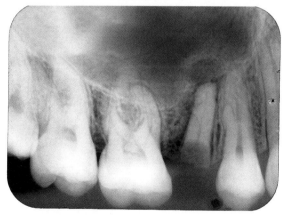

277 Periapical granuloma. P.

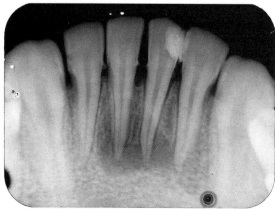

278 Periapical granuloma. P.

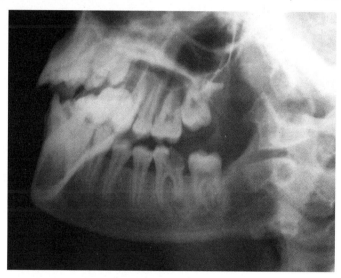

279 Periapical granulomas. OLM.

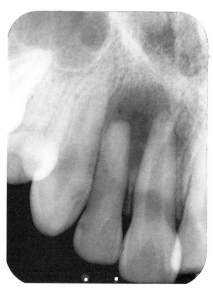

280 Periapical granuloma. P.

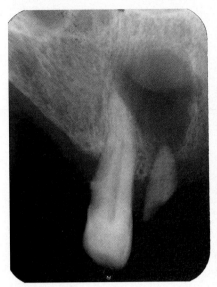

281 Radicular cyst. P.

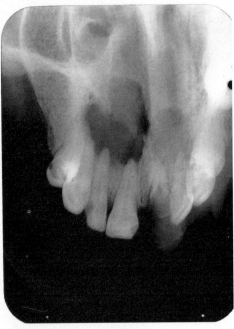

282 Radicular cyst. USO.

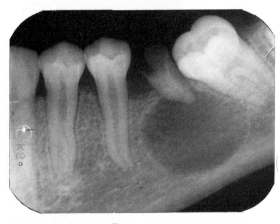

283 Radicular cyst. P.

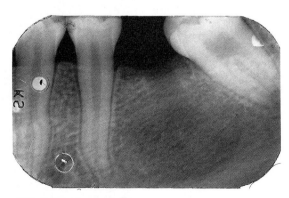

284 Radicular cyst. P.

Radicular (periapical) cyst

Long-standing periapical chronic inflammatory lesions commonly progress to cyst formation; such cysts are called radicular cysts.

It is unusual for periapical granulomas to be larger than 1.5–2.0 cm in diameter, but radicular cysts may excede this size. As a consequence, radiographs larger than the periapical may be required to show their full extent. Radicular cysts arise most commonly in the maxilla, particularly in association with the anterior teeth and are most frequent between the third and sixth decades of life. They enlarge by expansile growth, to produce an approximately circular or pear-shaped radiolucency at the apex of a non-vital tooth. Typically, the outline is well defined with a thin radio-opaque cortical margin, which is continuous with the lamina dura of the affected tooth. As the cyst enlarges it causes expansion and thinning of the alveolar cortical plates, resulting in an increase in the radiolucency of the cystic defect.

In the lesion (**281**) associated with 2⌋ root fragment, there is a clearly defined, periapical radiolucency surrounded by a thin, radio-opaque lamina and containing a circular, more radiolucent area centrally where the buccal cortical bone has been perforated. The lamina dura is absent apically. The radio-opaque shadow, with a distinct, curved lower margin superimposed upon the upper part of the lesion, is the soft tissue outline of the nose.

Another example on an upper standard occlusal radiograph (**282**) is shown in which there are bilateral cysts associated with the maxillary incisors. The larger of the two, on the right, appears as a dark radiolucency, approximately circular in outline with a well defined margin; the lamina dura apically 321⌋ is missing. There is a cavity distally 2⌋ and a fracture of the mesial incisal tip 1⌋, both of which could have lead to pulpal necrosis of the respective tooth. The radio-opaque bony outline of the lateral wall of the nose runs obliquely over the radiolucent area, approximately bisecting it, and the upper half is less radiolucent because of the superimposition of the nasal structures. The lesion on the patient's left, which is not so clear, is associated with a grossly carious ⌊1 .

In the lower jaw, radicular cysts are most commonly associated with first permanent molars, as in **283**, associated with a carious ⌊6 root. The circular radiolucency is well defined and shows the typical features of a radicular cyst. The radiograph (**284**), taken six months after treatment, demonstrates normal healing of the bony defect, which is mostly infilled with fine radio-opaque trabeculae of bone apart from the area of the socket, the outline of which persists. The periapical cortical lamina around the cyst has also resolved.

In the next example (**285**) radicular cysts are shown in both sides of the maxilla and in the left side of the mandible in a patient with gross dental neglect. Radicular cysts associated with 6| roots and |7 roots have formed circular radiolucent defects surrounded by a thin, radio-opaque lamina of cortical bone. On each side, the cyst projects into the floor of the antrum, but is separated from it. In addition, there is a third radicular cyst associated with |4 root, although this lesion is not well displayed. The radiolucent defect in the right body of the mandible appeared to be continuous with the inferior alveolar canal suggesting the possibility of a neoplasm of neural origin. However it was found to contain granulomatous tissue.

Periapical osteosclerosis (sclerosing osteitis)

Sometimes chronic irritation will lead to bone formation, or osteosclerosis, rather than bone resorption; in these circumstances, the bony changes appear radio-opaque. Periapical osteosclerosis may arise as a consequence of chronic pulpal inflammation (sclerosing osteitis), but sometimes has no obvious cause (osteosclerosis). In **286** there is an extensive area of radio-opaque osteosclerosis periapically |6 extending from the distal aspect |5 to the mesial root |7 . |6 contains a large, mesio-occlusal amalgam restoration. There is apical resorption of the distal root |6 , although the periodontal ligament space is present around both roots. The periphery of the sclerotic area blends into the adjacent unaffected bone.

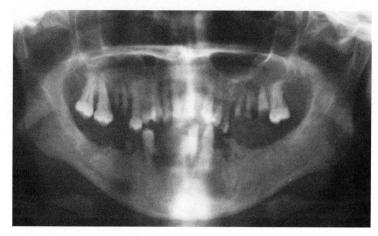

285 Radicular cysts. DPR.

Osteosclerosis is unusual in the maxilla but **287** shows an approximately circular radio-opaque area of osteosclerosis more clearly defined from the surrounding bone than in the previous illustration. The associated 4| bears a gold crown, which forms the abutment to a bridge. The dense radio-opaque area overlying the apices 7| is the root of the zygoma.

Another example (**288**) shows an area of osteosclerosis apical to 76| less clearly associated with the apices of these teeth, as the radio-opaque lesion is separated from them by a narrow zone of apparently normal bone. Note the dense radio-opacity distal to 4| caused by a fragment of amalgam in the tissues.

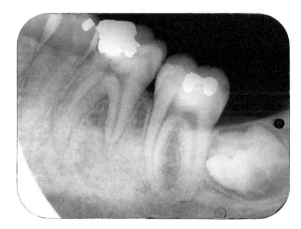

286 Periapical osteosclerosis. P.

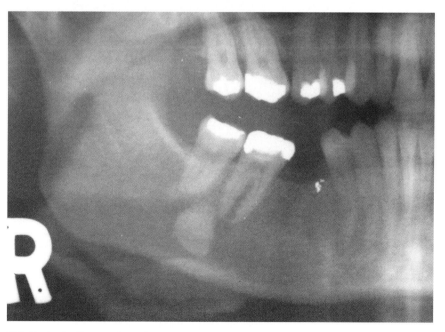

288 Periapical osteosclerosis. DPR.

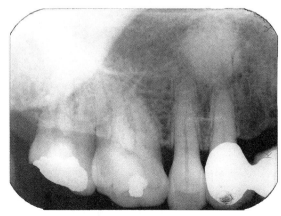

287 Periapical osteosclerosis. P.

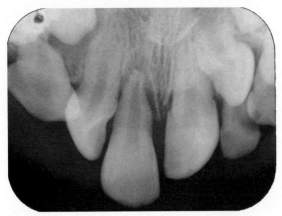

289 Tooth subluxation. P.

Traumatic conditions and their sequelae

Trauma to the teeth occurs commonly, either accidentally – as in the school playground – or following road traffic accidents or physical assault. The teeth may undergo partial (subluxation) or total displacement, or become fractured.

Subluxation of teeth

Subluxation 1| is shown in an eight-year-old child (**289**) following trauma. The tooth is displaced incisally from its socket, resulting in widening of the periodontal ligament space laterally and apically. The lamina dura is intact.

Tooth fracture

Fractures may involve any part of the tooth, either the crown or the root, at any level. In the crown, any or all of the three principle tissues of the tooth (enamel, dentine and pulp) may be involved. Intra-oral radiographs play a critical role in the assessment and diagnosis of these conditions, particularly when the root is involved. Fractures most commonly affect the maxillary incisors, frequently the central incisors.

In **290**, an oblique fracture passes through the crown |1 , involving the distal portion of the incisal edge. The fracture extends into the dentine close to the coronal pulp chamber; the incisal fragment is missing. Note the inverted, conical supernumerary tooth (mesiodens) in the midline.

Another example (**291**) in a nine-year-old child shows an approximately horizontal fracture 1| involving the coronal pulp chamber. Here the incisal fragment is retained and on its mesial aspect the fracture line is subgingival. In root fractures there may be displacement of the coronal fragment, and as a result, the fracture line appears wider.

In the comminuted oblique fracture of the coronal third of the root 1| (**292**) there is displacement, with fragments visible within the fracture line.

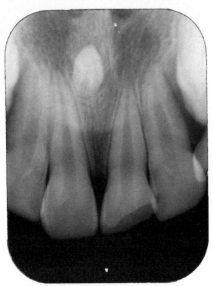

290 Tooth fracture. P.

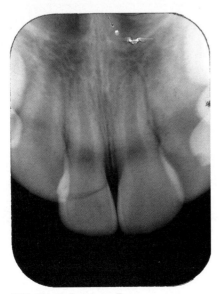

291 Tooth fracture. P.

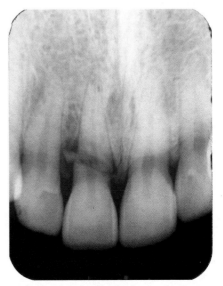

292 Tooth fracture. P.

In the next example (**293**), there are bilateral, horizontal fractures of the apical third of the roots 1|1 with displacement of the coronal fragments, hence the fracture lines appear to be widened.

Healing of fractured teeth may be achieved successfully if the coronal fragment is realigned and adequately immobilized, with or without endodontic treatment. In the horizontal fracture of the middle third of the root |1 (**294**) in a 14-year-old child, there is slight displacement of the coronal fragment but the crown is intact. One year after endodontic treatment of the coronal fragment (**295**) the lamina dura around both portions of the tooth remains intact. After a further year (**296**), there is bone formation in the fracture line indicative of healing.

Tooth fractures are less common in the mandibular incisors. In **297** the fracture line runs obliquely in an apical direction from the distal to the mesial aspect 1| in the cervical part of the root and is partly subgingival. Again, the coronal fragment is displaced incisally.

A second radiograph (**298**), taken with the X-ray beam aligned more obliquely to the plane of the fracture, projects it, misleadingly, as two separate fracture lines. The incorrect angulation of the beam in this radiograph is confirmed by the elongation of the tooth roots.

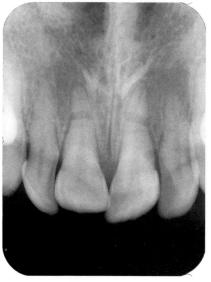

293 Fractured teeth. P.

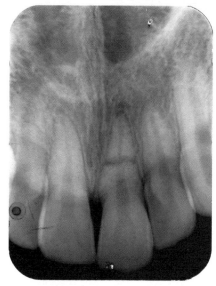

294 Tooth fracture. P.

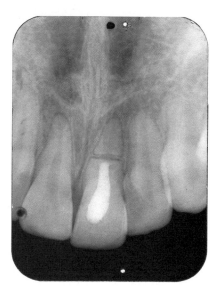

295 Tooth fracture. P.

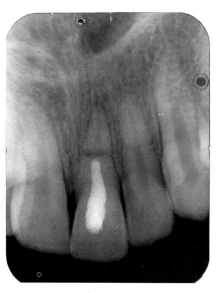

296 Tooth fracture. P.

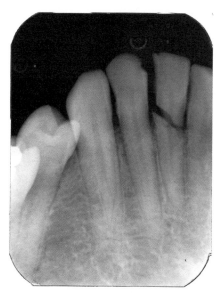

297 Tooth fracture. P.

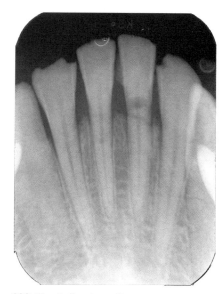

298 Tooth fracture. P.

Pulpal sclerosis

When trauma to the teeth does not result in fracture or subluxation, there may be damage to the apical vessels, resulting in altered cellular activity of the pulp cells, which may then produce excessive mineralized tissue. In **299** there has been pulpal sclerosis 1|12 with obliteration of the pulp chambers and the root canals by deposition of atypical, reparative dentine. There has also been slight root resorption, the apices appearing blunted, but the lamina dura remains intact. An attempt has been made to root fill and restore |1 .

In a further example (**300**) there is pulpal sclerosis 1| and apical root resorption 21|12 following trauma. The pulp chamber and the root canal 1| are totally occluded. The apical resorption is particularly advanced 1|1 . Bony repair has accompanied the root resorption so that there is a normal lamina dura and periodontal ligament space around the roots.

299 Pulpal sclerosis. P.

Regressive conditions

Pulp stone

Pulp mineralization can occur in young people but increases with age, and also in the presence of chronic inflammation. It may be diffuse or focal in nature. Focal masses of dentine or dentine-like tissue, pulp stones, may become sufficiently large and dense to be visible on radiographs. Their presence has practical significance if endodontic treatment is contemplated. In **301**, a discrete radio-opaque mass is present in the pulp chamber |7 coronally and in the incompletely formed root canal |8 .

In the second example (**302**), a larger pulp stone |3 is shown lying in a dilatation of the root canal cervically (arrow). There is, in addition, a root fragment near the surface of the alveolus, just mesial to |5 .

300 Pulpal sclerosis. P.

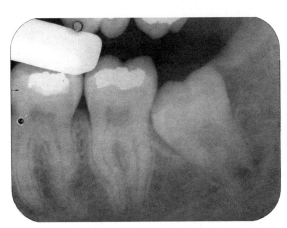

301 Pulp stones. P.

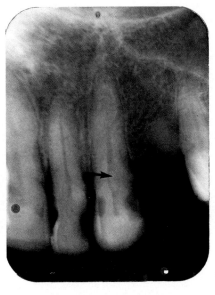

302 Pulp stone. P.

Root resorption

Resorption of the root surface is common microscopically under conditions of chronic periapical inflammation, trauma or the rapid orthodontic movement of teeth. Less frequently such resorption may progress to the stage where it is visible radiographically, especially when it occurs on the mesial, distal or apical aspects of the root surface, but less commonly with buccal or lingual lesions, due to the superimposition of normal tissue. Sometimes such resorption arises for no apparent reason (idiopathic root resorption), usually on the external surface of the tooth in the cervical region, spreading extensively into the crown and the apical part of the root. It may become so extensive as to lead to tooth fracture.

In **303**, large, carious cavities are present ⌐67 with exposure and necrosis of both pulps. There has been extensive resorption of the apices of both roots ⌐6 and compensatory reparative bone formation, so that only small areas of periapical radiolucency are present with the absence of a clearly defined lamina dura. There is also a small radiolucent granuloma at the apex of the mesial root ⌐7 .

Another example (**304**) shows apical resorption ⌐6 with a large amalgam restoration obscuring an exposure of the distal pulp horn. The pulp has undergone necrosis and there is a clearly defined, periapical radiolucency (probably a granuloma) on the mesial root, with loss of the lamina dura apically and also on the distal aspect of the root. There is apical resorption of both roots, more marked on the distal root. Note the pronounced clip mark overlying the pulp chamber ⌐5 .

The resorptive process on the distal roots ‾76 (**305**) has no obvious cause. On ⌐6 the process is now quiescent and reparative bone formation has occurred around the root surface so that it is clearly defined. On ⌐7, however, the process is still active, as demonstrated by the less sharply defined boundary of the apical part of the root surface.

In the next example (**306**), trauma to the lower incisors has resulted in pulpal necrosis ‾21 and development of a well-circumscribed, clearly defined, radicular cyst involving the apices ‾211 . In addition, ‾2 has irregular external resorption of the root surface. There is also an apparent irregular enlargement of the cervical two-thirds of the root canal, due to superimposition of the area of external resorption. The continuity of the resorbed area with the root surface is demonstrated in the middle of the distal aspect of the root (arrow). There is also resorption of the apex ‾2. On the basis of the radiographic appearance it is often difficult to distinguish this pattern of resorption from idiopathic internal resorption, which occurs only rarely.

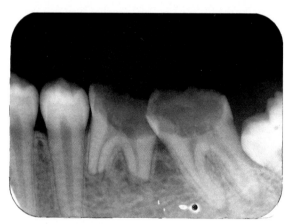

303 Root resorption. P.

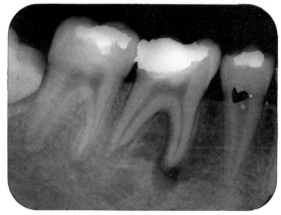

304 Root resorption. P.

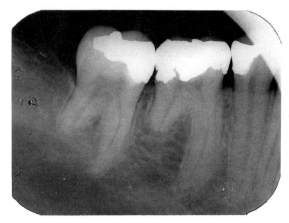

305 Idiopathic external root resorption. P.

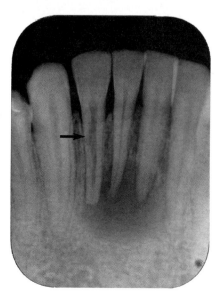

306 Idiopathic external root resorption. P.

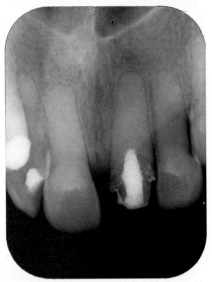

307 Idiopathic external root resorption. P.

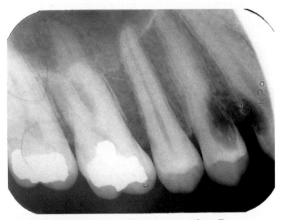

308 Idiopathic external root resorption. P.

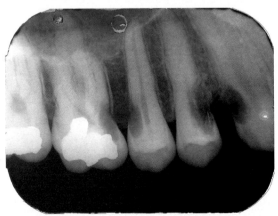

309 Idiopathic external root resorption. P.

In **307** the process started on the palatal aspect of the root 2⌋, casting an approximately circular radiolucent shadow over the cervical part of the root canal. The retention of the normal outline of the root canal is an important diagnostic feature in determining the external origin of the resorptive process.

Although idiopathic external resorption usually involves only one tooth, sometimes a number of teeth may be affected. In **308** there is an early lesion 5⌋ at the amelocemental junction distally, where a small semicircular radiolucency is present. In addition there are more advanced lesions 4⌋ mesially and 3⌋ distally, both of which show scalloped radiolucencies and undermining resorption of the enamel. Adjacent to the lesions there is evidence of early resorption of the interdental bone crests. The process of resorption is intermittent and may be accompanied by periods of repair by bone-like tissue. The lesion 4⌋ contains speckled radio-opacities, evidence of this repair process. Fifteen months later (**309**) there is considerable enlargement of the distal lesion 5⌋ and development of a new lesion 6⌋ mesially. 4⌋ and 3⌋ appear essentially unchanged.

Tumorous conditions

True neoplasms of enamel, dentine or cementum alone, without other odontogenic hard or soft tissues, are rare. However lesions of cementum (cementifying fibroma; benign cementoblastoma) and dentine (dentinoma) are recognized. The choice of radiograph required to demonstrate these conditions will depend upon their size and position; the resulting appearance varies according to the proportion of mineralized tissue. These lesions are illustrated elsewhere in Chapter 6.

Iatrogenic conditions

Tooth restorations

Much dental treatment involves the replacement of diseased or lost tooth tissue by inert materials. These materials are usually radio-opaque, although the density of the radio-opacity varies according to the nature of the material. As a consequence, most fillings, crowns and bridges can be readily demonstrated on radiographs. This is particularly useful if the filling or part of the filling is not directly visible in the mouth, as in root canal therapy or more complex intracoronal restorations. Their presence limits the value of future radiographic examination of the tooth as the dense radio-opacity of their image obscures the recognition of any tissue upon which it is superimposed. In addition to restoring decayed or damaged teeth by a variety of filling materials or crowns, missing teeth may be replaced by bridges using adjacent standing teeth as abutments. A few examples of the restorations themselves and some of the techniques applied during their insertion are illustrated below. However, since restorative dentistry is so widely practised, many of the radiographs in this book will coincidentally contain examples of restorative dentistry.

In the first illustration, a variety of restorative materials of different radiodensities are shown (**310**) varying from the radiolucent composites to the more radiodense metallic materials such as amalgam or gold. The distal surfaces of 1|1 and the mesial surface of |2 contain radiolucent composite fillings, and 2| has been restored with a porcelain crown fitted over a cast gold core and post. 7| bears a porcelain to gold crown. The missing |5 has been replaced by a bridge consisting of a gold pontic and gold inlay abutments on |4 and |6 .

The next example (**311**) shows a bridge replacing 5| consisting of porcelain to gold crowns 6| and 4| supporting a porcelain -to-gold pontic.

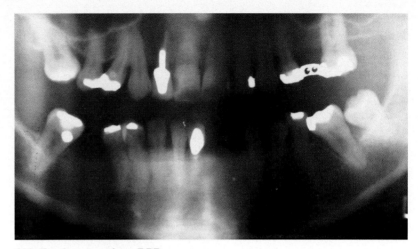

310 Tooth restorations. DPR.

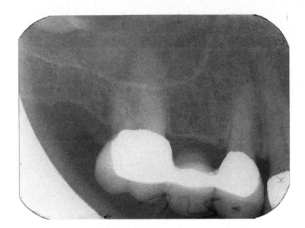

311 Tooth restorations. P.

Root canal therapy (endodontic therapy)

The clinical management of pulpal inflammation, necrosis and their sequelae usually involves the removal of the pulp with replacement by an inert filling material sealing the apex of the tooth root. Since the roots lie within the alveolar bone, radiographs are used to monitor the preparation and sealing of the root canals.

In the first example (**312**), 5| had become non vital after unsuccessful treatment of a carious lesion with subsequent development of an apical radiolucency. Access to the root canal has been obtained occlusally by removing part of the amalgam restoration, and a diagnostic plain broach (with an occlusally placed rubber stop) has been inserted to assess the length of the root canal prior to preparation and filling. The mechanical preparation of the canal is monitored by check radiographs to determine the position reached by the tip of the reamer.

In **313** it is shown in the correct position, 1 mm short of the apex 1| , prior to root filling. Compare the corrugated appearance of the reamer with the smooth outline of the diagnostic broach in the previous illustration. A radio-opaque rubber dam clip obscures most of the crowns of the adjacent teeth. 2| , which has been root filled previously with a gutta percha point, has a small, residual apical radiolucency with absence of lamina dura.

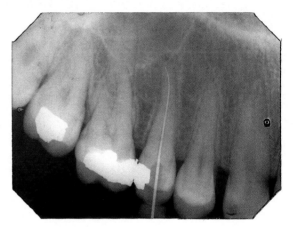

312 Root canal therapy. P.

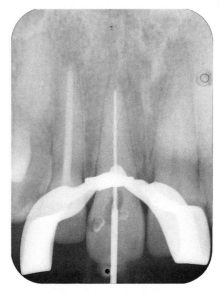

313 Root canal therapy. P.

314 Root canal therapy. P.

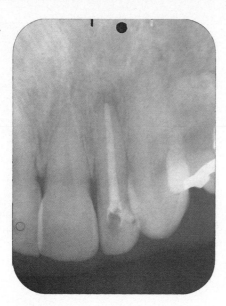

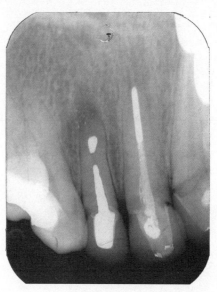

315 Root canal therapy. P.

A check radiograph is usually taken to determine that a root filling has been placed correctly (**314**). The root canal |2 contains a freshly cemented gutta percha point but the palatal access cavity has not yet been filled.

The next example (**315**) illustrates an alternative form of root filling using a sectional silver point, in the apical third of the root 1|. Compare the greater radio-opacity of this filling with that of the gutta percha in the previous illustration.

Periapical healing after root canal therapy

Following successful endodontic therapy, periapical granulomas and abscesses usually resolve, with progressive diminution in size of the periapical radiolucency and, ultimately, full restoration of the normal periapical radiographic anatomical appearance.

Sequential radiographs (**316**, **317**, **318**) of 2|, taken over a period of three-and-a-half years, demonstrate the periapical changes on a successfully root filled tooth. Prior to root canal therapy, there is loss of the lamina dura apically and an oval-shaped radiolucency with an ill-defined margin, probably a periapical granuloma (**316**). One year after root filling (**317**) the radiolucency is smaller, and a further two-and-a-half years later (**318**) bony repair is complete, with re-establishment of an intact lamina dura.

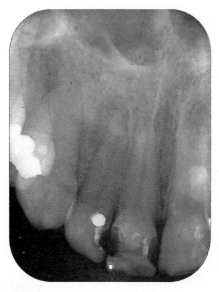

316 Periapical healing after root canal therapy. P.

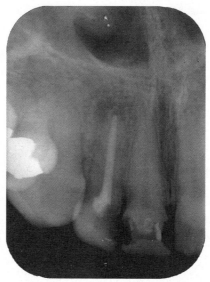

317 Periapical healing after root canal therapy. P.

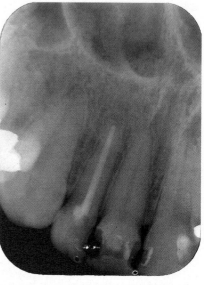

318 Periapical healing after root canal therapy. P.

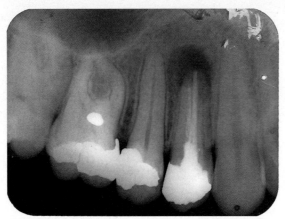

319 Periapical healing after root canal therapy. P.

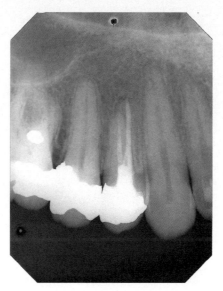

320 Periapical healing after root canal therapy. P.

The same changes occur periapically in successfully treated multirooted teeth. The first example (**319**) shows a radiolucent periapical lesion 4|, probably a granuloma, with a poorly defined outline and an absence of lamina dura immediately after completion of root canal therapy. Each root canal contains a separate gutta percha filling. After three years (**320**) bone repair is complete and a normal trabecular pattern and continuous lamina dura now surround the apices.

Complications of root canal therapy

There are several complications that can occur during root canal treatment; these include lateral perforation of the root, inadequate filling of the root canals and extrusion of the filling material into the periradicular tissues.

In the first example (**321**) the access to the root canal 2| was incorrectly placed, so that the instrumentation was mesially inclined and a lateral perforation of the mesial aspect of the root has occurred. A plain broach has been introduced through the perforation into the surrounding tissues. There is also a lateral root canal half-way along the distal aspect of the root.

Another example (**322**) of a laterally perforated root 1| shows a gutta percha point protruding from the perforation, with its apical portion being hooked and lying within the periapical lesion.

A second radiograph (**323**) taken with the X-ray tube in a more mesial position shows the hooked point more distally placed, indicating that the perforation is labial (parallax).

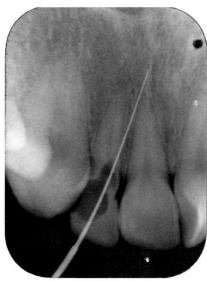

321 Laterally-perforated root canal. P.

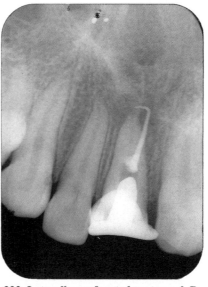

322 Laterally-perforated root canal. P.

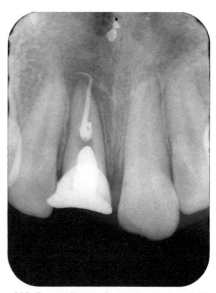

323 Laterally-perforated root canal. P.

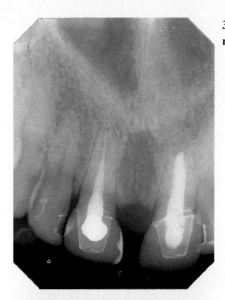

324 Inadequate root filling. P.

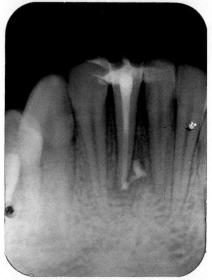

325 Excess root filling material. P.

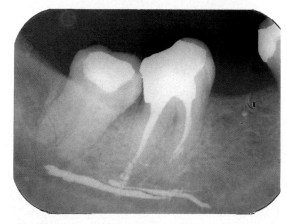

326 Excess root filling material. P.

In the next example (**324**) both maxillary central incisors have been root filled and bear porcelain jacket crowns. In 1⌋, the apical third of the root canal is inadequately filled and radiolucent defects are apparent at each side of the gutta percha point, whereas the root canal ⌊1 is correctly filled. Note the diastema 1⌋1 and the radiolucent incisive foramen.

Root canal cements and fillings in paste form may be extruded beyond the root apices (**325**). Unusually, the paste may be forced into adjacent structures, particularly if injected as in **326** where radio-opaque material is present along a considerable length of the inferior alveolar canal.

Apicectomy

Under certain circumstances, for endodontic therapy to be successful, removal of the root apex or apicectomy is necessary in addition to root canal filling. The exposed apical part of the root canal may then be sealed with a retrograde amalgam filling. When successful, the periapical bony defect resulting from this procedure heals (as in **327**) where, after one year, the apices ⌊12 are both encased in normal bone and surrounded by a thin, radiolucent periodontal ligament space and radio-opaque lamina dura. The apically positioned amalgam fillings are well condensed; both teeth have porcelain-faced gold crowns and contain gutta percha root fillings, that in ⌊1 being poorly condensed against the walls of the root canal.

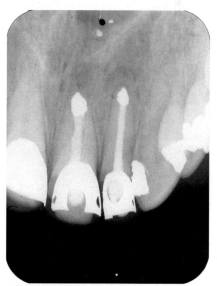

327 Apicectomy. P.

If retrograde root filling is performed improperly, excess filling material may be left in the periapical tissues (**328**) and may persist indefinitely. Sometimes the apex, although sectioned, is inadvertently left *in situ* and persists as a separate radio-opaque structure in the periapical tissues as shown above <u>|1</u> (**329**). <u>|2</u> has also undergone apicectomy and retrograde root filling with radio-opaque particles of amalgam present in the periapical tissues.

Dental implants

A wide variety of implants is available for the replacement of missing teeth. Those most frequently used become closely integrated with the host bone (osseo-integration) and may be used to replace single teeth (**330**) or support dentures (**331**).

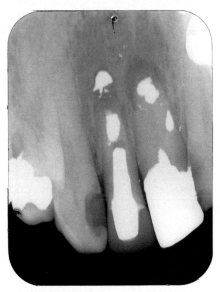

328 Apicectomy. P.

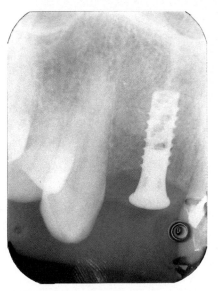

330 Dental implant. P.

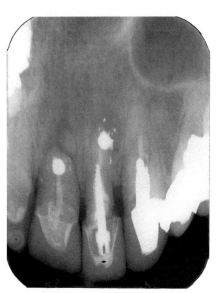

329 Apicectomy. P.

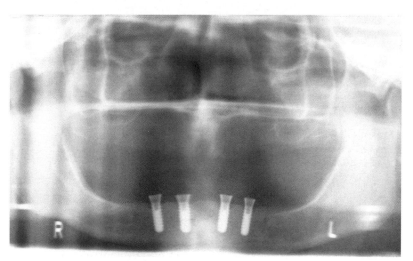

331 Dental implant. DPR.

117

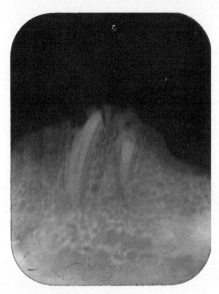

332 Retained roots. P.

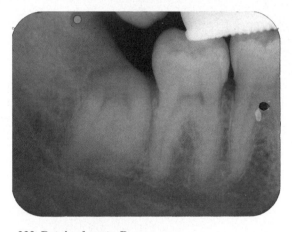

333 Retained roots. P.

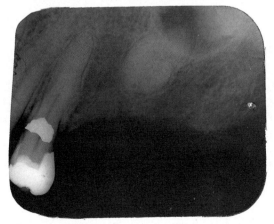

334 Retained roots. P.

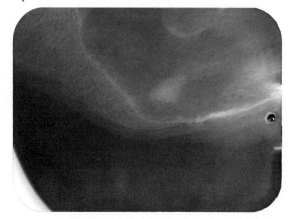

335 Retained root. P.

Retained roots

Portions of the roots of teeth may be retained in the jaws as a consequence of advanced dental caries or the incomplete extraction of teeth. They provide a potential focus for infection, and the resulting pain and swelling may lead to their discovery. In many instances, however, healing may occur without incident and the roots are found only when radiographs are taken for other purposes. Under these circumstances the distinction between a focus of bone sclerosis and a fragment of tooth root may be difficult.

In the first example (**332**), two roots are retained in the mandible following attempted extractions. There is a markedly oblique fracture of the coronal aspect of the root $\overline{3|}$ passing deeply into the socket mesially with a small retained fragment at the alveolar crest distally. The fracture surface is irregular at the coronal aspect of the $\overline{4|}$ root. There is a normal periodontal ligament space and lamina dura around both roots. The root canal is clearly present in $\overline{3|}$ root, although not so readily demonstrable $\overline{4|}$.

During the attempted removal $\overline{8|}$ (**333**) the roots were retained following fracture of the crown. The tooth is disto-angularly impacted and there is a marked distal curvature of the apex of the mesial root. The roots are surrounded by a normal lamina dura and periodontal ligament space, and their image is superimposed upon – but does not intrude into – the inferior alveolar canal, which runs uninterruptedly across both root apices.

When retained root fragments remain uninfected, the coronal part of the socket will heal fully, with complete remodelling of the overlying bone, as in **334**. The root fragments $\underline{|7}$, fractured at the time of extraction some years previously, are surrounded by a thin, radio-opaque cortical lamina and a radiolucent periodontal ligament space. Their root canals are obliterated, as is that in the apical part of the root $\underline{|5}$. The antral cavity is superimposed upon the apical part of the palatal root $\underline{|7}$. The radio-opacity overlying the antrum is formed by the root of the zygomatic process.

Another deeply-placed, retained root apex (**335**) is shown lying in an edentulous alveolus, many months after the extraction of $\underline{|6}$. There has been alveolar resorption so that the radio-opaque lamina marking the floor of the antrum passes close to the surface of the edentulous ridge. The root is therefore superimposed upon the antrum but is not actually within it. Its position within the bone is confirmed by the presence of a normal periodontal ligament space and lamina dura around the apex.

The 7| roots (**336**) were retained following attempted extraction a few weeks previously. |5 was extracted at the same visit, and the radio-opaque outline of the socket is already indistinct but several fragments of tooth debris are present within the socket. The circular radiolucency of the mental foramen lies antero-inferiorly to the |5 socket and there is a supernumerary tooth (paramolar) between |67 .

In the next example (**337**) there is a retained distal root |6 . The radiolucent mesial root socket is surrounded by a continuous, radio-opaque lamina dura and contains some radio-opaque zinc oxide dressing material. A radio-opaque area of osteosclerosis surrounds the apex of the distal root.

The attempted extraction |6 (**338**) in a young adult was complicated by the fracture of the crown, leaving the roots *in situ*; in addition there was fracture and retention of one blade of the forceps, which is superimposed upon the mesial root.

In the past, localizing plates (**339**) containing radio-opaque material such as stainless steel wire were used to aid the localization of embedded root fragments. The small radio-opaque root fragment is not surrounded by a lamina dura, suggesting the presence of inflammation.

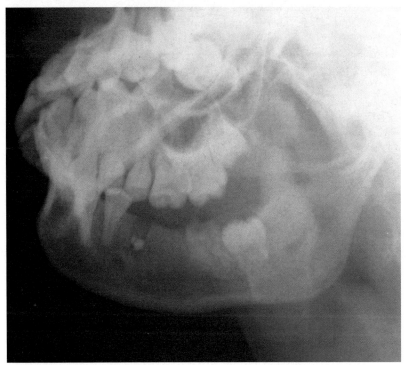

336 Retained roots. OLM.

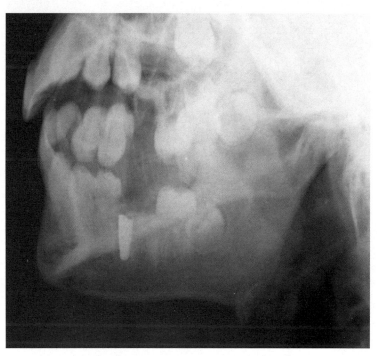

338 Retained roots. OLM.

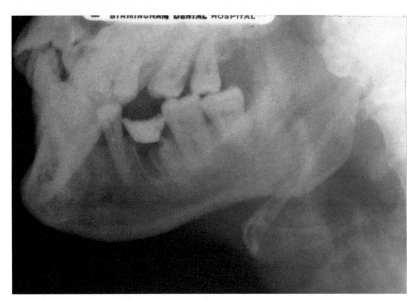

337 Retained root. OLM.

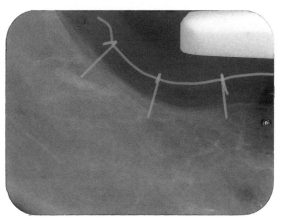

339 Retained roots. P.

Rarely, during attempted extraction, in particular of mandibular third molars, the tooth may be displaced into the adjacent soft tissues. The horizontally impacted 8| (**340**) was displaced into the lingual soft tissues so that its image is superimposed upon that of the ramus of the mandible. The radiolucent socket is clearly demonstrated and the displaced tooth is inverted. Prior to this incident an attempt was made to divide the crown with a bur, as indicated by the irregular area of radiolucency running across the cervical part of the tooth. The radio-opaque tip of the bur was broken and can be seen lying medially to the displaced tooth.

The next example (**341**) shows the attempted surgical removal of |6̄ roots, which exhibit marked apical curvature distally, particularly on the mesial root. There has been excessive and inaccurately directed removal of bone between |6̄7̄ where there is a large area of radiolucency, which, at its mesio-inferior corner, penetrates the cortical bone of the inferior border of the mandible.

Transplantation of teeth

Teeth may be surgically transplanted, the most common example being that of the unerupted maxillary canine. Transplantation usually involves the creation of a bony socket to accept the root of the transplanted tooth. This procedure may be followed by the re-establishment of a ligamentous attachment between the transplanted tooth and the surrounding bone. However, in a proportion of cases, the root may undergo resorption and/or ankylosis in the years following transplantation.

In the first example (**342**), |3 was transplanted eight years previously and there has been complete restoration of the alveolar bone with a normal periodontal ligament space and lamina dura around the entire root.

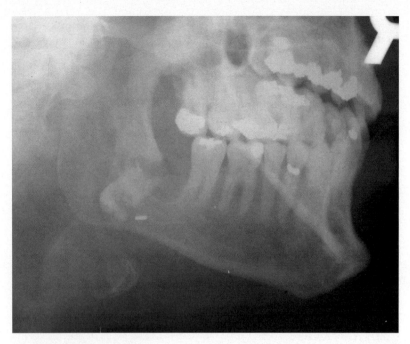

340 Displaced tooth. OLM.

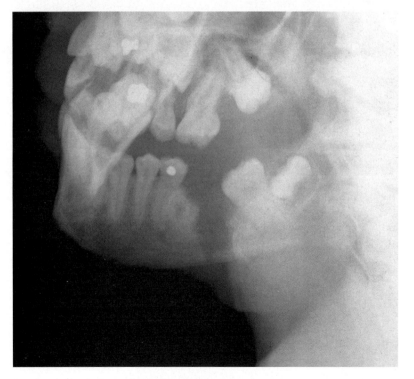

341 Attempted removal of roots. OLM.

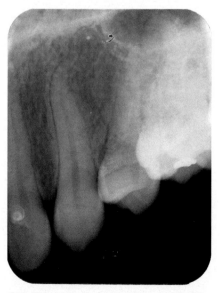

342 Transplanted maxillary canine. P.

In the next example (**343**), progressive resorption of the root of the transplanted 3| is demonstrated. A few months postoperatively, the radiolucent central area and surrounding indistinct cortical lamina of the original socket of the unerupted 3|, can still just be discerned above the apices 4|. There is as yet no obvious lamina dura around the root of the transplanted tooth. However, six months later (**344**), a distinct lamina dura is present around most of the root surface, although there is evidence of

early root resorption mesiocervically (arrows). By three years (**345**), the area of resorption has progressed to involve most of the root surface. The lamina dura is less clearly defined and there is flattening of the apex.

In another 3| (**346**), which was transplanted nine years previously, there is complete sclerosis and obliteration of the root canal; the periodontal ligament space is difficult to discern, suggesting that ankylosis may be taking place.

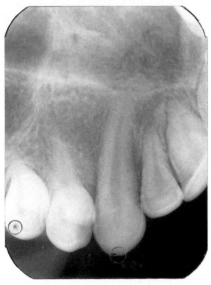

343 Transplanted maxillary canine. P.

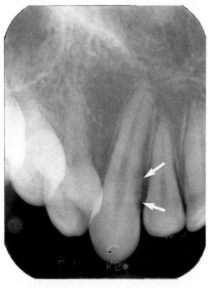

344 Transplanted maxillary canine. P.

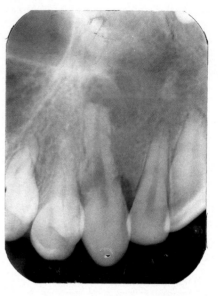

345 Transplanted maxillary canine. P.

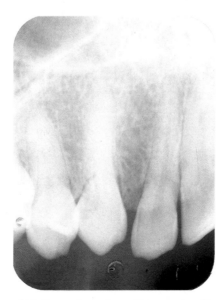

346 Transplanted maxillary canine. P.

IIrradiation-induced abnormalities

Developing tooth germs may be exposed to radiation used therapeutically for the treatment of malignant disease of the head and neck in children. As a consequence, tooth development may be disturbed or arrested according to the radiation dosage and the age of the child at the time of treatment.

In the nine-year-old (347) who received radiotherapy some 18 months previously, there is arrested development of the roots of the mandibular teeth, at the approximate stage that they had reached at the time of irradiation. The roots are stunted and blunted and the apical foramina narrowed. The periodontal ligament space is widened and the lamina dura is indistinct around some of the teeth. The nature of the apical changes is more clearly demonstrated on the intra-oral radiograph (348). The apical foramina of the incisors are almost completely obliterated. There are also numerous interstitial and labial cavities in the mandibular incisors (irradiation caries), partly as a result of reduced salivary secretion. Contrast the appearance of the mandibular teeth with that of the maxillary teeth, which were not affected by the irradiation.

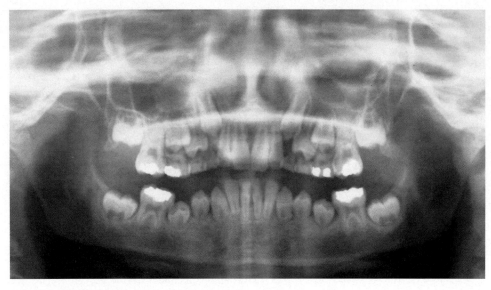

347 Irradiation-induced developmental anomaly. DPR.

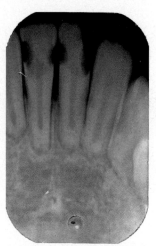

348 Irradiation-induced developmental anomaly. P.

5

The periodontium

Introduction

Radiographic examination of the supporting tissues of the teeth is widely used to determine the extent and pattern of bone destruction in patients with disorders of the periodontium. It also helps to identify localized predisposing factors in inflammatory diseases, such as overhanging restorations. In chronic periodontitis, which is the main indication for radiographic examination of the periodontium, bone loss starts in the crestal part of the interdental septum and is usually most advanced in this area of the alveolar bone. The extent of the bone loss can therefore be conveniently assessed on conventional dental radiographs. Bone loss on the buccal (labial) and lingual (palatal) aspects of the teeth is less clearly displayed because of the superimposition of the image of their roots. Whereas DPRs provide a convenient overview of the bony changes, they do not provide a good image of all the teeth, particularly the incisors, and other views are preferred for the more detailed assessment of bone loss. Bitewing radiographs and/or full mouth, periapical films taken with the paralleling technique provide an accurate analysis of the relationship of the crestal level of the alveolar bone to the root surface, particularly when the bone loss is not excessive. Localized areas of bone destruction occur more rarely, either due to cysts or tumours arising within the periodontium, by the involvement of the alveolar bone by lesions developing in adjacent tissues, or as part of a more generalized disease process. Most of these conditions are dealt with elsewhere in this book.

Developmental conditions

Lateral periodontal cyst

Rarely, developmental cysts may arise from residues of odontogenic epithelium within the gingiva (gingival cyst) or periodontal ligament (lateral periodontal cyst). Being within soft tissue, the gingival cyst does not produce any radiological changes, although slight 'cupping' of the underlying bone surface is occasionally present. However, a lateral periodontal cyst is usually visible on radiographs of the dental supporting tissues and is usually diagnosed after it has become infected or as an incidental radiographic finding. The first example (**349**) shows a pear-shaped lateral periodontal cyst occupying the interdental septum between |23 . The lesion is well defined and partly overlies the adjacent teeth whose apices are slightly displaced.

In the second example (**350**), there is an oval radiolucency overlying the roots of a noncarious, vital |4 , around much of which there is a thin cortical lamina. The lamina dura distally and apically is absent, and the two roots are displayed clearly. The absence of bony trabeculae overlying the

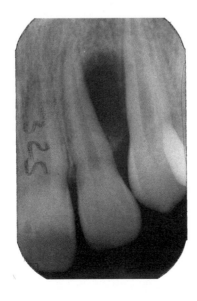

349 Lateral periodontal cyst. P.

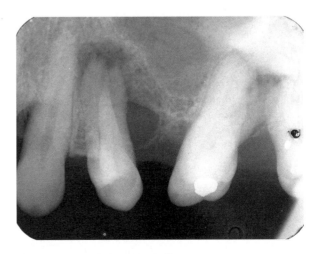

350 Lateral periodontal cyst. P.

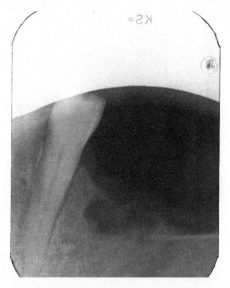

351 Lateral periodontal cyst (botyroid cyst). P.

more occlusal part of the lesion indicates that the cortical plate of the alveolus has been perforated. Occasionally, lateral periodontal cysts are multilocular in form and have been likened to a bunch of grapes (botyroid cyst). The cyst has the same relationship to the teeth as in the unilocular type and is most common in the mandibular premolar region, although in **351** the teeth have been extracted leaving the lesion behind in the edentulous bone. There is a well-defined, multilocular radiolucency in the left mandibular premolar region, surrounded by a thin, radio-opaque cortical lamina.

Microbial conditions and their sequelae

Chronic adult periodontitis

Periodontal disease is a common progressive inflammatory disease of the gingiva and underlying supporting tissues of the teeth, caused by the accumulation and persistance of dental plaque at the gingival margin. In its early stages it is limited to the soft tissues of the gingiva (chronic gingivitis) and so there are no radiographic changes of significance, but as the condition spreads to involve the alveolar bone, there is a progressive loss of the bony support of the tooth starting from the alveolar crest and spreading apically.

Although the condition often starts in childhood, it progresses slowly with intermittent phases of active disease, so that destruction of the alveolar bone is not apparent until adulthood (chronic adult periodontitis). The disease usually effects all quadrants of the mouth producing a characteristic pattern of horizontal bone loss, but is sometimes more localized and may be exacerbated in some less common forms of systemic disease (e.g. avitaminosis C).

Advanced loss of alveolar bone, leading to loosening and eventually shedding of the teeth, does not usually occur until later life. In some individuals, the disease is particularly aggressive (rapidly progressive periodontitis) and reaches the terminal stage at a much earlier age. In a small number of patients the bone destruction occurs in childhood. These are clinically distinct forms of the disease (prepubertal periodontitis; juvenile periodontitis) and are associated with specific underlying abnormalities of the host or with particular micro-organisms.

The first example (**352**) shows an early stage of chronic adult periodontitis in a 35-year-old, with loss of the cortical outline of the crests of the interdental septa; this is more marked on the right side of the mouth. Prominent overhanging margins are present on the amalgam restorations 7| mesially and 6| distally; 6| bears a porcelain crown.

At a more intermediate stage (**353**), there is generalized irregular destruction of the bone at the crests of the interdental septa, showing a loss of their cortical outline together with craterform radiolucency. The bone destruction is more advanced between the maxillary central incisors, where there is also a diastema and in the four molar quadrants, where, in the lower jaw, there are infrabony pockets 76|67 . In addition, there is some radiolucency inter-radicularly |6 , indicating early root bifurcation involvement.

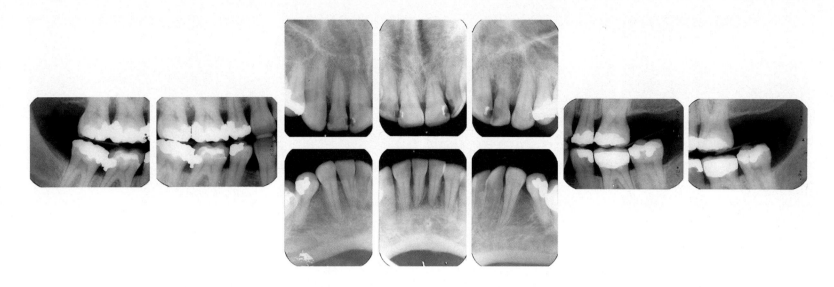

352 Chronic adult periodontitis. P, BW.

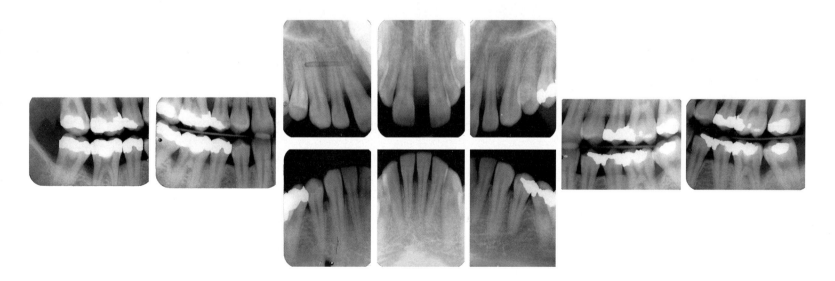

353 Chronic adult periodontitis. P, BW.

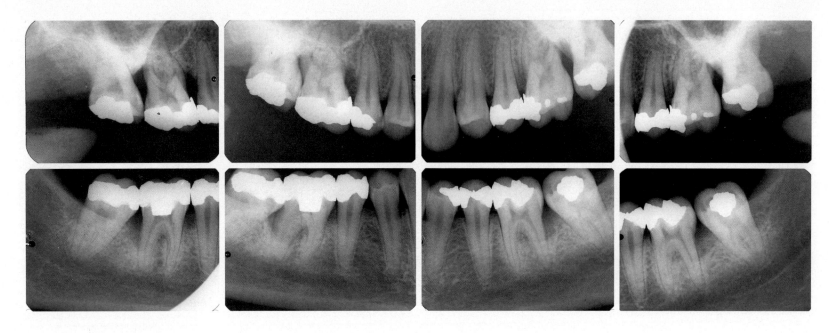

354 Chronic adult periodontitis. P.

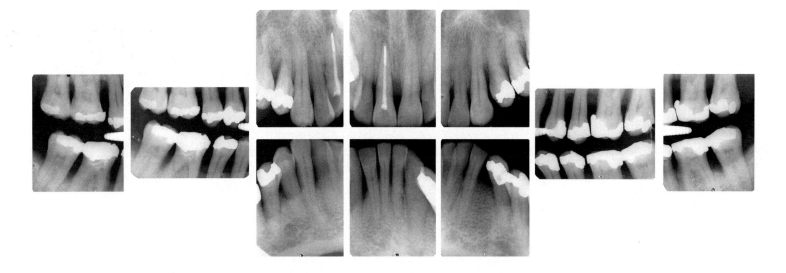

355 Chronic adult periodontitis. P, BW.

Periapical radiographs (**354**) of the same patient, taken by the bisecting angle technique, illustrate how an inaccurate picture of the bone loss may be obtained due to the angulation of the film relative to the X-ray tube, and how the image of the zygomatic process and arch may be projected over and obscure the roots of the maxillary molars, making interpretation difficult.

At a more advanced stage of the condition in a 57-year-old (**355**), the disease is particularly marked bilaterally in the molar region. The bone loss is so advanced that its full extent is not evident on conventional bitewing films, but is revealed when the films are positioned vertically. There are a number of restorations with overhanging cervical margins.

356 Chronic adult periodontitis. DPR.

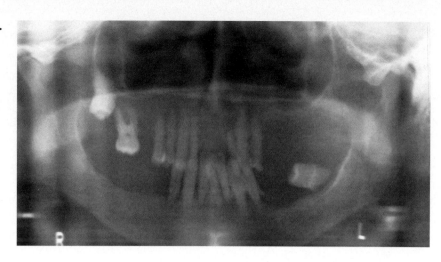

In the terminal stages, there is loss of most or all of the alveolar bone so that the teeth have no functional support and are ultimately shed naturally. In the badly neglected mouth of a 62-year-old (**356**) there has already been loss of many of the teeth; those that remain have little or no alveolar support. Indeed, there is total loss of bone $\overline{8}$, which appears to be floating in soft tissue. Most of the teeth show a radio-opaque collar of calculus around the middle of their roots.

In rapidly progressive periodontitis (**357**), the rate of bone destruction is much greater in spite of reasonable standards of oral care and reaches a terminal stage in much younger patients. In this 32-year-old patient there is little evidence of calculus deposition on the teeth and a generally good standard of restorative treatment and yet the alveolar bone destruction has progressed to the apical third of the roots of most of the teeth. Some molars have already been lost and there is marked irregularity of the surface of the edentulous ridge in the left maxillary molar region.

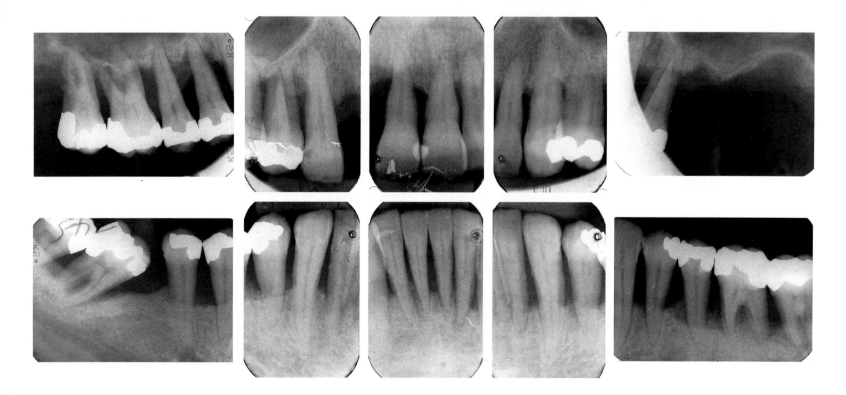

357 Rapidly progressive periodontitis. P.

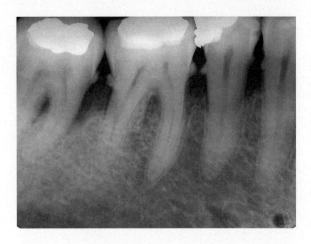

358 Calculus. P.

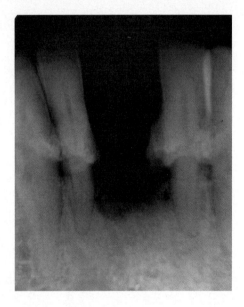

359 Calculus. P.

and may be a local factor in the progress of the disease. When sufficiently large they are readily visible on radiographs, as in **358** showing heavy deposits of supragingival calculus, forming projecting, radio-opaque spurs on the cervical surfaces of the mandibular premolar and molar teeth. There is loss of the cortical outline of the interdental crests together with irregular radiolucent loss of the bone. The bone loss interdentally $\overline{76|}$ has progressed at different rates on each root surface, forming two infrabony pockets separated by a residual spur of bone towards the interdental crest. There is also early bifurcation involvement of $\overline{76|}$ as demonstrated by the small areas of inter-radicular radiolucency.

Another example (**359**), in the anterior part of the mouth, shows heavy deposits of supragingival calculus cervically on the interstitial and lingual surfaces of the mandibular anterior teeth, except $\overline{1|1}$ which are missing. The deposits are of varying radio-opacity and are layered, suggesting formation in successive increments. There is advanced loss of the alveolar bone and absence of cortical lamina, particularly in the edentulous part of the ridge.

Prominent cervical margins of restorations predispose to plaque formation and are one of many factors that may account for localized disease. In **360** there is an area of localized periodontitis associated with the overhanging cervical margin on the large amalgam restoration $\overline{6|}$ distally. The underlying alveolar crest has a craterform radiolucency with loss of cortical outline; a small spur of radio-opaque calculus projects from the mesiocervical surface $\overline{7|}$. There are fillings in the two separate canals of the mesial root and in the pulp chamber $\overline{6|}$.

Another example (**361**) shows a more advanced, localized lesion interdentally $\underline{|67}$ associated with gross excess of amalgam cervically on the mesio-occlusal filling $\underline{|7}$. There is bone destruction up to the apical third of the root $\underline{|7}$ although it is much less advanced in the other interdental spaces.

In chronic adult periodontitis, the rate of bone loss is usually similar around all the affected teeth (horizontal bone loss).

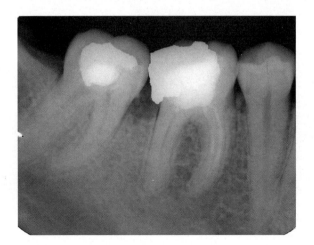

360 Overhanging restoration. P.

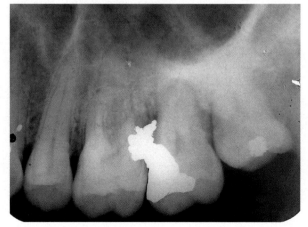

361 Overhanging restoration. P.

In **362** only the apical half of the roots remain supported by bone. There are irregular radiolucent defects in all the interdental crests with loss of the cortical lamina. The bone loss is a little more advanced interdentally 7̅6̅, in association with the extra root of the three-rooted molar, which exhibits early trifurcation involvement. The marked occlusal attrition indicates that an occlusal factor may have contributed to the pattern of the disease in this case.

Although, in chronic adult periodontitis, the overall rate of bone destruction is similar throughout the affected parts of the mouth, individual teeth may show more advanced disease, as in the molar in **363** where the bone loss has reached the apex. Radiolucent areas of bone destruction are present mesially, distally and apically, there being a deep, infrabony pocket mesially, which is in close proximity to the thin cortical lamina of the antral floor. Projecting from the mesial root surface are numerous radio-opaque spurs of calculus. Calculus is also present distocervically ∣5̅ .

Note the coronoid process of the mandible in the lower right corner of the illustration and the shadow of the thick mucoperiosteum covering the tuberosity.

Another advanced lesion 7̅∣ is shown (**364**) in a patient suffering from generalized periodontitis with destruction of the periodontal ligament, adjacent lamina dura and alveolar bone extending around the entire surface of the root. The root is surrounded by a wide, radiolucent defect, which is clearly defined mesially. In addition, the patient had an acute lateral periodontal abscess ∣7̅ where the periodontal ligament space is widened and the tooth is slightly protruded from its socket.

The periapical radiograph **365** shows these changes more clearly, and in addition demonstrates a diffuse radiolucency in the surrounding alveolar bone, particularly mesially. Note that in addition to the coronoid process of the mandible, the pterygoid hamulus is displayed clearly.

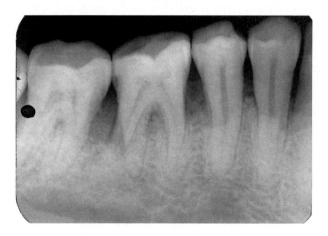

362 Overhanging restoration. P.

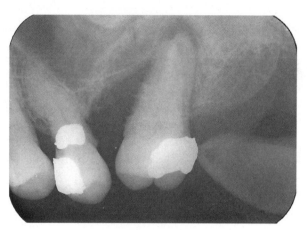

363 Chronic adult periodontitis. P.

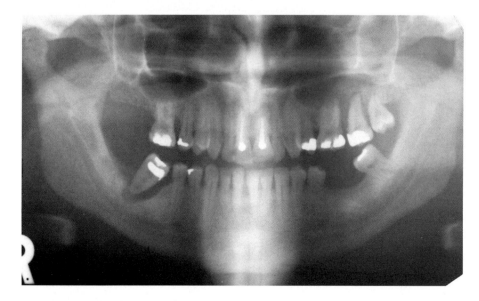

364 Chronic adult periodontitis. DPR.

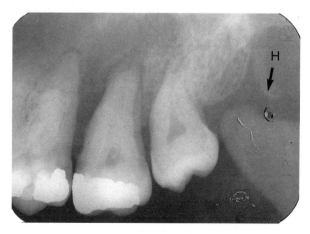

365 Chronic adult periodontitis. P. H: pterygoid hamulus.

Juvenile periodontitis

This form of periodontitis is usually diagnosed in the second decade of life and results in rapid bone loss with loosening and drifting of the teeth. It is more common in people of African origin and may affect many teeth of the permanent dentition (**366**), although the changes are often most marked in association with the incisor and molar teeth. In this example, the radiolucent area of bone loss 2̲ has progressed almost to its apex, and that around the molar roots involves their furcations. More localized forms of the disease also occur, as in **367** where 6̲ has an obvious lesion and the other three first molars have been extracted as a consequence of the disease.

Prepubertal periodontitis

Rarely, advanced periodontitis is diagnosed in the first decade of life and usually these patients have some underlying systemic disease, such as Langerhans' cell histiocytosis or hereditary hypophosphatasia. As a consequence it may affect the primary and/or permanent dentitions. In the 15-year-old patient (**368**) with the Hand–Schüller–Christian type of Langerhans' cell reticulosis, there are localized, punched-out areas of bone loss associated bilaterally with the premolars and first molars in the mandible. The condition of the alveolar bone elsewhere is healthy.

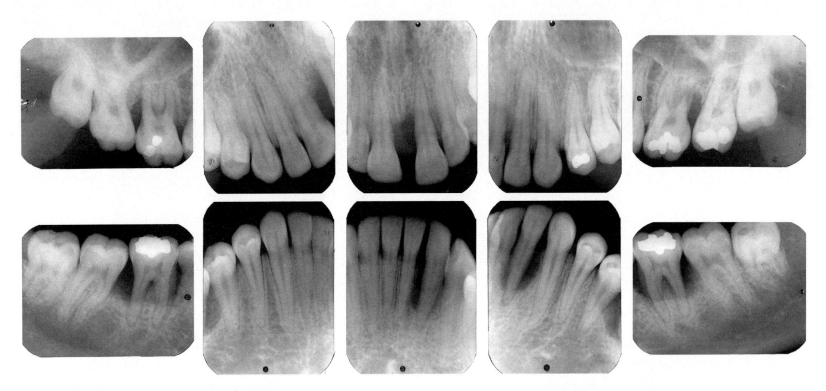

366 Juvenile periodontitis. P.

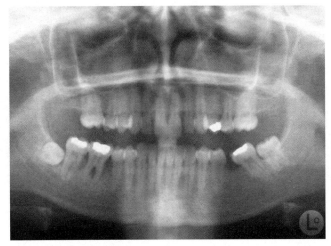

367 Juvenile periodontitis. DPR.

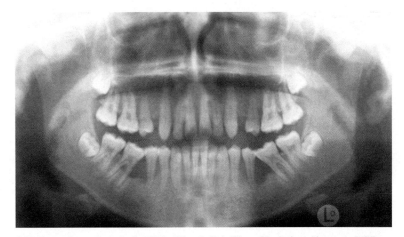

368 Prepubertal periodontitis (Hand–Schüller–Christian disease). DPR.

Laterally-positioned radicular cyst

Although radicular cysts occur typically in the periapical region of a tooth, they may develop laterally in association with a lateral root canal, or lateral root perforation. In the lesion **369**, which has arisen as a result of a lateral perforation of the root 2|, there is a pear-shaped, radiolucent defect in the interdental septum 32| extending from the crest inferiorly towards the apices superiorly. There is loss of the lamina dura mesially 3| and distally 2|, and displacement of both tooth apices away from the lesion. The metal tip of the post crown is projecting through the perforation and some radio-opaque cement is lying within the adjacent soft tissues. The root filling is deficient apically and is poorly condensed. In the past, lesions in this location and with this appearance may have been designated as globulomaxillary cysts.

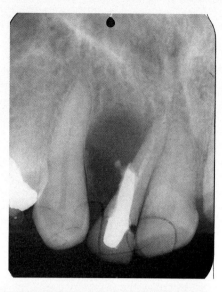

369 Laterally-positioned radicular cyst. P.

Paradental cyst

Typically, these cysts arise in young adults in association with partially erupted, impacted mandibular third molars where there is a history of recurrent pericoronitis. They most commonly occur buccally and distally in relation to the associated tooth and hence their image is partly superimposed upon that of the affected molar. The example (**370**) shows an oval, radiolucent cystic area surrounded by a thin, radio-opaque lamina. The lesion extends to the roof of the inferior alveolar canal and overlaps part of the distal root of the tooth, although the apices are not involved. The darker radiolucency occlusally indicates that there is marked thinning of one of the cortical plates of the alveolus.

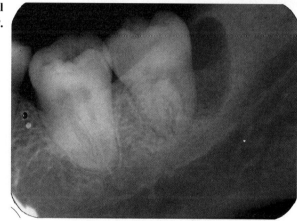

370 Paradental cyst. P.

Fibrous epulis

These hyperplastic soft-tissue masses, which arise as local gingival swellings in response to irritation, do not normally show well on radiographs, but may be better demonstrated by reduced exposure. However, a proportion, approximately 25%, contains areas of mineralization. The soft-tissue outline (arrows) of the lesion (**371**) on the lingual aspect of the lower anterior teeth extends from 5| to |2 , describing a smooth curve. It contains several irregularly shaped mineralizations, which are faintly radio-opaque, many of them running at right angles to the surface of the mandible.

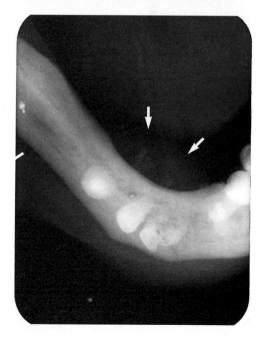

371 Fibrous epulis. LTO.

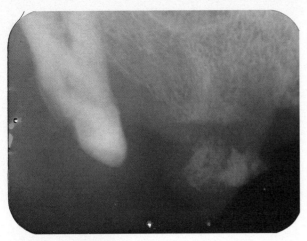

372 Fibrous epulis. P.

Another example (**372**) shows an inflammatory hyperplasia in the maxillary right molar region, containing numerous radio-opaque trabeculae of abnormal mineralization towards the centre. There is no obvious continuity between the metaplastic bone and the underlying maxillary bone, the two being separated by radiolucent soft tissue, although there is a poorly-defined area of radiolucency in the alveolus suggesting some bone resorption has occurred. The metaplastic bone lacks the fine trabeculation characteristic of normal bone. 8| is extensively carious with loss of the distal cusps and a deep infrabony pocket is present mesially.

Traumatic conditions and their sequelae

Occlusal traumatism

This occurs when the masticatory forces exceed the normal physiological limits of tooth support, as may occur if a restoration is high on the bite or in bruxism. The condition is exacerbated when the alveolar support for the tooth is reduced in chronic periodontitis and indeed persistent occlusal traumatism will accelerate further bone loss in this condition. The radiograhic appearance of occlusal traumatism is of an overall increase in the width of the periodontal ligament space, which appears more prominent than normal. In addition, there may be loss of definition of the lamina dura. In the example (**373**, **374**) there is generalized loss of bone from the crests of the interdental septa, which are blunted and exhibit irregular radiolucencies due to the chronic adult periodontitis. The bone loss is particularly advanced |1 . In addition, the radiolucent periodontal ligament space is widened around most of the teeth so that it is seen more clearly than usual. This widening has arisen from the excessive movement of the teeth in their sockets, as a result of the occlusal trauma.

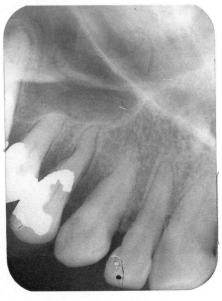

373 Occlusal traumatism. P.

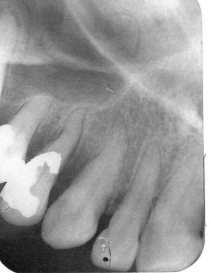

374 Occlusal traumatism. P.

Metabolic conditions

Avitaminosis C (scurvy)

This may occur in individuals whose diets lack fresh fruit and green vegetables. In this condition – because of the widespread incidence of chronic periodontal inflammation and the more rapid metabolic turnover of the collagen fibres in the periodontium compared with those in other tissues – there may be early involvement of the periodontal ligament leading to its rapid destruction. In the example (**375**), there is advanced loss of the interdental bone around the mandibular incisors and the periodontal ligament space; the lamina dura persists only in the periapical regions of the teeth. Deposits of calculus are present on the cervical parts of the roots of the teeth projecting laterally and forming more densely radio-opaque collars where they are superimposed upon the roots.

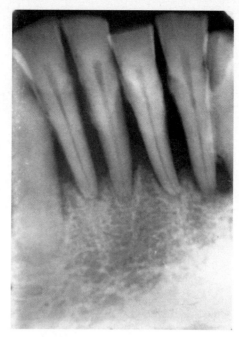

375 Avitaminosis C (scurvy). P.

6

The facial bones

Introduction

The jaws can be affected by the whole range of diseases that involve the other bones of the skeleton, but they are unique in that they contain the teeth and the odontogenic tissues. Therefore, they are also affected by conditions arising from these tissues. As with the remainder of the skeleton, radiographs and other imaging techniques form part of the diagnostic procedure. They support or confirm the provisional clinical diagnosis, but the definitive diagnosis frequently depends upon a combination of clinical, radiological and laboratory findings.

Although there is a variety of imaging techniques that can be applied to the investigation of disorders of the jaws and facial skeleton, radiographic views form the basis of the initial examination. Radiographs not only reveal the presence of the bony abnormality, sometimes unsuspected, but also its nature, extent and effect on adjacent structures. The jaws are well displayed on the DPR which demonstrates both sides on one film, though it may be complemented with intra-oral views to show

lesions in the alveolus in greater detail. For the investigation of disorders affecting the middle third of the facial skeleton, other standard radiographic views are required, with the occipitomental being particularly useful.

The facial skeleton may also be investigated by CT and MRI. These investigations are indicated for traumatic and neoplastic disorders or when the condition is not completely demonstrated on plain radiographs. The use of intravenous contrast media or of **3D** CT scanning may further improve the diagnostic information that can be obtained from these investigations.

Radionuclide scanning using technetium methylene diphosphonate may also be used in the investigation of disorders affecting the facial skeleton. The main indications include the assessment of tumours, the evaluation of bone grafts and the determination of areas of active bone growth.

Developmental conditions

Torus palatinus

Perhaps the most common developmental malformations of the jaws are localized bony protuberances, occurring on the midline of the palate or the lingual aspect of the mandible. These are referred to as torus palatinus and torus mandibularis respectively. Torus palatinus arises in the midline of the palate and affects up to 20% of the population in a minor form. Only when large does it appear on radiographs, forming a projection of dense cortical bone which may be lobulated or smooth in outline. In **376**, a uniformly dense radio-opaque mass is present superimposed upon both sides of the nasal septum (arrows), although mostly on the right side. It has a smooth, clearly defined outline.

376 Torus palatinus. USO.

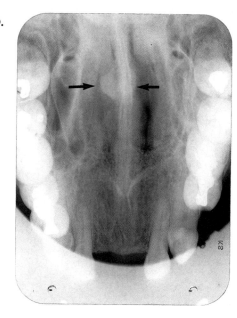

135

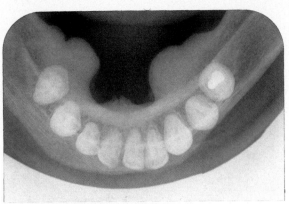

377 Tori mandibularis. LTO.

Torus mandibularis

This developmental abnormality of the mandible usually consists of bilateral bony exostoses lingual to the mandibular premolar teeth. They are composed of dense cortical bone, are often nodular and when large are displayed on occlusal radiographs, as in **377**. The genial tubercles are also clearly seen in the midline lingually. On a periapical radiograph, the images of the tori may be projected over the apices of the mandibular premolars, as in **378**, thus simulating an area of periapical osteosclerosis.

Cleft palate

Clefting of the lip and palate may occur separately or in combination. These are primary structural defects caused by localized disturbances in morphogenesis resulting in a failure of fusion of the palatal processes. They may be associated with more complex developmental abnormalities of the craniofacial skeleton.

The incidence of cleft palate varies widely, but in some communities may be as high as 1:2,500 individuals. Cleft palates vary in severity, involving the midline of the palate posteriorly and extending into the alveolus anteriorly, usually in the lateral incisor region, where they may be unilateral or bilateral. Unerupted and/or supernumerary teeth may be associated with the alveolar cleft; one or both permanent lateral incisors are often missing.

The first example (**379**) shows a unilateral radiolucent cleft running between B| and C|, continuous with the nasal cavity. On the mesial side of the cleft, 1| is slightly retroclined, as indicated by its foreshortening and 2| is missing. In addition, two conical supernumerary teeth are present in the upper right quadrant.

The second example (**380**, **381**, **382**) shows a bilateral cleft through the maxillary lateral incisor region. The lateral incisors are absent and the central incisors are present in the central block of bone of the premaxilla. There is discontinuity in the outline of the floor of the nose bilaterally, where the clefts extend superiorly.

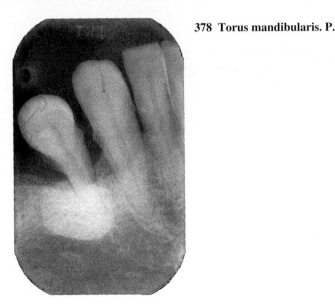

378 Torus mandibularis. P.

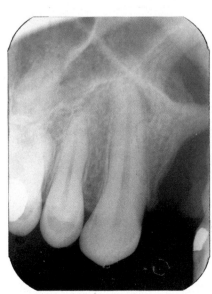

379 Unilateral cleft palate. P.

380 Bilateral cleft palate. P.

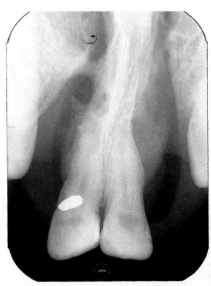

381 Bilateral cleft palate. P.

The majority of patients with cleft palate have underdevelopment of the maxilla producing a characteristic soft tissue outline. The tip of the nose (**383**) is depressed and blunted and the upper lip retruded, so accentuating the lower lip. Note the prominence of the soft palate which forms an approximately vertical, radio-opaque image, just posterior to the molar teeth.

Craniofacial anomalies

Differentiation of the cranium is complex and commences early in human development with nearly 60% of its ultimate growth present at birth. The craniofacial skeleton can be divided into three parts:

- The upper part consists of the forehead and the anterior part of the neurocranium.
- The middle part consists of the orbits, nose and maxilla, including the cranial base and the branchial arch components.
- The lower part is the mandible.

Disorders in growth and development (dysplasia) of any one of the three divisions of the face may affect the other two. These abnormalities can be classified into several broad groups:

- Cerebrocranial dysplasias, which result in anomalies such as microcephaly and anencephaly.
- Premature fusion of one or more cranial sutures, which gives rise to a variety of craniosynostoses, the resulting deformity and thus nomenclature depending upon which sutures are affected.
- Midface deformities, such as Apert's syndrome, which may also be associated with cranial suture synostoses.

Facial malformations may be relatively simple or complex with the primary defect producing a series of secondary and tertiary anomalies. Some of these malformations are genetic in origin, with dominant or recessive traits, whilst others are the result of spontaneous mutation. Growth disorders may affect one or both jaws, and one or both sides of the affected jaws producing a variety of malocclusions. Unilateral facial deformities include hemihypertrophy, hemifacial microsomia and first branchial arch syndrome. Bilateral facial deformities include conditions such as mandibulofacial dysostosis (Treacher Collins syndrome). The various forms of facial deformity are sometimes associated with clefting.

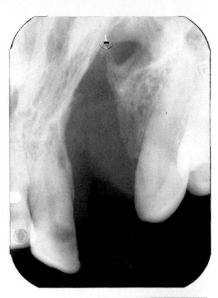

382 Bilateral cleft palate. P.

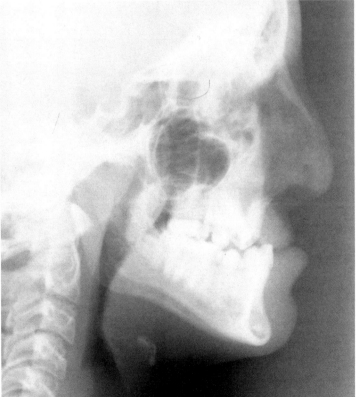

383 Cleft palate. LC.

CRANIOSYNOSTOSIS

The first example (**384**, **385**) is of an infant in whom there has been premature fusion of some of the cranial sutures. The coronal suture remains faintly visible (**384**) but the metopic suture has closed. The classic 'copper beaten' appearance of the skull (**385**) has arisen as a result of increased intracranial pressure.

The next example (**386**, **387**) shows a case of complex multiple synostoses resulting in severe deformity of the skull. The abnormalities are well displayed in the 3D CT scan (**387**), which has particular application in the evaluation of these growth disorders.

APERT'S SYNDROME

In the example (**388**) there is closure of the coronal suture and cranial deformity, with a small anterior cranial fossa (turribrachycephalic). The anteroposterior diameter of the vault of the skull is shortened and there is evidence of midface retrusion. Cranial markings, or convolutions, are visible in the occipital region. Note the outline of the adult carpal bones of the fingers supporting the infant's chin.

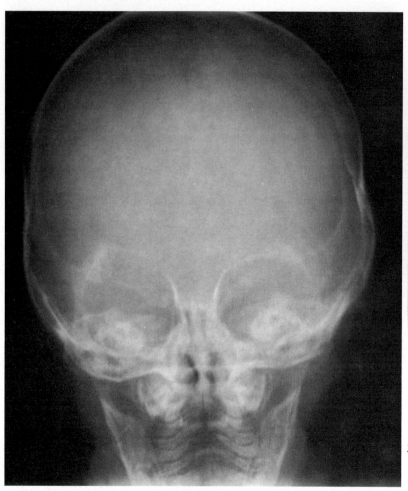

384 Craniosynostosis. PA.

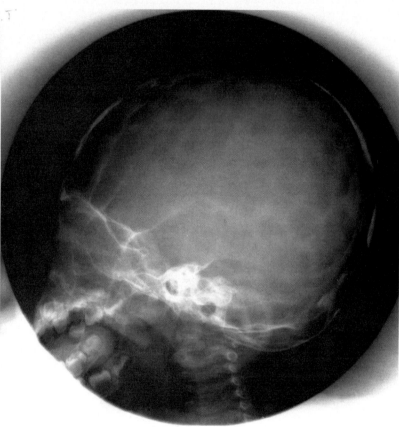

385 Craniosynostosis. L.

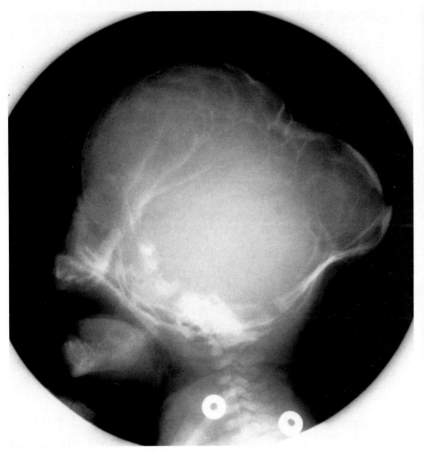

386 Craniosynostosis. L.

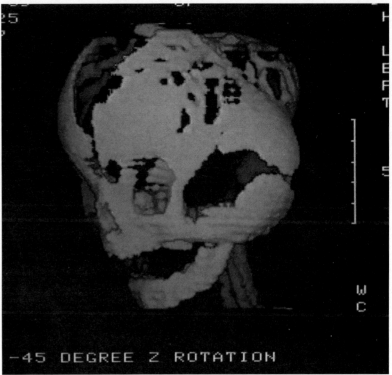

387 Craniosynostosis. CT.

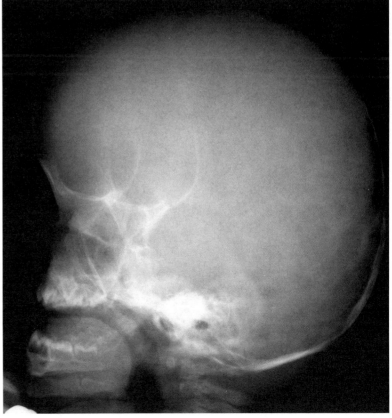

388 Apert's syndrome. L.

FIRST ARCH SYNDROME

This syndrome is associated with abnormal vascularization of the first arch during embryonic development. It is variable in its presentation and severity.

In the example (**389**) there is a complete absence of the condyle and ramus of the mandible resulting in pronounced micrognathia. $\overline{ED|}$ have erupted but $\overline{6|}$ is missing and the developing $\overline{7|}$ is displaced forwards, its crown lying horizontally and pointing posteriorly. $\overline{5|}$ is also displaced anteriorly, lying beneath the unerupted $\overline{4|}$. In addition, the external auditory meatus was deficient, but this is not clearly demonstrated on this radiograph.

In the second example (**390**), the defect is less severe, there being hypoplasia of the right mandibular ramus and condyle. The affected ramus is more medially placed and the condylar head and coronoid process are less well developed than on the normal side. There is deviation of the point of the chin to the affected side, although the mandibular and maxillary incisors are in a normal relationship. The patient is partially deaf on the right side and the pinna is deformed.

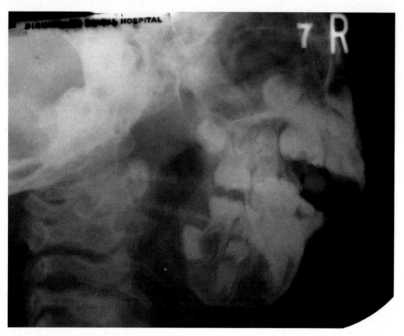

389 First arch syndrome. OLM.

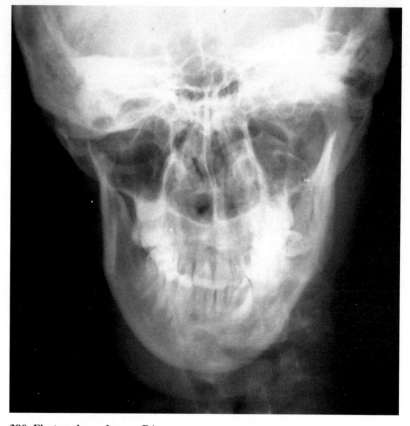

390 First arch syndrome. PA.

MANDIBULOFACIAL DYOSTOSIS (TREACHER COLLINS SYNDROME)
In mandibulofacial dysostosis, the maxilla, mandible and zygoma are all underdeveloped producing a characteristic facial appearance with flattening of the midface and retrusion of the chin. In the example (**391**, **392**), the maxilla and mandible are both underdeveloped, the latter markedly so, producing a receding chin and a steep mandibular angle (**391**). The underdevelopment of the supra-orbital ridges, the zygomatic bones and the zygomatic arches are difficult to identify on this radiograph. There is a malocclusion with proclination of the maxillary and mandibular incisors and overall crowding of the teeth (**392**). The inferior border of the mandible is concave with pronounced antegonial notching and, in this example, the right maxillary antrum is less well developed. The pinna of the ear on the right (arrow) is underdeveloped and abnormally shaped.

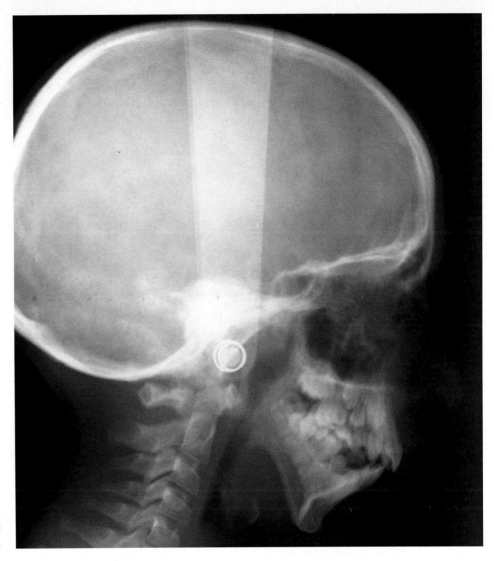

391 Mandibulofacial dysostosis (Treacher Collins syndrome). LC.

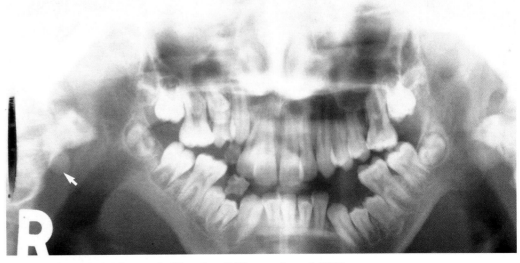

392 Mandibulofacial dysostosis (Treacher Collins syndrome). DPR.

A second example (**393**) shows marked underdevelopment of both rami of the mandible with absence of the condyles, extreme bowing of the inferior border of the mandible with pronounced antegonial notching and absence of the zygomatic complexes. Note the unerupted, incompletely developed, supplemental premolar on the left side of the mandible.

Surgical treatment of this condition may involve the use of bone grafts, as illustrated in **394**. There has been onlay grafting to both zygomas in addition to surgical advancement of the chin.

Cleidocranial dysplasia (dysostosis)

This is an autosomal dominant disorder producing both skeletal and dental anomalies. The former includes the absence of the clavicles, the presence of additional small bones within the cranial sutures (wormian bones), frontal bossing and maxillary retrognathism. The main dental anomalies include delayed or failed eruption of the permanent teeth with retention of the primary dentition, and the presence of supernumerary teeth. In the 14-year-old (**395**) there are several unerupted supernumerary teeth which can be identified because their stage of development is behind that of the normal dentition.

In the next example (**396**) there are several wormian bones within the sagittal suture of the vault of the skull, as indicated by the complex suture pattern. In some individuals supernumerary teeth are not particularly numerous, as in **397** in which, in addition to the presence of many unerupted teeth of the normal dentition, there are only two supernumerary teeth in the anterior maxilla. Also, a dentigerous cyst is present in the |34 region.

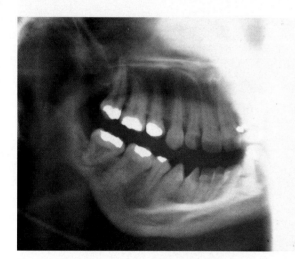
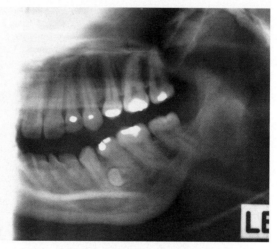

393 Mandibulofacial dysostosis (Treacher Collins syndrome). DPR.

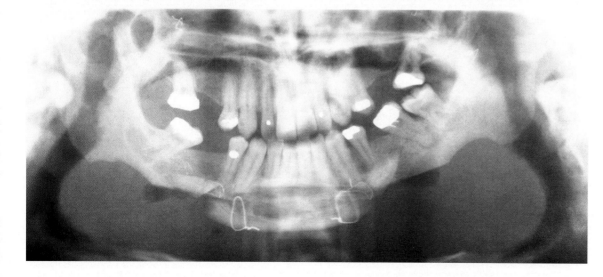

394 Mandibulofacial dysostosis (Treacher Collins syndrome). DPR.

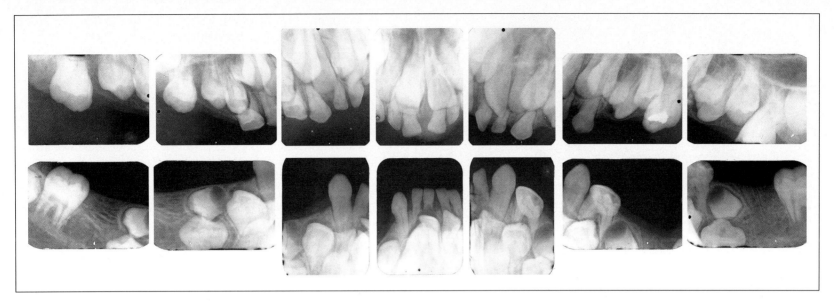

395 Cleidocranial dysplasia. P.

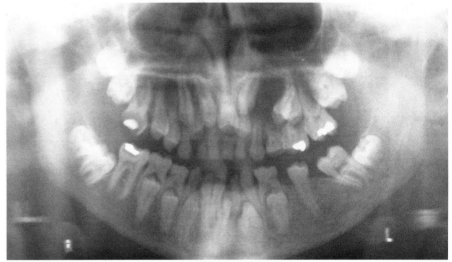

397 Cleidocranial dysplasia. DPR.

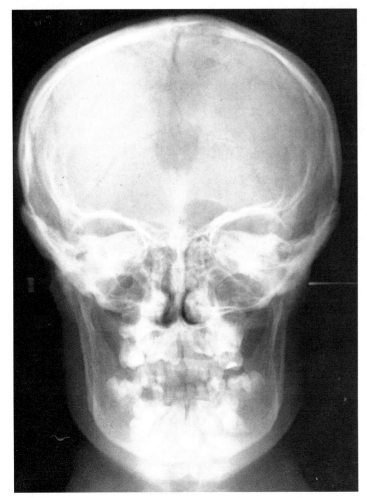

396 Cleidocranial dysplasia. PA.

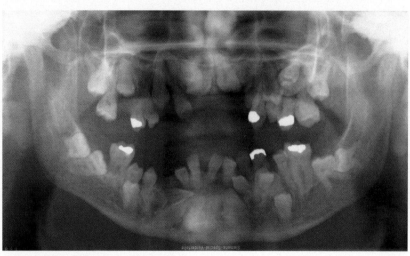

398 Cleidocranial dysostosis. DPR.

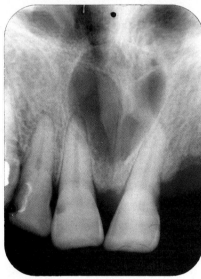

399 Nasopalatine cyst. P.

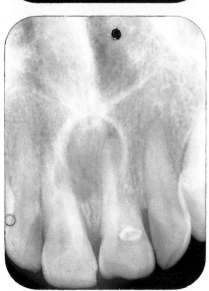

400 Nasopalatine cyst. P.

Many of the permanent teeth may fail to erupt, as demonstrated in the radiograph of a 28-year-old patient (**398**).

Developmental cysts

These cysts may arise in the jaws as a consequence of cystic breakdown in epithelium either at lines of fusion of embryonic processes or from residues left behind after odontogenesis. There are therefore two groups of developmental cysts: the inclusion cysts and the odontogenic cysts.

INCLUSION CYSTS

Most commonly, inclusion cysts develop in the nasopalatine (incisive canal) area of the maxilla, but they may also arise elsewhere in the midline of the maxilla or the mandible. Previously it was believed that cysts occurring between the maxillary lateral incisors and canines, 'globulomaxillary' cysts, were developmental in origin. However, closer study of the embryonic development of this part of the jaws precludes such a pathogenesis and these lesions can now be ascribed to other types of pathological entity such as laterally positioned radicular cysts or odontogenic keratocysts.

Nasopalatine (incisive canal) cysts Nasopalatine (incisive canal) cysts produce a radiolucent defect in the anterior part of the midline of the maxilla and may be circular, pear-shaped or bilobed in outline. The example (**399**) showing a pear-shaped lesion is bounded by a thin, radio-opaque lamina and has caused slight divergence of the roots 1|1 . The lamina dura and the periodontal ligament space are continuous apically 1|1 . Note the images of the anterior nasal spine and the anterior border of the floor of the nose superimposed upon the radiolucent lesion.

Small inclusion cysts may present difficulty in diagnosis for two reasons. Firstly, they are difficult to differentiate radiologically from a large incisive foramen, although a radiolucency greater than 6.0 mm in width is likely to be cystic. Secondly, the area may be superimposed upon the roots 1|1 , thus simulating a periapical lesion. In the next example (**400**), there is a circular radiolucency surrounded by a thin, radio-opaque lamina in the midline, superimposed upon the apical half of the roots 1|1 . A second radiograph (**401**), taken with the X-ray tube to the left of the midline, confirms the palatal position of the lesion (by parallax), which is now overlying the apex |1 resembling a periapical inflammatory lesion. However, the periodontal ligament space and the lamina dura remain intact apically.

Example **402** shows a large, clearly defined, circular, radiolucent lesion bounded by a radio-opaque lamina in the midline of the anterior part of the maxilla in which 1|1 are absent. The teeth have been missing for several years and the resulting gap has become narrowed. In the absence of 1|1 the radiological differentiation between a nasopalatine cyst and a residual cyst may be difficult but as a general rule a cyst arising from a tooth tends to occur rather more to one side of the midline. The images of the nasal spine, the anterior border of the floor of the nose, and the anterior part of the nasal septum are superimposed upon the lesion.

Another circular, radiolucent lesion (**403**) is shown in the anterior region of the midline of the palate of an edentulous patient. It is bounded by a thin, radio-opaque lamina and has expanded the labial aspect of the ridge. Superimposed upon the lesion, the anterior part of the nasal septum is breached and the cyst has expanded into the nasal cavity. Note the shadow of the soft tissues of the nose.

'Globulomaxillary' cyst Example **404** shows the typical appearance of what was previously called a 'globulomaxillary' cyst. There is displacement of the roots of the lateral incisor and canine mesially and distally, respectively. The radiolucent cyst has a clearly defined margin and is pear shaped, the bell of the pear lying superior to the roots of the teeth. There is slight expansion upwards of the cortical lamina of the floor of the nose and, despite the size of the lesion, the crestal bone interdentally |23 remains intact. |4 root has also been displaced distally.

ODONTOGENIC CYSTS

A number of different types of odontogenic cysts are believed to be developmental in origin and these include dentigerous cysts, odontogenic keratocysts, lateral periodontal cysts, paradental cysts and glandular odontogenic cysts. Lateral periodontal cysts and paradental cysts have been described in Chapter 5.

Dentigerous cyst This type of cyst forms by the breakdown of the reduced enamel epithelium around the crown of an unerupted tooth and therefore most frequently arises in association with teeth which commonly fail to erupt, such as third molars and maxillary canines. However, any unerupted tooth may be involved. The cyst enlarges in a manner that produces an approximately circular lesion around the crown of the affected tooth. A typical example (**405**) shows a circular, radiolucent cyst encompassing the

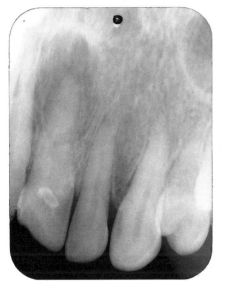

401 Nasopalatine cyst. P.

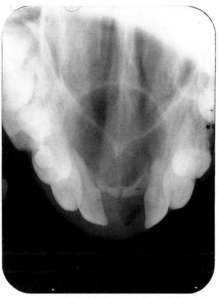

402 Nasopalatine cyst. USO.

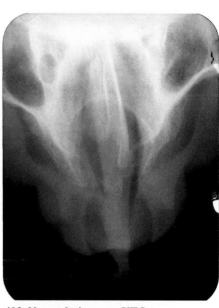

403 Nasopalatine cyst. UTO.

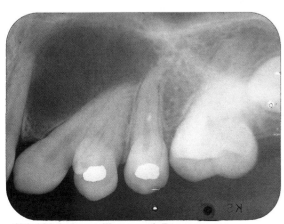

404 'Globulomaxillary cyst'. P.

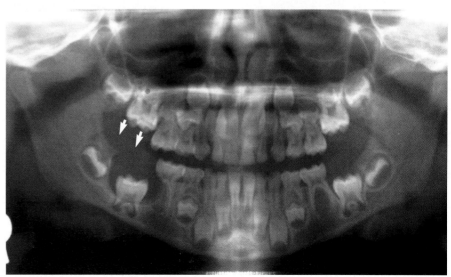

405 Dentigerous cyst. DPR.

crown 6| in a six-year-old. The cortical bone is perforated with expansion of the overlying soft tissues (arrows) but the remainder of the lesion is bounded by a thin, radio-opaque lamina. The associated tooth is displaced inferiorly and only its crown projects into the cyst cavity. There has been resorption of the whole of the distal root E| . Note the failure of 5|5 to develop, although faintly radiolucent follicular spaces are present inter-radicularly E|E .

In small lesions (406), radiological distinction from a large tooth follicle is impossible. The circular radiolucent lesion is surrounded by a thin radio-opaque lamina and envelops the whole of the crown |5 symmetrically. There are diastemas to each side of |4 .

The next example (407) shows a large, well-circumscribed, approximately circular, radiolucent cyst extending from the midline of the palate medially to the margin of the expanded alveolus laterally, where only a thin lamina of bone remains. This lesion has arisen in an eight-year-old, on the crown of the unerupted 3| (arrow) which is displaced posteriorly. DCB1| are erupted normally, although the root 1| is displaced mesially. 2| and 4| are unerupted and displaced medially and buccally, respectively.

Another smaller cyst is shown (408) lying eccentrically around the crown of a disto-angularly impacted 8| . Because of the position of the tooth, the majority of the radiolucent cyst cavity lies postero-inferiorly. The cyst is surrounded by a thin, radio-opaque lamina and has caused expansion of the overlying alveolus.

In 409 there is a cyst associated with 7| forming an approximately circular, well-defined radiolucency extending from the mesial aspect 6| to the distal aspect 8| , with the appearance of an entire tooth being situated within the cyst lumen. The mandible is expanded and thinned superiorly and inferiorly. There is a thin, radio-opaque corticated margin and the tooth has been displaced with a disto-angular inclination.

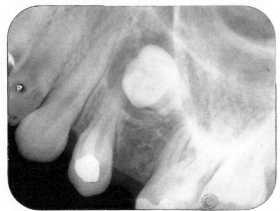

406 Dentigerous cyst. P.

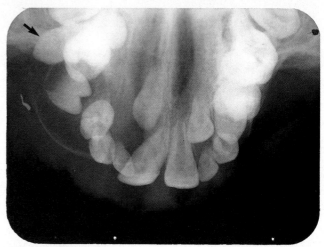

407 Dentigerous cyst. USO.

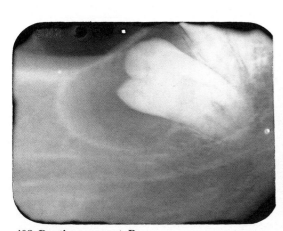

408 Dentigerous cyst. P.

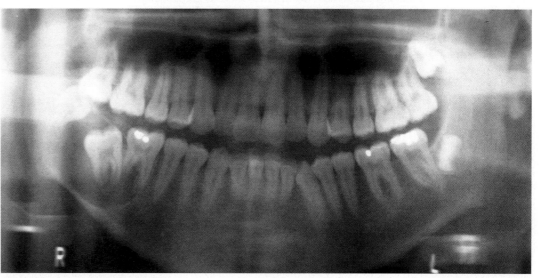

409 Dentigerous cyst. DPR.

With larger lesions, the shape of the cyst may be more elongated and can give a radiographic image which is similar to that of a number of other conditions. In the large cyst (**410**, **411**) in an otherwise edentulous mandible, a clearly defined radiolucency extends from the coronoid notch of the ramus posteriorly to the $\overline{5|}$ region anteriorly. The alveolar surface of the mandible and the anterior aspect of the ramus up to the base of the coronoid process have been perforated, and only a thin layer of cortical bone remains inferiorly, although there is no evidence of a pathological fracture. In the posterior part of the lesion there are several radio-opaque flakes which are probably remnants of the cortical bone. The images of the hyoid bone and the bodies of the atlas and axis vertebrae overlie the cyst defect (**410**). There is lingual expansion (arrows) of the ramus (**411**) and $\overline{8|}$ lies transversely on the buccal side of the cyst.

Rarely, more than one tooth may be associated with the same cyst. In **412**, the crowns of $\overline{7|}$ and $\overline{5|}$ project into a radiolucent cyst cavity. A thin, radio-opaque lamina surrounds the lesion inferiorly and anteriorly. $\overline{8|}$ is horizontally impacted and its crown is surrounded by a radiolucent follicular space of normal size. $\overline{6|}$ is missing.

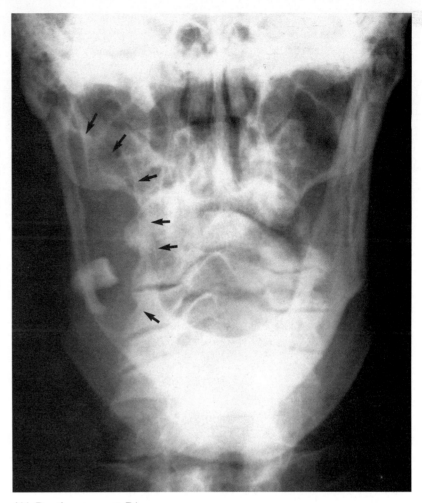

411 Dentigerous cyst. PA.

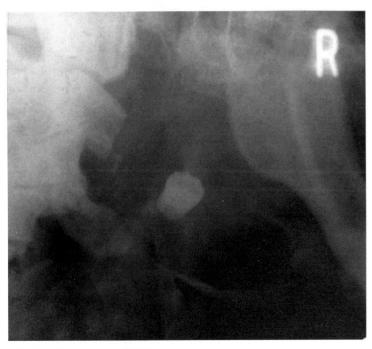

410 Dentigerous cyst. OLM.

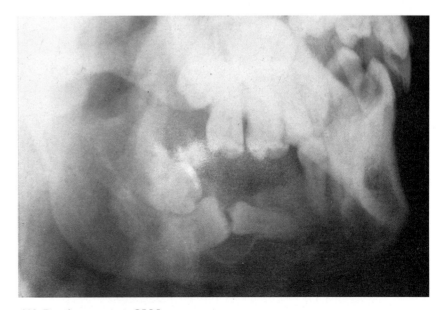

412 Dentigerous cyst. OLM.

Odontogenic keratocyst Odontogenic keratocysts occur most commonly in the second and third decades, but can be diagnosed at any age. There is controversy over the tissue of origin but most lesions probably arise from proliferation of the epithelial residues of the dental lamina, the glands of Serres. They are frequently associated with unerupted teeth, but these are usually displaced by the lesion rather than being part of it. Occasionally they may develop instead of a tooth when they have been described as primordial cysts. They occur most commonly in the posterior part of the body and ascending ramus of the mandible, although they may arise in any part of both jaws. Because odontogenic keratocysts enlarge by both a physicochemical expansile mechanism and primary epithelial growth, their outlines are often less regularly shaped, with a scalloped periphery; they grow preferentially in an anteroposterior direction through the cancellous bone. Radiologically they may resemble some other types of odontogenic cysts or tumours, particularly dentigerous cysts and ameloblastomas. If they arise in relation to the anterior and premolar teeth they may have the appearance of a lateral periodontal cyst, forming a well-circumscribed radiolucency somewhat pear shaped in outline, with a thin, radio-opaque

cortical lamina. In the example (413), $\overline{5|}$ root is displaced mesially and is vital.

If one of the adjacent teeth has been extracted previously, the cyst may remain in the edentulous part of the jaw, as in 414, where there is an ovoid radiolucency distal to $\overline{|3}$, with a clearly defined lower margin and loss of lamina dura and alveolar bone distally.

The next example (415) shows a medium sized lesion in the molar region and ramus of the right side of the mandible. It has a slightly scalloped outline which is demarcated by a thin, radio-opaque lamina, except superiorly distal to $\overline{7|}$. The anterior extremity of the lesion overlies the distal root $\overline{7|}$ and the inferior margin approximates to the inferior alveolar canal. Note the absence of $\overline{8|}$ indicating the probable primordial origin of the cyst.

Because their main direction of growth is in an anteroposterior direction, keratocysts can reach considerable sizes without causing marked bony expansion. The first clinical signs of the lesion may be intra-oral discharge or infection. In a 19-year-old patient with such symptoms in the $\overline{|7}$ region, the periapical radiograph (416) revealed a disto-angularly

413 Odontogenic keratocyst. OLM.

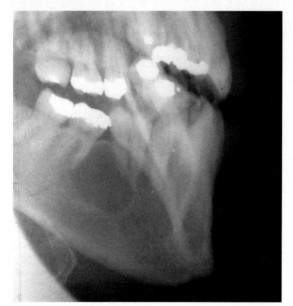

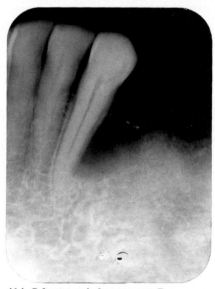

414 Odontogenic keratocyst. P.

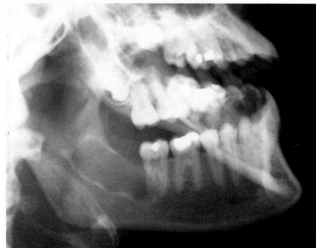

415 Odontogenic keratocyst. OLM.

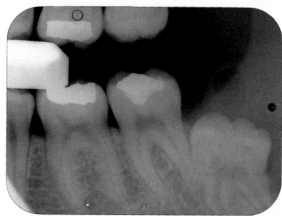

416 Odontogenic keratocyst. P.

impacted 8̶ and a radiolucency in the bone distally. A further radiograph (**417**) revealed the full extent of the lesion occupying most of the left ramus of the mandible, related to the crown and distal aspect of the roots 8̶ which has been displaced inferiorly. Despite its size there was little evidence of expansion of the mandible, the cyst having an almost complete, loculated, clearly defined margin composed of a thin, radio-opaque lamina.

Occasionally the associated unerupted tooth is markedly displaced from its normal position in the jaw (**418**). Here, in a 13-year-old, there is a large, radiolucent lesion in the left ramus associated with an unerupted 8̶ which has been displaced into the neck of the condyle. The ramus is expanded buccally and lingually, with marked thinning of the cortical bone; the cyst has a smooth outline with a thin, radio-opaque lamina. The relationship of the cyst to the crown of the tooth could lead to the interpretation of a dentigerous cyst, but closer examination indicates that the cyst does not envelope the entire crown, suggesting that the tooth is outside the lesion. Furthermore, the early stage of development 8̶ associated with a cyst of this size, makes the diagnosis of a dentigerous cyst unlikely. The interior alveolar canal is well shown.

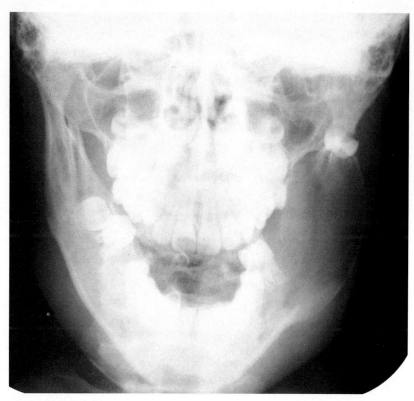

418 Odontogenic keratocyst. PA.

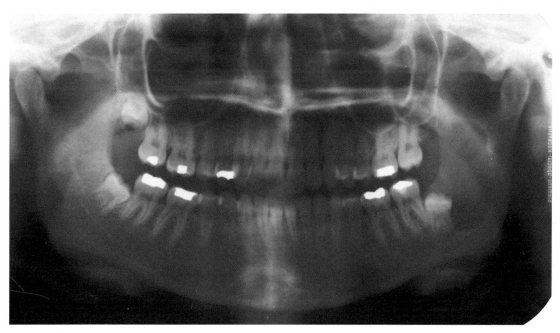

417 Odontogenic keratocyst. DPR.

149

Odontogenic keratocysts may reach a considerable size, particularly in edentulous jaws. The large radiolucent lesion (**419**) in the left body and ascending ramus of the mandible is loculated, with a distinct radio-opaque corticated outline and has caused expansion of the ramus anteriorly. There are several thin, radio-opaque, bony septa within the lesion, particularly inferiorly. Overall the mandible is more radiolucent than normal, with thinning and lack of density of the inferior cortical plates and loss of definition of the inferior alveolar canal, suggesting the presence of osteoporosis. Note that there is apparent asymmetry of the mandible and prominence of the outlines of the tongue, soft palate and epiglottis on the side of the lesion, probably as a consequence of incorrect positioning of the patient during exposure.

Another example (**420**) shows a large, multilocular cyst in the left body and ramus of an edentulous mandible, extending to the midline. At the periphery of the cyst there is thinning of the cortical bone; despite its size there is only slight expansion of the lingual aspect of the mandible. Bony septa divide the lesion into locules, giving an appearance similar to that of ameloblastoma.

When odontogenic keratocysts occur in the maxilla, similar radiological changes are produced although they may not be as clearly displayed. The first example (**421**, **422**) shows a cyst of the left side of the maxilla with a loculated outline partly surrounded by a radio-opaque lamina, extending from the |1 to |6 region to the midline of the palate. There is displacement of the roots |2 and |3 mesially and distally, respectively. The variation in the degree of radiolucency of the lesion indicates a variable amount of thinning and possibly perforation of the cortical plates. The exact outline of the cyst is difficult to determine because of the superimposition of the images of the maxillary antrum, nasal cavity and zygomatic process. There is resorption of the apical part of the root |2 and an absence of lamina dura disto-apically |2 and mesio-apically |3 .

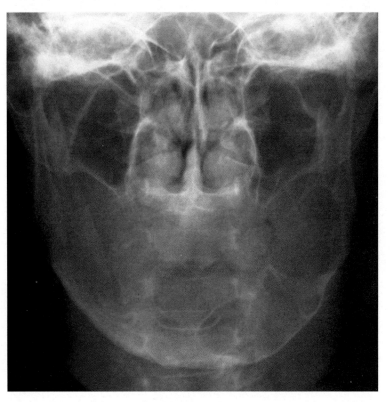

419 Odontogenic keratocyst. DPR.

420 Odontogenic keratocyst. OLM.

Large lesions in the maxilla encroach upon the antrum so that the maxilla may become expanded to a variable degree. The next example (**423**) shows a large lesion of the left side of the maxilla which occupies the majority of the antrum, with displacement of the unerupted ⌊8 superiorly and medially. The full extent of the cyst is difficult to determine as the outline is indistinct, but the antrum is relatively radio-opaque and there is destruction of the lateral wall. The intact roof of the antrum and the infra-orbital foramen (arrow) are clearly visible.

Another example (**424**) in an edentulous maxilla shows a cyst which has expanded the lateral wall (arrows) and the floor of the antrum, forming

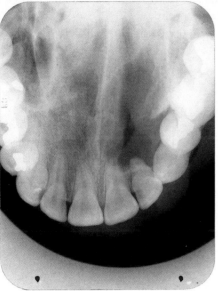

421 Odontogenic keratocyst. USO.

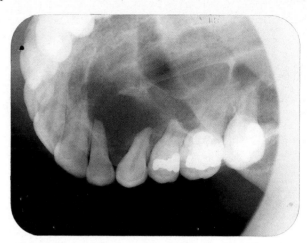

422 Odontogenic keratocyst. UOO.

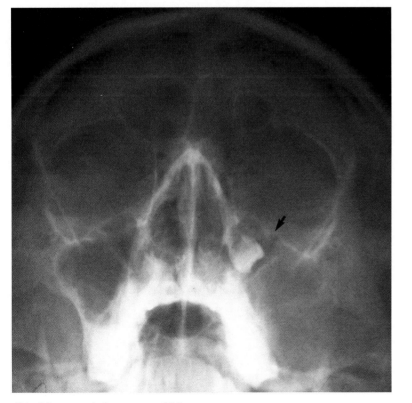

423 Odontogenic keratocyst. OM.

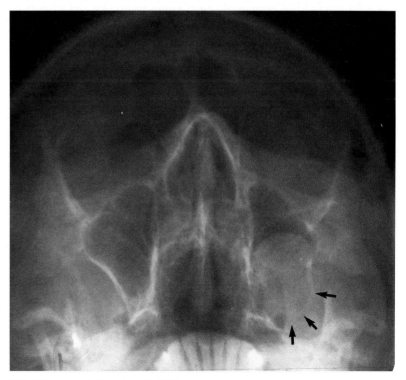

424 Odontogenic keratocyst. OM.

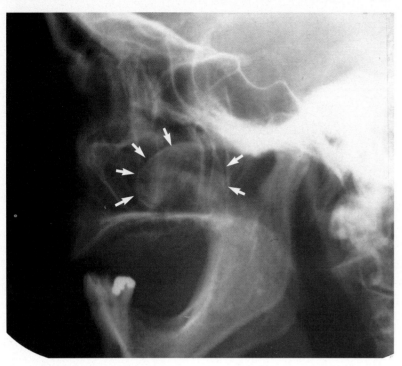

425 **Odontogenic keratocyst. L.**

a relatively radio-opaque, dome-shaped mass. The overall radio-opacity of the lesion (**425**), together with the thin, radio-opaque lamina around the periphery (arrows), indicate that it is surrounded by a thin layer of bone and is thus separate from the antral cavity. Note the vertical, radiolucent, pterygomaxillary fissures at the posterior aspect of the mass, each bounded by thin, radio-opaque laminae. The apparently more anterior fissure is projected from the opposite side of the jaw and is superimposed upon the cyst, the profoundly radiolucent pterygopalatine foramen being at the upper end of the fissure.

Naevoid basal cell carcinoma syndrome (Gorlin and Goltz syndrome)
Patients with naevoid basal cell carcinoma syndrome have odontogenic keratocysts as well as a number of other abnormalities, including multiple basal cell naevi of the skin, bifid ribs, bifid vertebral spines, mineralization of the falx cerebrae and intracranial neoplasms. As the syndrome is inherited as an autosomal dominant with variable expressivity, the range of abnormalities in each patient is varied. The skin naevi usually progress to become basal cell carcinomas. Odontogenic keratocysts are usually multiple, often present at the same time, but sometimes appearing in a chronological sequence. The presence of multiple odontogenic keratocysts may be the first indication that a patient is affected by the syndrome. Example **426** shows cysts in all four quadrants in a young patient with this syndrome. The coincidence of odontogenic keratocysts and unerupted teeth in a young patient may simulate the appearance of dentigerous cysts as in this example.

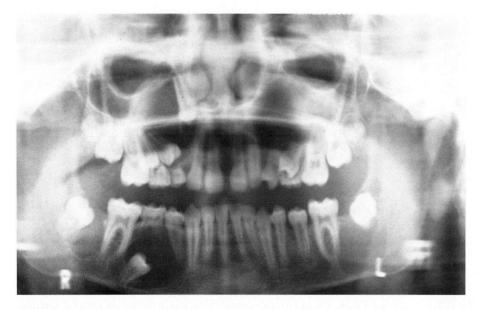

426 **Multiple odontogenic keratocysts in a patient with naevoid basal cell carcinoma syndrome. DPR.**

Dystrophic mineralization of the soft tissues, notably of the falx cerebri (arrow) (**427**) and diaphragmatica sellae are common in this syndrome. In this illustration there is also a generalized opacity of the right antrum due to the presence of a cyst.

The next example (**428**) shows a postoperative radiograph taken after the removal of multiple odontogenic keratocysts. The cysts in the mandible have been packed with ribbon gauze incorporating a radio-opaque marker. The cyst in the upper right maxilla has been enucleated but not packed. Note the segmentally mineralized, stylohyoid ligaments which are present bilaterally. Odontogenic keratocysts tend to recur so long-term postoperative radiographic review is particularly important.

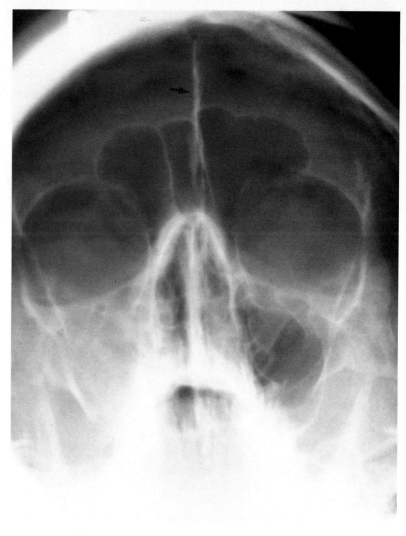

427 Naevoid basal cell carcinoma syndrome. OM.

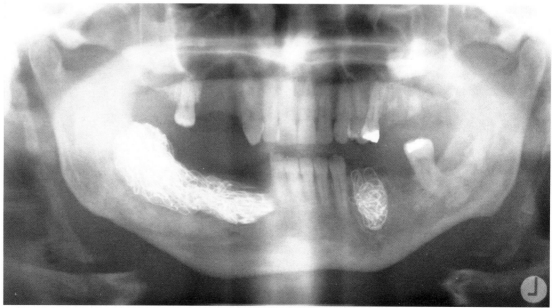

428 Odontogenic keratocysts in a patient with naevoid basal cell carcinoma syndrome (treated by enucleation and packing). DPR.

Glandular odontogenic cyst (sialo-odontogenic cyst) This rare condition, of unknown origin, occurs most commonly in the anterior region of the mandible and is typically multilocular. The radiographic appearance is similar to that of several other odontogenic lesions, in particular the odontogenic keratocyst and ameloblastoma. In the example (429) there is a loculated, radiolucent lesion extending from the midline to $\overline{5|}$ with thinning of the lower border of the mandible. The lesion is well defined, contains some incomplete bony septa and reaches into the interdental bone between $\overline{|345}$.

Another example (430) shows a larger, loculated radiolucent lesion in the anterior region of the mandible, extending from $\overline{6|}$ to $\overline{|6}$. It is surrounded by a thin, radio-opaque lamina of bone and has a clearly defined, scalloped boundary overlying the apices of the related teeth superiorly and encroaching upon the cortical bone of the mandible inferiorly. There is resorption of the apices of many of the adjacent teeth. The darker, clearly defined area beneath $\overline{|456}$ indicates an area of perforation of the cortical bone. The mental foramen on the left is visible beneath this area and on the right side the distal part of the inferior alveolar canal approaching the mental foramen

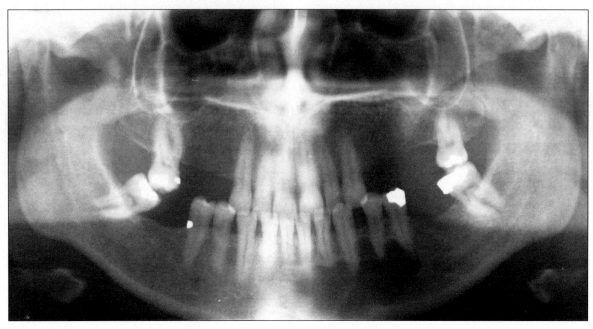

429 Glandular odontogenic cyst. DPR.

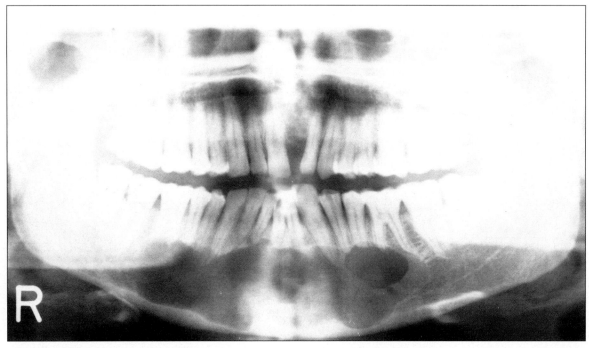

430 Glandular odontogenic cyst. DPR.

is also clearly seen. The lesion was excised and a thin section of the inferior cortical plate of the mandible was preserved (**431**). The defect was reconstructed with a rib graft, secured by titanium miniplates.

Hamartomatous lesions

Hamartomatous lesions are abnormalities of development which result in tumours appearing during the period of normal growth and development. They are composed of tissues which are normally present at the site in which they form and tend to become inactive when general body growth ceases. A number of different lesions may occur in the jaws including odontogenic tumours (ameloblastic fibro-odontome; ameloblastic fibrodentinoma; odonto-ameloblastoma), neuro-ectodermal-derived tumours (neuro-ectodermal tumour of infancy), vascular tumours (haemangioma) and bone tumours (fibrous dysplasia; cherubism).

AMELOBLASTIC FIBRO-ODONTOME

In its early stages prior to deposition of mineralized tissue, this lesion is predominantly radiolucent, but as increasing numbers of centres of odontogenesis arise, more and more radio-opacities develop within it. In the example (**432**) of a lesion at an intermediate stage of development in a 16-year-old, there is a well-defined, ovoid radiolucency in the alveolar part of the $\overline{678|}$ region which is expanded occlusally. Around its periphery there is a thin, radio-opaque lamina posteriorly; the anterior margin is superimposed upon $\overline{6|}$ roots and is not well demonstrated. The lesion contains numerous, irregular radio-opacities randomly scattered throughout the mass, some of them, particularly superiorly, being larger than the others and having the appearance of denticles. $\overline{7|}$ is displaced towards the inferior border of the mandible and its roots are curved distally but not yet completely formed. A radiolucent follicular space surrounded by a thin, radio-opaque lamina, is still visible around the crown mesially and occlusally. $\overline{8|}$ is absent, and the unopposed $\underline{|7}$ has overerupted.

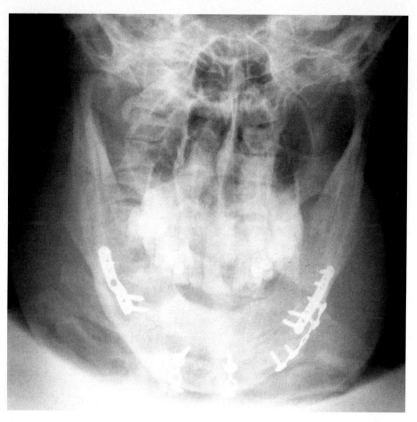

431 Glandular odontogenic cyst following resection and reconstruction. PA.

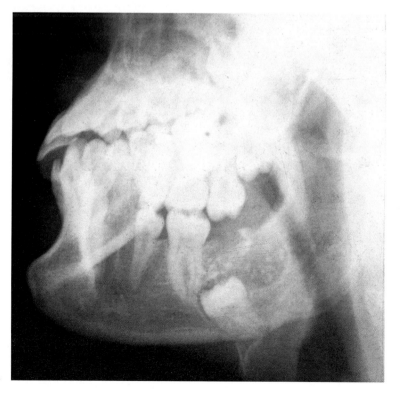

432 Ameloblastic fibro-odontome. OLM.

Another example (**433**) arising in the right side of the maxilla of an eight-year-old, consists of a mass which contains numerous small, rounded, radio-opaque structures which resemble denticles. The lesion projects into the antrum and the antral floor is raised. It has a clearly defined margin and around the anterosuperior aspect there is a thin, radio-opaque lamina of cortical bone and a radiolucent capsular space. E|, 654| and 7| are unerupted and have been displaced by the mass, E| lying over its centre, 6| posteriorly, 7| inferiorly and 54| mesially.

ODONTO-AMELOBLASTOMA

These tumours with the combined histological features of an ameloblastoma and a composite odontome usually occur in the first two decades of life. There is uncertainty as to whether they are a distinct form of odontogenic tumour, or represent a developing stage of an odontome when there is still much of the odontogenic soft tissue present, although the recent WHO classification regards them as neoplasms. In **434** the lesion occupies the lower part of the left ramus of the mandible and forms a well-defined, approximately circular mass which is radiolucent peripherally and radio-opaque centrally. The radio-opacity is mottled in some areas and in others it is arranged in a radial pattern. The developing |8 is displaced inferiorly and the thin cortical lamina outlining the lesion is continuous with the lamina around the tooth. The bone at the lower end of the anterior margin of the ramus of the mandible is expanded.

NEURO-ECTODERMAL TUMOUR OF INFANCY (PROGONOMA)

This lesion which originates from neuroectodermal elements arises in the anterior part of the maxilla of young infants, producing an expansile, soft tissue mass. In the example (**435**), in a two-month-old infant, an approximately circular radiolucent mass occupies the incisor region causing displacement of A| labially and B| distally. The labial alveolus is expanded and eroded, leaving only a small, thin remnant of radio-opaque cortical plate. The deep margin of the tumour can just be determined and the soft tissue outline of the lip is displaced anteriorly.

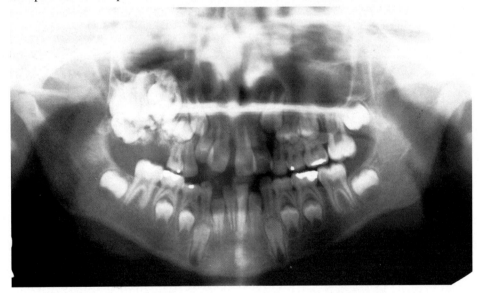

433 Ameloblastic fibro-odontome. DPR.

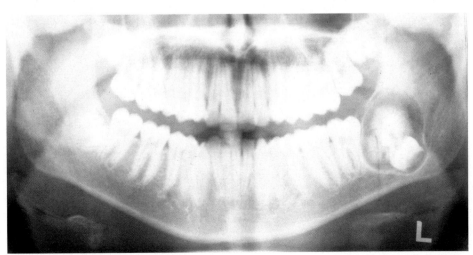

434 Odonto-ameloblastoma. DPR.

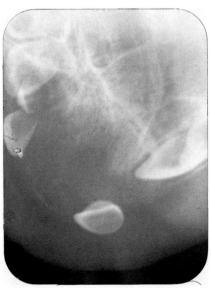

435 Neuro-ectodermal tumour of infancy. P.

HAEMANGIOMA

Haemangiomas are composed of masses of blood vessels, either capillaries, or larger cavernous vessels, most frequently lying in the skin. Sometimes they arise in deeper tissues, including bone, where they may or may not be associated with a more obvious superficial lesion. When bone is involved, the condition is usually apparent on radiographs as a radiolucent area, but may be poorly defined. Some lesions cause an enlargement of the intertrabecular spaces whereas others have a multicystic or soap bubble form. Most haemangiomas are hamartomas and are usually diagnosed in the first two decades of life. In the example (436) of a cavernous haemangioma arising centrally in the mandible, there are several radiolucent defects, noticeably in the regions of the third molar, ramus and mental foramen, although most of the bone shows abnormal structure. Generally, the trabecular pattern has an indistinct appearance and throughout the bone there are randomly arranged, pinhead sized radiolucencies probably arising from vessels lying within the bone in the direction of the X-ray beam. There are also several, irregular, longitudinal, radiolucent channels running between the two main parts of the lesion. Note the recent extraction socket ⌐6 which was the site of profuse haemorrhage. The nature of the lesion was confirmed by carotid angiography (437). The radio-opaque contrast medium defines the lesion in the molar/ramus region, although the more anterior part has not yet filled.

FIBROUS DYSPLASIA

This hamartomatous lesion of bone is characterized by an overgrowth of cellular fibrous tissue which becomes progressively replaced by bony trabeculae and can occur in any part of the skeleton. There is painless enlargement of the affected bone which may reach a considerable size. The condition usually affects only one bone (monostotic), but several bones (polyostotic) may be involved. When the jaws are involved, the maxilla is more commonly affected. Although usually diagnosed in the first two decades of life, the condition may remain silent in its early stages and not be diagnosed until later. The radiographic appearance depends upon the degree of maturation of the lesion. Immature lesions are generally radiolucent due to a preponderance of fibrous tissue to bone. With maturation, more bone is laid down and the tissue becomes increasingly radio-opaque, although the radio-opaque areas may initially be randomly arranged. Fibrous dysplasia is usually poorly demarcated from the surrounding bone.

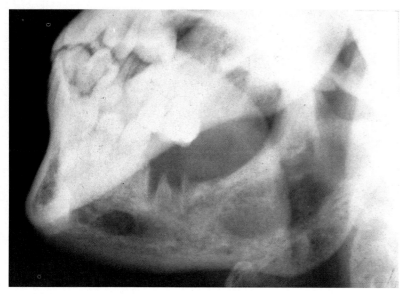

436 Haemangioma. OLM.

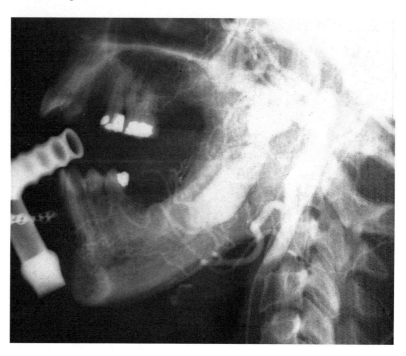

437 Haemangioma. L.

The example (**438**, **439**, **440**), in the mandible of an 18-year-old shows a monostotic lesion that is variably radiolucent and radio-opaque, the radio-opacities being randomly scattered throughout and irregularly shaped. The mass which had been present for at least eight years has prevented the eruption of $\overline{54|}$ which are displaced, their crowns being surrounded by normal radiolucent follicular spaces. The overlying alveolar ridge is expanded but the cortex remains intact. The inferior part of the lesion is more radiolucent with an irregularly-loculated appearance (**439**). There is expansion of the buccal cortical plate (**440**) which is also intact. Much of the margin of the lesion is poorly defined and irregularly shaped and blends imperceptibly with the adjacent normal bone. Note the retained roots $\overline{6|}$ and the small, periapical radiolucency beneath the mesial root.

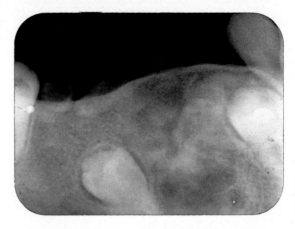

438 Fibrous dysplasia. P.

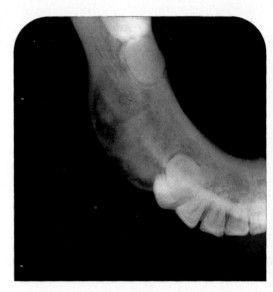

440 Fibrous dysplasia. LTO.

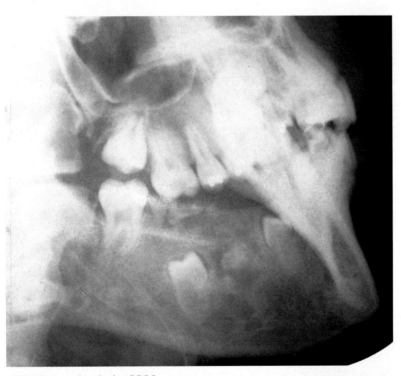

439 Fibrous dysplasia. OLM.

In the next example (**441**) of a mature lesion in the maxilla in an adult there is a granular radio-opacity above the teeth in the $\underline{|3-8}$ region. The mass has raised the antral floor, which remains intact, and has obscured the apices of the teeth. There is no distinct margin between the lesion and the adjacent normal bone. The interdental bone between the molar and the premolar teeth is less severely affected but the tuberosity and the alveolar bone anterior to $\underline{|3}$ appear normal.

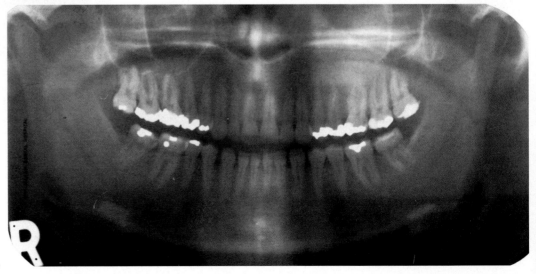

441 Fibrous dysplasia. DPR.

Another example (**442**) of a lesion in the maxilla of a 19-year-old shows how the normal trabecular pattern of the alveolar bone has been replaced by a diffuse radio-opacity of uniformly stippled appearance. The alveolar bone is expanded and |5 is displaced distally. The normal anatomical features of the region have been partly obscured and both the lamina dura around the roots |45 7 and the boundaries of the maxillary antrum are indistinct.

The mature lesion becomes uniformly radio-opaque throughout and displays the typical 'orange peel' appearance. In the example (**443**) in the edentulous maxilla of an adult, there is also marked expansion of the alveolar ridge as demonstrated by the increased distance between the floor of the antrum and the bone surface.

FAMILIAL FIBROUS DYSPLASIA (CHERUBISM)

This rare, inherited condition affects the jaws in early childhood and results in their expansion by a mass of fibrocellular tissue in which relatively little bone formation occurs. It very often involves all four quadrants of the jaws which exhibit a multicystic pattern of radiolucency with varying numbers of radio-opaque septae running between the locules. Bilateral expansion of the maxilla tends to displace the lower eyelids inferiorly, so revealing more sclera beneath each cornea and giving the eyes an apparent upward looking gaze. The overall result is the classic cherubic appearance. In the example (**444**), only the mandible is affected and there are bilateral lesions in the rami and posterior part of the body. They appear as 'soap bubble' radiolucencies and have caused displacement of the second and third molar teeth, and expansion and thinning of the cortical bone of the anterior aspect and of the inferior border of the rami.

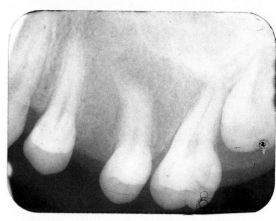

442 Fibrous dysplasia. P.

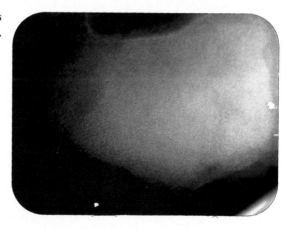

443 Fibrous dysplasia. P.

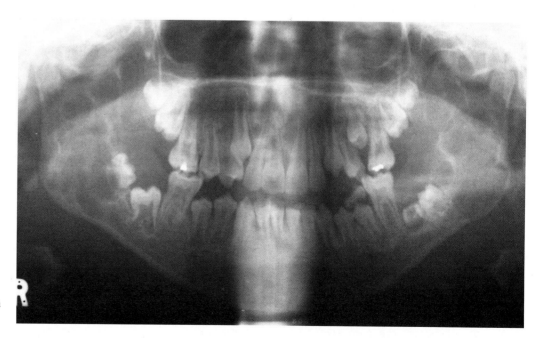

444 Familial fibrous dysplasia (cherubism). DPR.

Stafne's bone cavity

This developmental defect of the mandible is believed to arise from the inclusion of aberrant submandibular salivary gland tissue; it typically occurs beneath the inferior alveolar canal, at the base of the ramus. It is uncommon and appears as a well-defined, circular radiolucency (**445**) surrounded by a thin, radio-opaque lamina of cortical bone. Although this abnormality is usually discovered as an incidental finding, it may reach a considerable size (**446**), but seldom exceeds 3 cm in diameter.

While the radiographic appearance of the lesion is usually characteristic, sialography may help in confirming the diagnosis. In **447**, a lateral branch of the main submandibular duct can be seen overlying, and possibly entering, the radiolucent defect. A further radiograph taken at right angles to this view would be helpful to confirm the exact relationship. These defects are believed to be soft tissue invaginations into the lingual aspect of the mandible, as is well illustrated in the next example (**448**). The defect on the left side is occupied partly by glandular tissue and partly by tissue of low attenuation, e.g. fat.

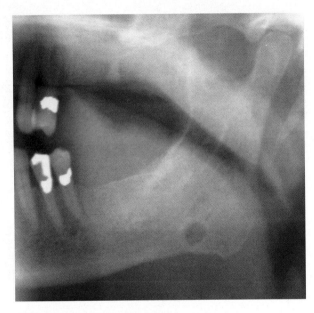

445 Stafne's bone cavity. DPR.

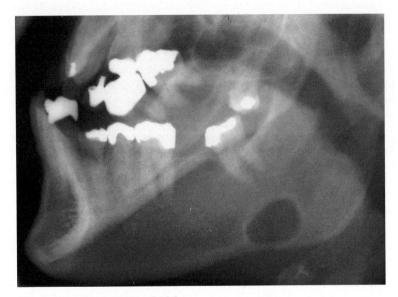

446 Stafne's bone cavity. OLM.

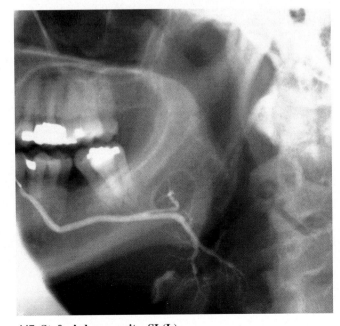

447 Stafne's bone cavity. SL(L).

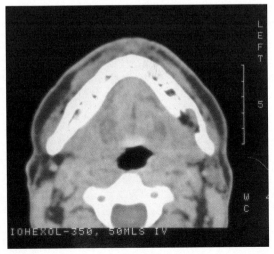

448 Stafne's bone cavity. CT.

Infantile cortical hyperostosis (Caffey–Silverman syndrome)

Symmetrical, bilateral enlargement of the mandible by cortical thickening, especially of the lower border, is the classical feature of this disorder, although other bones may also be involved. The extent of the changes may vary on the two sides. The condition, which is often associated with a fever, usually arises during the first three months of life, as in the two-month-old child (**449**) in whom there has been considerable formation of additional periosteal bone, particularly along the inferior border of the mandible. A faint 'onion skin' layering of the bone can be discerned, presumably as a consequence of successive increments of bone deposition. As the child develops, the excess bone usually undergoes resolution.

Microbial conditions and their sequelae

The presence of teeth provides a potential pathway for micro-organisms and/or their products to spread into the underlying bone. Such lesions are usually clearly associated with the teeth and most of them have been fully described in Chapters 4 and 5. Although inflammatory lesions of the jaws are most commonly a consequence of dental infection, they may more rarely be the result of specific infections such as tuberculosis and syphilis. These may effect the bone surface alone, as in a periostitis where reactive bone is formed subperiosteally, or spread through the marrow spaces, as in osteomyelitis. Radiographic changes are not usually apparent before ten

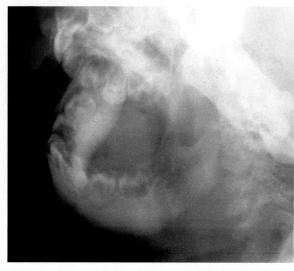

449 Infantile cortical hyperostosis (Caffey–Silverman syndrome). OLM.

days, but subsequently provide a good indication of the extent of such lesions and may show the presence of localized areas of separated necrotic bone or sequestrae. Bone necrosis may also occur in other situations, e.g. following radiation or exposure to phosphorus.

Residual cyst

Residual cysts are radicular cysts that persist in the jaws after the extraction of the causative tooth. They are often symptomless and may be diagnosed as an incidental radiographic finding. They sometimes continue to enlarge, but usually undergo regression. The example (**450**) in the 54| region shows a small, circular, clearly defined, radiolucent cyst, which is surrounded by a thin, radio-opaque lamina. The remnants of the 54| sockets are present and the alveolar bone is expanded and markedly thinned.

The next example (**451, 452**) in the right side of an edentulous maxilla shows a clearly defined, circular radiolucency which is surrounded – except on the alveolar surface – by a thin, radio-opaque lamina. There are several, small, irregular, radio-opaque areas in the alveolar aspect of the lesion, indicating deposits of dystrophic mineralization. As residual cysts age, such deposits become increasingly common. The image of the root of the zygomatic arch is superimposed upon the cyst in both radiographs. Note the incisive fossa (arrow).

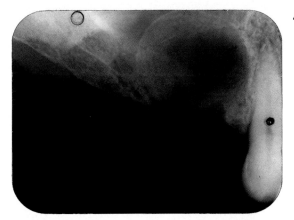

450 Residual cyst. P.

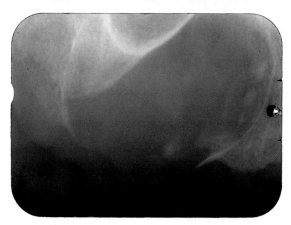

451 Residual cyst. P.

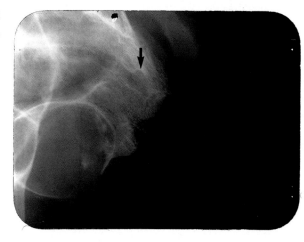

452 Residual cyst. UOO.

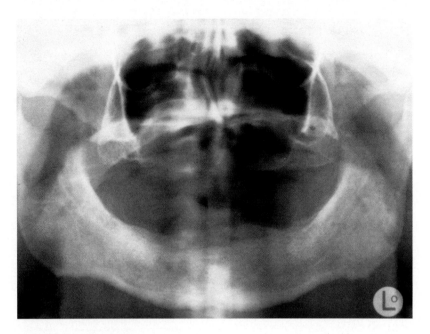

A further example (**453**) shows a well-circumscribed radiolucency in the anterior part of the right side of an edentulous maxilla, occupying the alveolar part of the bone and expanding into the antral cavity and the floor of the nose. It is bounded by a thin, radio-opaque cortical lamina around most of the periphery. There is deviation of the nasal septum, although it is not possible to determine from this radiograph if this is a consequence of the cyst growth. Involvement of the antral and nasal cavities is confirmed on the coronal (**454**) and axial (**455**) CTs, together with the extent of the anterolateral expansion of the maxilla. In a lower tomographic slice, the extent of the destruction of the alveolar part of the maxilla is also clearly seen (**456**).

453 Residual cyst. OPG.

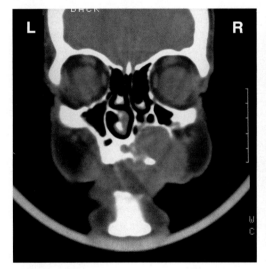

454 Residual cyst. CT.

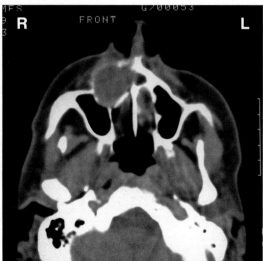

455 Residual cyst. CT.

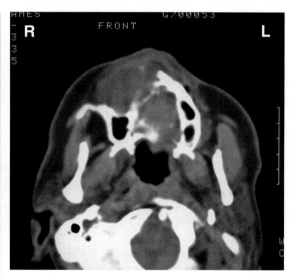

456 Residual cyst. CT.

A bone window setting on a CT will usually demonstrate the extent of the resorption of bone more clearly, as in **457**, where the thin, bony plate still separating the cyst from the antral and nasal cavities is more accurately displayed (arrows).

A further example (**458**) of a residual cyst in the $\overline{8-6|}$ region of an edentulous mandible shows thinning of the cortical bone at the inferior border. The approximately circular radiolucency is surrounded by a thin, clearly defined, radio-opaque lamina and contains an ovoid, more radiolucent area centrally, indicating thinning of the lingual or buccal cortical plates.

Healing cyst

Following removal of cysts from the jaws, the bone cavity normally becomes slowly filled with new bone centripetally. There is loss of the cortical outline and a gradual reduction of the radiolucent defect. The next three radiographs (**459**, **460**, **461**) illustrate the sequence of events following enucleation of a residual cyst in the $|2\,$ region with primary closure of the wound. One week postoperatively (**459**), the residual radiolucent bony defect has a poorly defined outline, and although the lamina dura around the roots of $|1-3\,$ is indistinct apically, the teeth remained vital. Four months postoperatively (**460**), the lamina dura and the periodontal ligament space $|1-3\,$ are present and much of the cavity has been filled from the periphery by fine trabeculations arranged radially, particularly in the nasal aspect of the defect. After twelve months (**461**) the defect is filled completely, although there is still some radial arrangement of the trabeculae.

457 Residual cyst. CT.

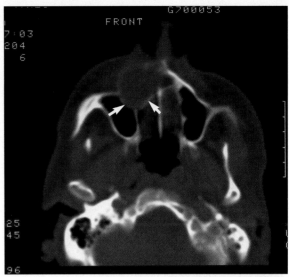

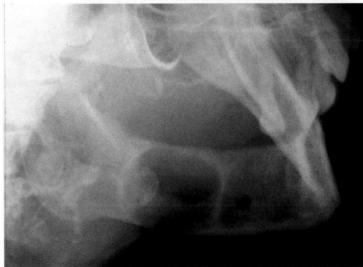

458 Residual cyst. OLM.

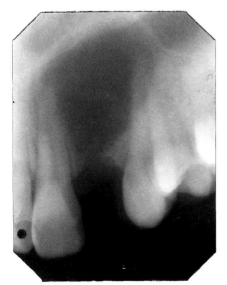

459 Healing bone cavity following cyst enucleation. P.

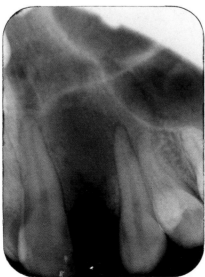

460 Healing bone cavity following cyst enucleation. P.

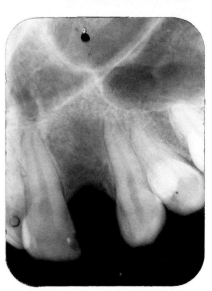

461 Healing bone cavity following cyst enucleation. P.

Sometimes the bony defect is not completely filled by bone and a scar of fibrous tissue persists, forming a persistent area of radiolucency smaller than the original defect. In **462, 21⌋** had been treated some two years previously by apicectomy. The persisting radiolucent defect is punched out and irregularly shaped, typical of a fibrous scar. These sometimes arise from failure of the cortical plates to be completely repaired, usually on the palatal side, resulting in an area of more intense radiolucency.

Twelve months after the treatment of a large cyst of the right body and ramus of the mandible by enucleation and primary closure (**463**), there are radially arranged trabeculae of reparative bone around the periphery of the defect, the outline of which can still be determined. A keyhole-shaped area of radiolucency remains where bony repair is not complete. At this stage of healing, substantially more trabeculae than are necessary for normal function have been deposited, so the tissue is relatively radio-opaque.

Another example (**464**) shows a residual cyst in the right body of the mandible eighteen months after treatment by enucleation and primary closure.

The outline of the original bony defect is indistinct, especially anteriorly. The defect is now completely filled with bone which, at its centre in the more recently healed part of the lesion, is more radio-opaque with a radial arrangement of the trabeculae. Peripherally, the process of bone remodelling is further advanced and a more normal trabecular pattern is present. The inferior alveolar canal has been displaced inferiorly by the original lesion.

Periostitis

Infection of the jaws may be accompanied by reactive changes in the adjacent periosteum, particularly in young individuals, when the osteogenic potential is at its greatest. In the mandible, this is often best displayed on occlusal radiographs, as in **465**, where a localized deposition of reactive bone is present buccally in the premolar/molar region. Several lamellae of new bone have been formed, giving an 'onion skin' appearance.

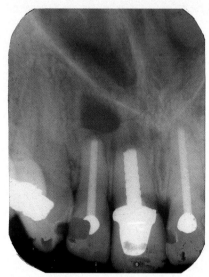

462 Periapical scar. P.

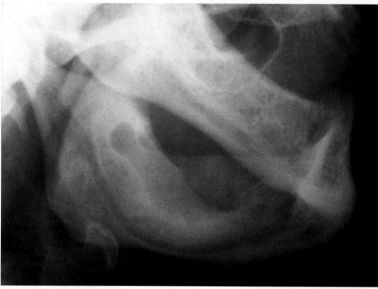

463 Healing bone cavity following cyst enucleation. OLM.

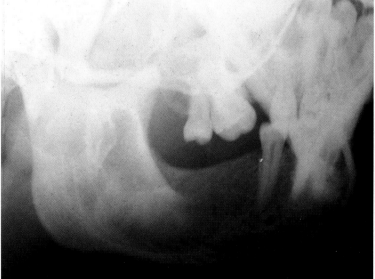

464 (left) Healing bone cavity following cyst enucleation. OLM.

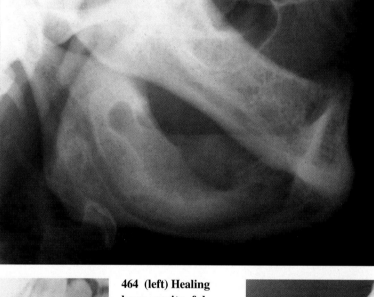

465 Periostitis. LTO.

Osteomyelitis

Osteomyelitis of the jaws is more common in the mandible than the maxilla and usually follows an episode where a portal of entry for micro-organisms has been provided, such as a local apical infection, tooth extraction, bone fracture or insertion of a bone plate. As with all inflammatory lesions arising *de novo* within bone, radiological changes are uncommon before ten to fourteen days and they are therefore usually entering a chronic phase before such sequelae are apparent.

In the lesion of the left side of the mandible twelve days after the extraction $\overline{6|}$ (466), there is a poorly-defined, indistinct, radiolucent defect with an irregular outline in the $\overline{2-8|}$ region, within which the margins of the inferior alveolar canal are indistinct. As the infection develops, local-ized areas of bone undergo necrosis (sequestra), producing apparent radio-opacities within a surrounding osteolytic zone. Several radio-opacities are present, together with a clearly-defined, elongated sequestrum at the inferior border of the mandible in the $\overline{345|}$ region. The radiolucent image of the $\overline{6|}$ socket is already indistinct, suggesting a more rapid process of bone resorption than would normally be expected. After four weeks of treatment (467), the condition is resolving and the trabecular bone pattern has become more distinct, but several clearly-defined, radiolucent defects are still present in the body of the mandible in the $\overline{456|}$ and $\overline{7|}$ regions. Distinct radio-opaque sequestra are present in the former site and disto-apically $\overline{5|}$. The sequestrum previously identified at the inferior border of the mandible has undergone rarefaction and there is evidence of periosteal new bone formation.

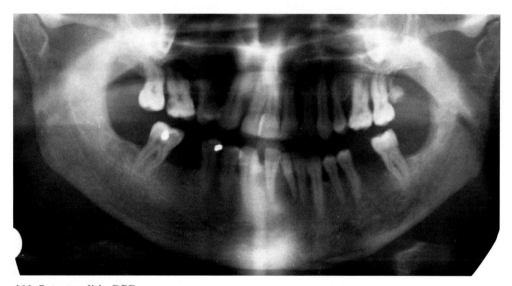

466 Osteomyelitis. DPR

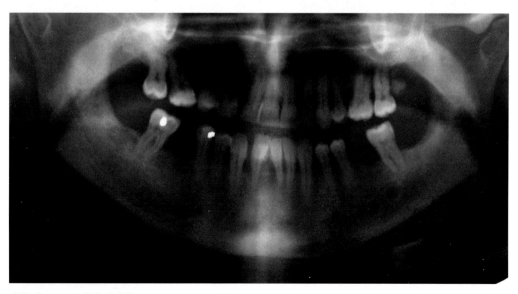

467 Osteomyelitis. DPR

A more chronic lesion is shown in the left side of the mandible (**468**) arising from a focus of infection associated with a root-filled |5̄ . Overall there is a sclerotic change extending from the mental foramen to the ascending ramus, containing areas of irregular radiolucency, which has resulted in a less clear definition of the trabecular pattern and the inferior alveolar canal. There is also some resorption of the bone of the inferior border of the left side of the mandible accompanied by a reactive periostitis, with formation of new periosteal bone (arrows).

Another example (**469**) is shown in a patient who developed a peri-apical abscess 5̄| on which an apical radiolucency is present. The tooth was extracted but five weeks later (**470**) there was a poorly defined radiolucency extending from 6̄–2̄| involving the full thickness of the mandible, with a pathological fracture in the premolar region (arrow). There are several irregularly shaped, radio-opaque sequestra in this area, the largest lying in the inferior part of the mandible.

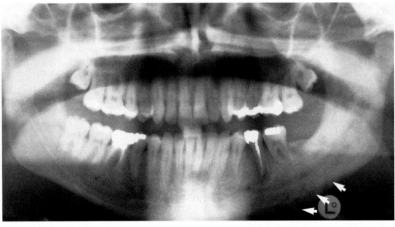

468 Osteomyelitis. DPR.

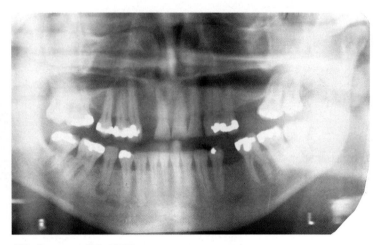

469 Osteomyelitis. DPR.

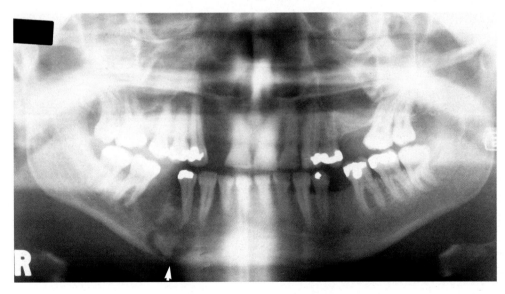

470 Osteomyelitis. DPR.

Example **471** shows a long-standing lesion in an edentulous mandible with a clearly defined, scalloped, radiolucent defect in the molar region, within which lie several irregularly shaped, radio-opaque sequestra. The slightly increased radio-opacity of the surrounding bone indicates the presence of reactive osteosclerotic bone. Although the condition appeared to involve the inferior alveolar canal, there was no disturbance of neural function.

Osteomyelitis occasionally occurs in the maxilla and in the small lesion localized to the alveolar part of the ⌊56 region (**472**); a diffuse, poorly defined area of radiolucency is present around the apices of the teeth and involves the interdental septa. There is loss of the lamina dura, and small radio-opaque sequestra are present interdentally ⌊45 and in the main part of the lesion. There is loss of bone mesially in the trifurcation ⌊6 and the thin, radio-opaque lamina, which outlines the floor of the antrum and dips down posteriorly overlying the apical half of the roots ⌊6, is less distinct than normal. The apical part of ⌊5 is irregular, indicating the presence of root resorption.

The next example (**473**) is a chronic case involving the premolar region of an edentulous maxilla, with a sequestrum that is clearly separated from the remaining bone. The sequestrum, which lies in a deep radiolucent defect in the alveolus, has the trabecular pattern of bone. Adjacent to the sequestrum, the bone is slightly more radio-opaque due to reactive osteosclerosis and there is a small tooth fragment anterosuperiorly (arrow).

Phosphorus necrosis

Although rare today, exposure to phosphorus may result in necrosis of the jaws, which can be persistent and progressive. Such lesions usually become secondarily infected.

In the example (**474**) in the incisor region of the mandible, a radiolucent area is present, which contains a clearly demarcated, radio-opaque sequestrum of bone. The sequestrum was removed, but six months later (**475**) the condition was still present, with evidence of further sequestration as demonstrated by the more indistinct outline containing numerous small radio-opacities.

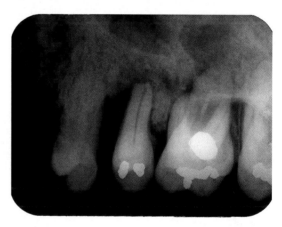

472 Osteomyelitis. P.

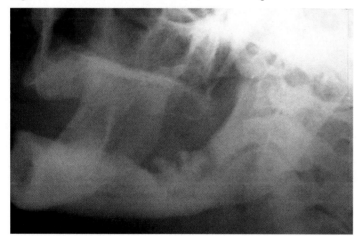

471 Osteomyelitis. OLM.

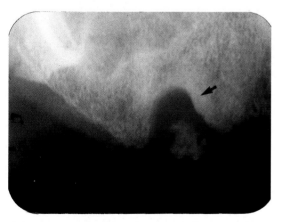

473 Osteomyelitis. P.

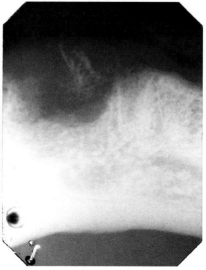

474 Phosphorus necrosis. P.

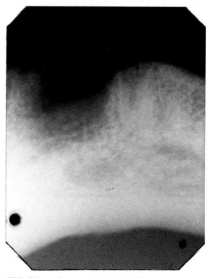

475 Phosphorus necrosis. P.

Traumatic conditions and their sequelae

A radiographic assessment is commonly required following maxillofacial trauma, particularly when bone fractures are suspected. Apart from confirming the presence of fractures, radiographs reveal the extent of the injury and the degree of displacement of the bone fragments. This may require a number of radiographic projections, often at right angles to each other. In addition to bone fractures, there may be damage to teeth (Chapter 4) or foreign material embedded in the soft tissues (Chapter 10).

Fractures of the mandible may be complete or incomplete, simple, compound or comminuted. They tend to occur at sites of potential weakness such as the neck of the condyle, the symphysis and the angle of the mandible. The presence of an unerupted lower third molar makes the latter site even more vulnerable. Displacement of bone fragments may be the direct result of trauma or a consequence of traction from the attached musculature. Hence some fractures, such as those at the angle of the mandible, are often termed favourable or unfavourable depending upon the direction of the fracture line and the distracting force of the muscles.

The zygomatic bone forms the prominence of the cheek and is therefore prone to trauma and fractures. The bone may be likened to a three-legged stool with the legs articulating at the temporal, frontal and maxillary bones respectively. Trauma may result in displacement at any one or all of these sutures, with rotation of the zygoma as a whole and consequent facial deformity. However, compared with the mandible, the zygoma is less robust and fractures are often comminuted. Occipitomental radiographs show this part of the facial skeleton well, with the SMV view being particularly useful for demonstrating zygomatic arch fractures.

Fractures of the middle third of the facial skeleton are of three basic types as described originally by Le Fort. The Le Fort I, II and III classification refers to the level and complexity of the injury (476, 477). However, in many instances, the situation may be one of a complex combination of fractures that is not always fully demonstrated on standard radiographs. In such cases, a combination of radiographic and CT scanning techniques provides a fuller assessment.

Fractures of the orbit may be confined to the orbital margin or may involve the complex of bones that form the orbital cavity. The floor and medial wall consist of relatively thin bone and the former may be fractured and displaced into the antrum following trauma to the globe of the eye. Such 'blow-out' fractures may be visible on occipitomental radiographs but are often better demonstrated by CT.

In common with other fractures, those of the facial bones are treated by reduction, apposition and fixation. The latter may be achieved by direct or indirect means.

476 (left) An anterior view of a dry skull showing the site of fractures of the middle part of the facial skeleton according to Le Fort. Type I: green. Type II: blue. Type III: red.

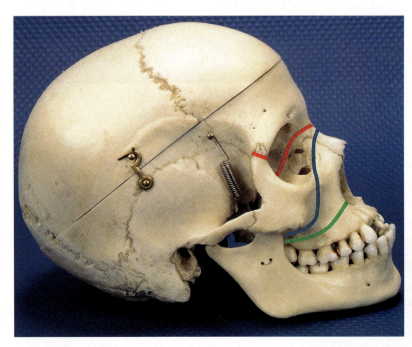

477 (above) A lateral view of a dry skull showing the site of fractures of the middle part of the facial skeleton according to LeFort. Type I: green. Type II: blue. Type III: red.

Fractures

MANDIBLE

Dento-alveolar fractures are confined to the tooth-bearing part of the jaws. They occur more commonly in the anterior part of the mouth and the fractured segment(s) often contains one or more teeth.

The first example (**478**) shows a comminuted dento-alveolar fracture of the left mandibular premolar and canine region. One radiolucent fracture line extends antero-inferiorly from the crest of the alveolus mesially $\overline{6}$ across the middle part of the roots $\overline{45}$. A second fracture runs more steeply in a similar direction, from the alveolar crest overlying $\overline{5}$ to cross the apices of the roots $\overline{34}$. The root of $\overline{5}$ is fractured with displacement of the crown and there is widening of the periodontal ligament space apically $\overline{34}$. The tooth-bearing fragment of the alveolus is minimally displaced.

A second example (**479**) shows a more unusual fracture in which the anterior lingual bony plate of the mandible has been separated and displaced posteriorly by contraction of the attached muscles. $\overline{21|12}$ have been avulsed and the trabeculations of the cancellous bone of the mandible are clearly visible. The scalloped outline of the alveolar crests is displayed on the displaced fragment together with the genial tubercles on its upper margin.

The next example (**480**) shows spontaneous fracture of the genial tubercles with displacement of the fragment posteriorly (arrow) due to muscle contraction.

Periapical radiographs may unexpectedly reveal a fracture when taken for the investigation of a patient complaining of a loosened and/or painful tooth. In **481** the radiolucent fracture line extends inferiorly from the base of $\overline{5|}$ socket and the tooth has been displaced occlusally with widening of the periodontal ligament space. Note the area of osteosclerosis associated with the apical part of the mesial root $\overline{6|}$. Further radiographs would be required to determine the full extent of the fracture.

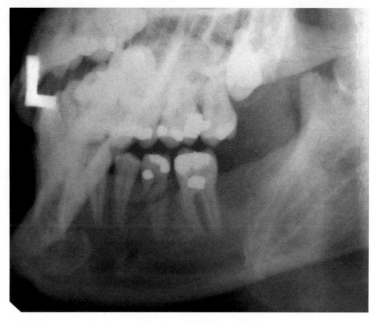

478 Dento-alveolar fracture of the mandible. OLM.

479 Cortical plate fracture of the mandible. LTO.

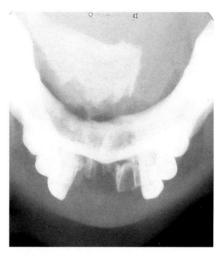

481 Fracture of the mandible. P.

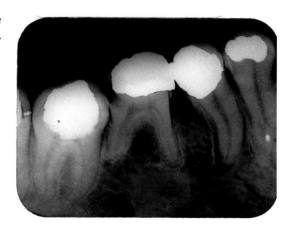

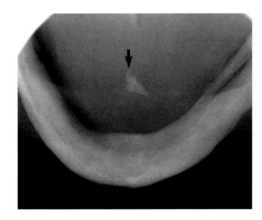

480 Fracture of the genial tubercles. LTO.

In the next example (**482**), there are bilateral fractures of the mandible with minimal displacement of the fragments. The fracture on the left passes obliquely backwards and downwards from the follicular space distal to the impacted 8̅ and that in the right canine region passes downwards through the interdental septum mesially and runs obliquely posteriorly to the inferior border of the mandible in the premolar region. The apex 3̅| has been separated from the tooth by the fracture.

Another example (**483**) of a bilateral fracture is shown in the right body of the mandible involving the mesial root 7̅| and in the left anterior region passing through the socket |3̅ . There is a step deformity in the occlusion on the left, due to the upward displacement of the posterior segment and also to a lesser extent on the right. The displacement of the segment on the left is confirmed by disruption of the normal contour of the inferior border of the mandible.

Illustrations **484** and **485** show a unilateral oblique fracture of the left body of the mandible running through the distal aspect of the |8̅ socket to

482 Fractures of the mandible. DPR.

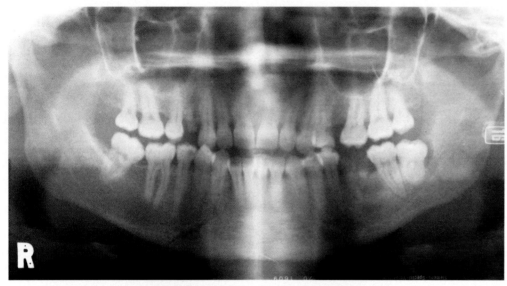

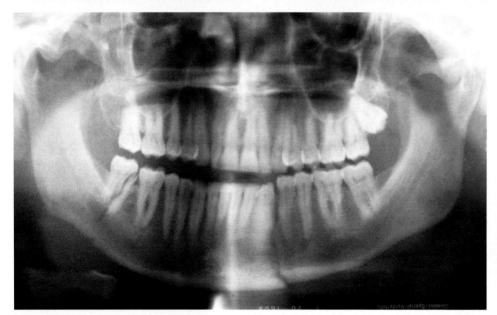

483 Fractures of the mandible. DPR.

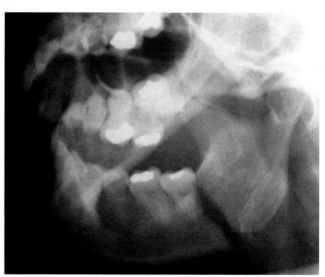

484 Fracture of the mandible. OLM.

the inferior border close to the angle. The posterior fragment has been displaced upwards and inwards (**485**) by contraction of the attached muscles as a consequence of the unfavourable plane of the fracture. The extent of the displacement can be assessed from the disparity in the levels of the inferior border and the inferior alveolar canal in the two fragments (**484**).

Direct violence to the facial bones sometimes results in comminuted fractures as in the lesion in the right side of the mandible (**486**). The posterior fragment has been displaced upwards, resulting in a step deformity

of the inferior border of the mandible. Oblique fractures running through the inner and outer cortical plates often give the appearance of a double fracture. Such an appearance is shown clearly in this example, together with duplication of the image of the mental foramen.

Direct trauma to the point of the chin may result in fractures not only of the anterior part of the mandible but also of one or both condyles. In **487**, $\overline{2|}$ has been avulsed and a fracture line runs through the wall of the socket towards the inferior border of the mandible. There is separation of

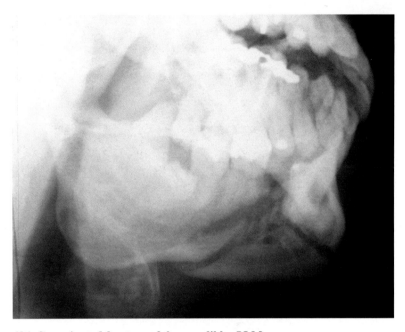

486 Comminuted fracture of the mandible. OLM.

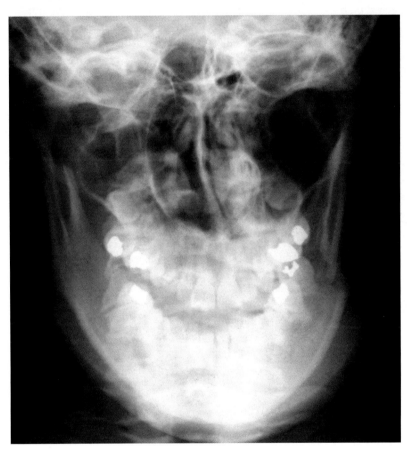

485 Fracture of the mandible. PA.

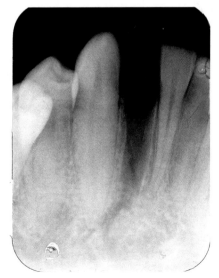

487 Fracture of the mandible. P.

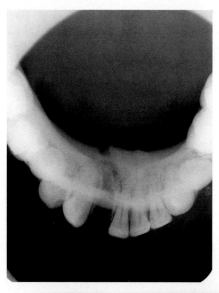

488 Fracture of the mandible. LTO.

the bone fragments, which is particularly well shown on the occlusal radiograph (**488**); both condyles (**489**) have been fractured through their necks by transmission of the force of impact through the mandible. There is, however, minimal displacement of the condylar heads.

In the crack fracture of the mandible shown in **490**, there are two distinct fracture lines running approximately parallel to each other, the more anterior extending inferomesially from the $\overline{4|}$ socket to the lower border, and the posterior from the $\overline{7|}$ socket in a similar direction. $\overline{4|}$ is slightly displaced from its socket as indicated by the widened periodontal ligament space distally. Also, there are bilateral condylar neck fractures with displacement of the condylar heads and gagging or opening of the bite. Note also the presence of multiple amalgam fragments in the lower left quadrant. The fractured condyles are also well demonstrated by the zonarc temporomandibular joint programme (TMJ(Z)) (**491**). Other examples of fractured condyles are shown in Chapter 7.

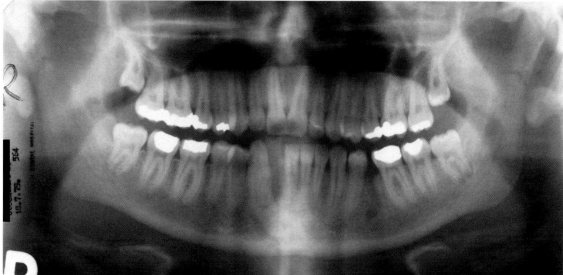

489 Fractures of the mandible. DPR.

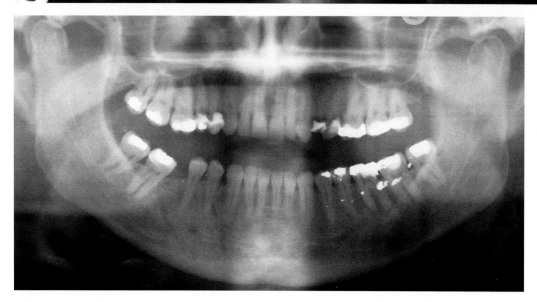

490 Fractures of the mandible. DPR.

A less common form of mandibular fracture, involving the base of the left coronoid process, is shown in **492**. The fracture line extends posterosuperiorly from the distal aspect $\overline{8}$ to the posterior part of the sigmoid notch. The fracture line is widened anteriorly due to the upward displacement of the coronoid process by contraction of the attached temporalis muscle. There is the suggestion of a fracture of the base of the left condyle. A further view (**493**) using the TMJ(Z) confirms the posterior extension of the fracture line (arrow) into the base of the condylar process.

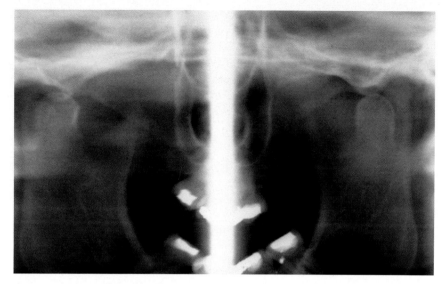

491 Fracture of the mandibular condyles. PZ(J).

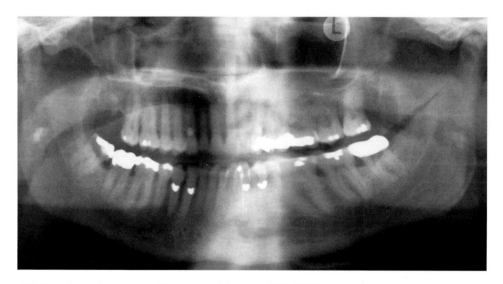

492 Fracture of the coronoid process of the mandible. DPR.

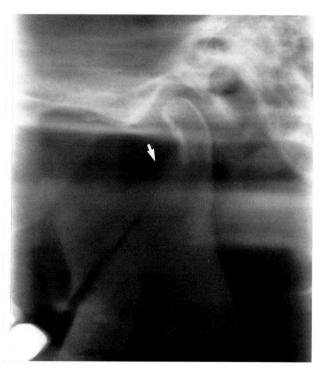

493 Fracture of the coronoid process of the mandible. PZ(J).

TREATED FRACTURES OF THE MANDIBLE

Mandibular fractures are treated by a variety of different techniques, three of which are illustrated. In the first example (**494**) bilateral fractures (arrows) through the right angle and left body of a partially dentate mandible have been immobilized by means of intermaxillary fixation. There are eyelet wires on many of the upper teeth and an acrylic plate with radio-opaque, metallic, L-shaped cleats has been secured to the mandible by two circumferential wires. There is also an upper border transosseous wire across the fracture line, distal to the carious $\overline{8|}$. The fracture of the left body of the mandible runs in the sagittal plane, with overlap of the fragments.

In the next example (**495**), the fracture on the left side of the mandible has been immobilized with a four-hole titanium miniplate. There

are fractures in the $\overline{5|}$ and $\overline{|8}$ regions, both of which have a double fracture line confirming the involvement of the buccal and lingual cortical plates. The fracture on the right passes through the $\overline{5|}$ socket. The long axis of the screws securing the plate is approximately in the same direction as that taken by the X-ray beam so that they appear end on as denser radio-opacities overlying the screw holes.

In the third example (**496**), the fracture of the right angle of the mandible involving the $\overline{8|}$ has been immobilized by a lower border trans-osseous wire; intermaxillary fixation has been achieved using upper and lower metal arch bars wired to the teeth. Note also the linear radio-opacity overlying the left body of the mandible, caused by the ghost image of the transosseous wire.

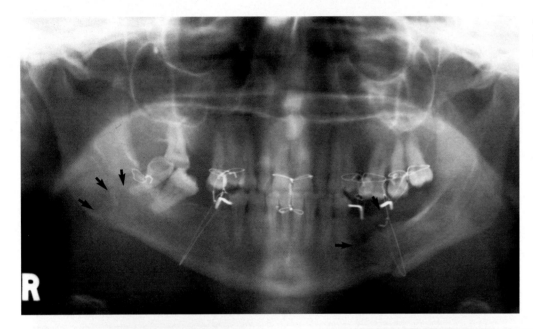

494 Fractures of the mandible treated by intermaxillary fixation. DPR.

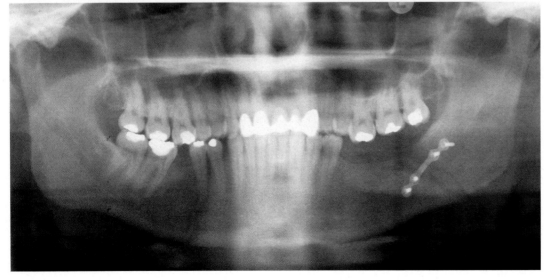

495 Fracture of the mandible treated by direct fixation. DPR.

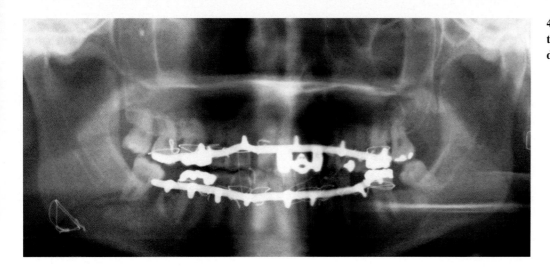

496 Fracture of the mandible treated by intermaxillary and direct fixation. DPR.

FRACTURES OF THE EDENTULOUS MANDIBLE

The edentulous state is, of course, found more commonly in elderly people. The edentulous mandible is weaker than the dentate jaw, partly because alveolar resorption follows the loss of the teeth, but also because a degree of osteoporosis is often present. These combined changes mainly affect the body of the mandible and hence fractures are more common in this part of the lower jaw. In the case of bilateral fractures of the body of the mandible (**497**), there is only slight displacement of the anterior fragment.

Due to the obliquity of the fracture on both sides, the radiolucent fracture lines of the inner and outer cortical plates appear separate but converge at the upper and lower borders, thus confirming that there is only a single fracture on both sides. Note the calcified lymph node beneath the angle of the mandible.

Another example (**498**) of bilateral fractures through the right and left body of an edentulous mandible, shows marked inferior displacement and rotation of the anterior fragment.

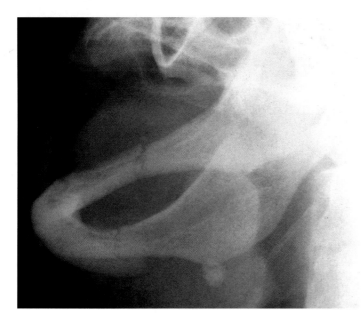

497 Fractures of the edentulous mandible. OLM.

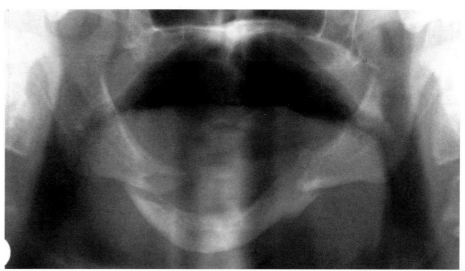

498 Fractures of the edentulous mandible. DPR.

Because of the absence of teeth from edentulous jaws, immobilization of fractures is mainly dependent upon direct fixation techniques. In the next case (**499**), the fractures have been treated by plating and transosseous wires. On each side, the plates lie on the inferior border of the mandible and the securing screws pass upwards into the bone.

As the edentulous mandible becomes increasingly atrophic, fractures are more likely following minor trauma. The example (**500**) shows a crack fracture of the left body of an atrophic mandible in an elderly patient, with minimal displacement of the bony fragments. There is swelling of the soft-tissue outline of the face overlying the fracture. Note that the atrophic changes are confined to the tooth-bearing part of the mandible.

The next example (**501**, **502**) shows a comminuted fracture in the body of a markedly atrophic mandible in an elderly patient. There are at least two small fragments, both of which are displaced and the posterior part of the mandible has been pulled upwards and forwards by the attached muscles.

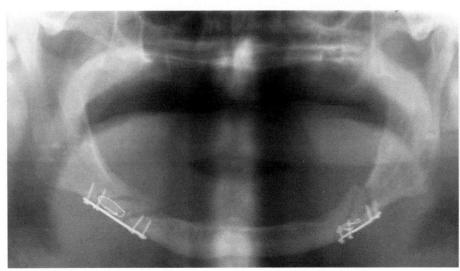

499 Fractures of the edentulous mandible treated by direct fixation. DPR.

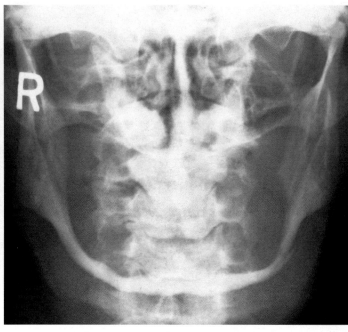

500 Fracture of an atrophic mandible. PA.

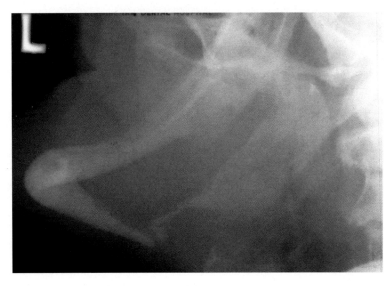

501 Comminuted fractures of an atrophic mandible. OLM.

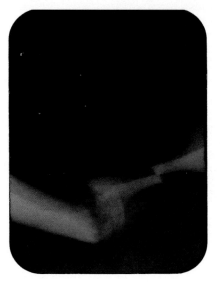

502 Comminuted fractures of an atrophic mandible. P.

Another example (**503**) demonstrates a fracture of the left body of an atrophic mandible, in which an attempt has been made to oppose the fracture ends by means of a transosseous wire (arrowhead) and further stabilization has been achieved with an acrylic splint (Gunning type) retained by three circumferential wires. There is also a fracture of the right condylar neck (arrows).

FRACTURES OF THE MANDIBLE IN CHILDREN

The bones of children are generally less brittle than those of adults and the jaws are no exception. Fractures are, therefore, relatively uncommon and may sometimes be incomplete (greenstick). The first example (**504**) shows an oblique fracture of the right side of the body of the mandible in a nine-year-old. There is displacement of the posterior fragment in an upward and forward direction, with alteration of the occlusion.

A second example (**505**) shows an oblique fracture at the base of the left condylar neck in a seven-year-old. The fracture (arrows) extends into the coronoid process anteriorly and there is displacement of the bone fragments. Interpretation of fracture lines in this site may be complicated by superimposition of the radiolucent shadow of the pharyngeal air space upon the ramus, as shown here.

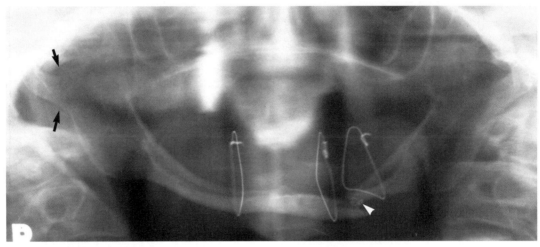

503 Fractures of an atrophic mandible treated with a Gunning splint. DPR.

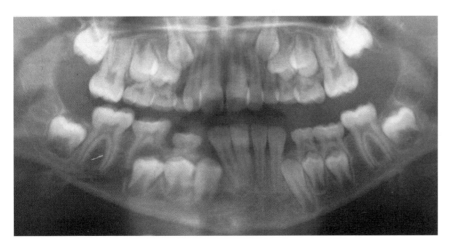

504 Fracture of the mandible in a child. DPR.

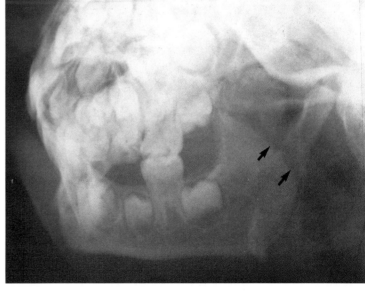

505 Fracture of the neck of the mandibular condyle in a child. OLM.

Another radiograph (**506**) reveals fractures of the anterior part of the mandible and the neck of the right condyle in a nine-year-old child resulting from a fall on the chin. The anterior fracture line runs approximately vertically, passing between ⌐12. The condylar fracture (arrow) has arisen indirectly from transmitted force and the condylar head has been displaced medially by the lateral pterygoid muscle.

FRACTURES OF THE MAXILLA

As with the mandible, fractures of the maxilla may be restricted to the dento-alveolar region or they may be more extensive, even involving adjacent facial bones. In the example of a dento-alveolar fracture (**507**), the radiolucent fracture line extends from the 2⌐ socket across the hard palate to the 6⌐ region. The fragment bearing 2345⌐ is displaced, resulting in widening of the fracture line and incisal displacement of the 2⌐ relative to 1⌐.

Fracture of the tuberosity may occur during extraction of maxillary molars, particularly single standing teeth when the alveolus has been weakened by pneumatization of the antrum. It may also occur during the removal of unerupted teeth or, more rarely, when there has been fusion (concrescence) between the root of the tooth to be extracted and an adjacent tooth.

In **508**, a radiolucent fracture line (arrow) runs antero-inferiorly from the mesial aspect of the apical part 7⌐, through the walls of the antrum, to its floor and the crest of the edentulous ridge. The more posterior part of the fracture line is obscured by the root of the zygoma. The course of the fracture line extending beyond the limits of the antrum, and also its jagged outline, distinguishes it from a vascular channel.

Fracture of the anterior nasal spine alone is unusual. In the soft-tissue exposure (**509**) such a fracture is demonstrated (arrow) and there is minimal displacement of the bone fragment.

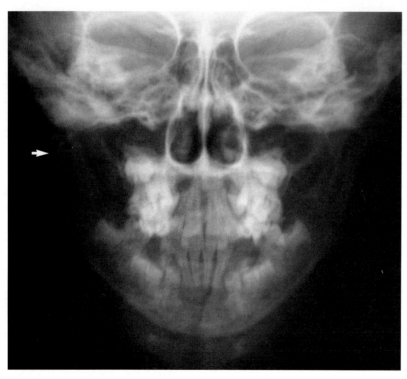

506 Fractures of the symphysis and condyle of the mandible of a child. PA.

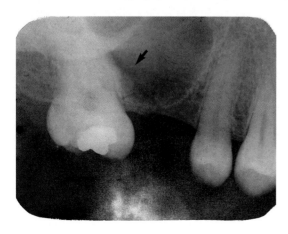

508 Fracture of the maxillary tuberosity. P.

507 (right) Dento-alveolar fracture of the maxilla. USO.

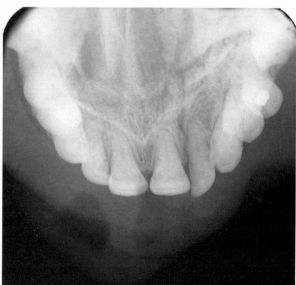

509 Fracture of the anterior nasal spine. L.

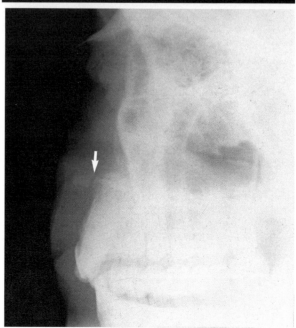

The sites of the different levels of fractures of the maxilla reflects the weakness of the individual bones of the middle part of the face. In the Le Fort Type I (**510**) there are bilateral fractures of the maxilla passing through the lateral wall of both antra and involving the floor of the nose, with resulting step deformities in the lateral walls of both antra (arrows). Both antra are partially radio-opaque due to haemorrhage: the right more diffusely so, the left having a distinct horizontal upper border to the opacity, indicating a fluid level. Note the vertical radio-opacity superimposed over the midline of the vault of the skull, caused by dystrophic mineralization in the falx cerebri. In the lateral view (**511**), the radiolucent fracture line is more clearly displayed and passes obliquely upwards and backwards through the lateral wall of the antrum from a point slightly superior to the anterior nasal spine.

Although fractures of the middle part of the facial skeleton have been classified into different types, the injuries are often complex and it is not always possible to categorize the fractures clearly into one type or another. The distribution of the fracture lines is often difficult to determine fully in the Le Fort Type II and III cases, making definitive interpretation of the radiographs imprecise.

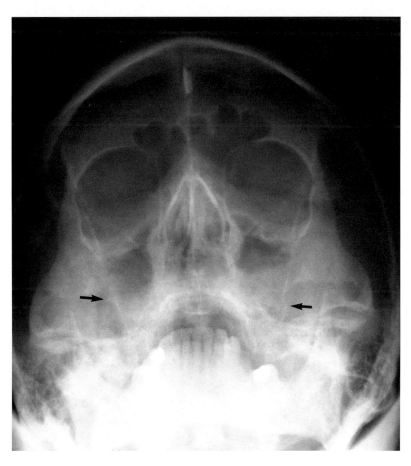

510 Fractures of the midfacial skeleton Le Fort Type I. OM.

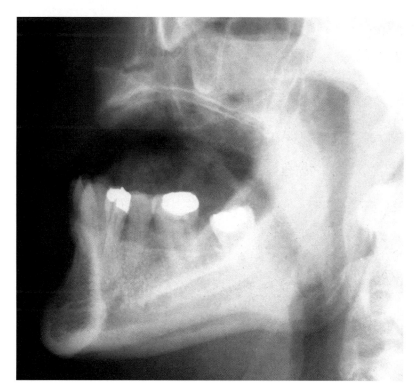

511 Fracture of the mid facial skeleton Le Fort Type I. L.

In examples **512–515** there are bilateral fractures (arrows) forming a pyramidal lesion involving the lateral walls of the maxillary antra, the infra-orbital margins, orbital floors and frontonasal part of the maxilla, typical of a Le Fort Type II injury. In addition, there are other fractures (arrowheads) producing widening of the zygomaticofrontal suture and discontinuity of the superior orbital bone margin on the left. There is opacity of both antra with that on the right showing a fluid level, and of the frontal sinuses on both sides, which also contain fluid levels. The mid-face zonarc programme (**513**) confirms that the fractures involve the upper and lower aspects of the orbits, and shows a fracture of the nasal septum and the presence of air within the left orbit, as demonstrated by the radiolucent, arcuate shadow (arrows) in its upper part. An axial CT scan (**514**), taken at the level of the middle of the maxillary antra, also demonstrates the fractures in the anterior and posterior walls of both antra, the fluid occupying the left antrum and, in addition, the presence of fluid in the ethmoidal air sinuses on both sides.

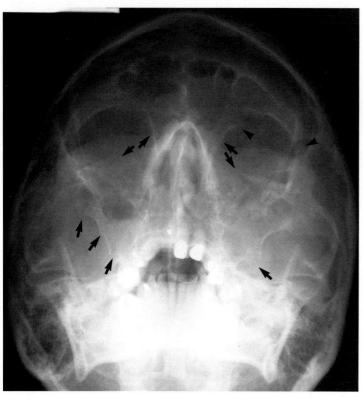

512 Fractures of the mid facial skeleton Le Fort Type II. OM.

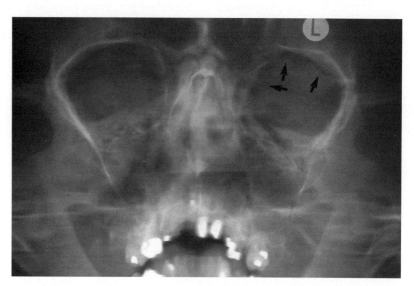

513 Fractures of the mid facial skeleton Le Fort Type II. PZ(F).

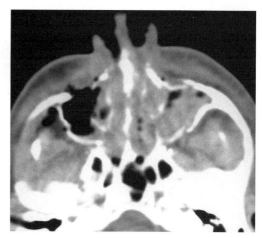

514 Fractures of the mid facial skeleton Le Fort Type II. CT.

Coronal CT scans show the extent of the injuries in another plane; the example **515** is one of a series of scans that shows fractures of the right infra-orbital margin, right medial wall of the antrum, left infra-orbital floor, with inferior displacement of the bone fragment (arrow) and of the left medial and lateral walls of the antrum.

FRACTURES OF THE NASAL BONES

Soft-tissue exposures are usually used to demonstrate fractures of the nasal bones as they demonstrate the relationship of the bone fragments to the soft-tissue profile. In the first radiograph (**516**) the anterior fragments have been displaced downwards, whilst in the next (**517**), a detached fragment has been displaced anteriorly and has penetrated the overlying skin.

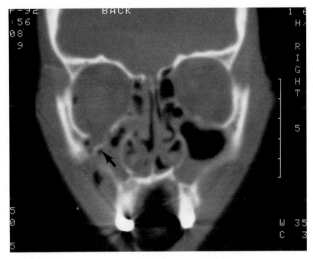

515 Fractures of the mid facial skeleton Le Fort Type II. CT.

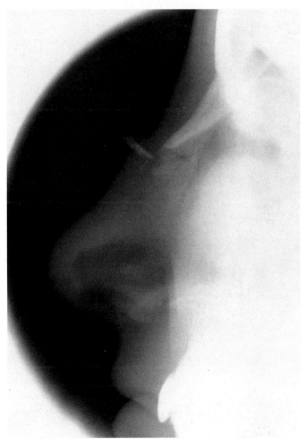

517 Fracture of the nasal bones. L.

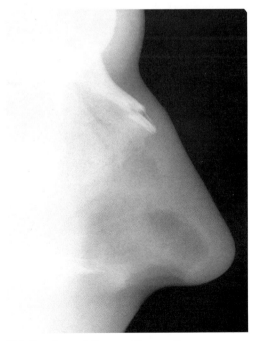

516 Fracture of the nasal bones. L.

FRACTURES OF THE FRONTONASO-ETHMOID COMPLEX

Trauma to this part of the facial skeleton often results in multiple comminuted fractures due to the weakness of the constituent bones and displacement of the fragments. The example (**518**) shows severely comminuted and depressed fractures of the frontonaso-ethmoid complex with loss of the right supra-orbital margin and gross distortion of the normal radiographic anatomy. A bone fragment has been displaced from the superomedial margin of the left orbit and is lying inferomedially within the orbital cavity (arrow). There are other fractures of the facial skeleton, particularly of the right side of the maxilla, which are poorly demonstrated on this radiograph.

Trauma that leads to fractures of the frontonaso-ethmoid complex is often severe and may be associated with multiple fractures of the skull. In the example (**519**) there is a reticular pattern of fractures of the frontal bones, particularly on the right, resulting in comminution and displacement of the lateral margin of the orbital rim superiorly (arrow). The fragments were realigned and stabilized with multiple narrow-gauge stainless steel wires (**520**) and the jaws were immobilized by means of archbars.

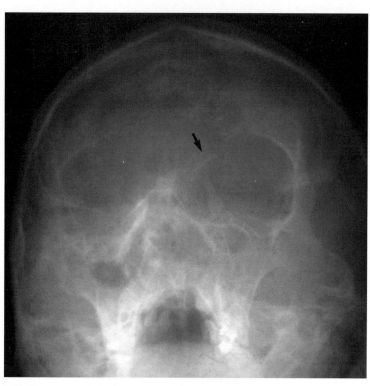

518 Fractures of the frontonaso-ethmoid complex. OM.

519 Fractures of the frontonaso-ethmoid complex. PA.

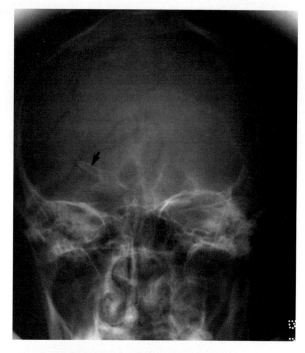

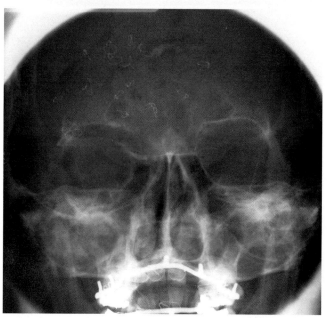

520 Treated fractures of the frontonaso-ethmoid complex. PA.

Another example (**521a,b**; **522**) shows the value of CT in the assessment of this type of injury. It demonstrates the extent of the fracture more clearly and will confirm the presence of brain damage when this is suspected clinically. This patient was struck on the right side of the forehead and has sustained a comminuted fracture, with displacement of the fragments. The sequential tomographic slices reveal depression of the supra-orbital ridge of the frontal bone (**521a**), with a separate bone fragment lying free in the superior aspect of the orbit and a further fracture of the frontal bone (**521b**), which has been displaced into the cranial cavity. The area of increased attenuation in the frontal lobe of the brain (arrow) indicates intracranial haemorrhage and haematoma formation. The fractures are more graphically demonstrated in the three-dimensional scan (**522**).

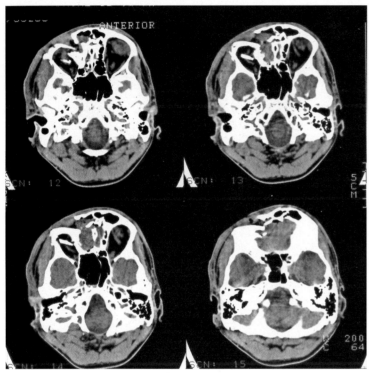

521a (above), b (top right) Fractures of the frontonaso-ethmoid complex. CT.

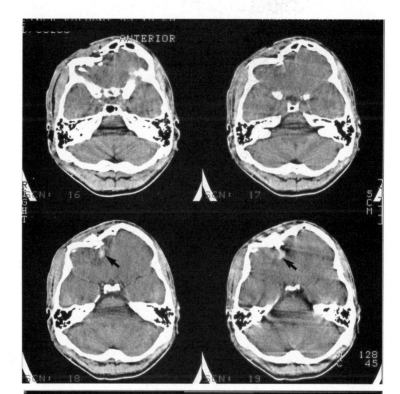

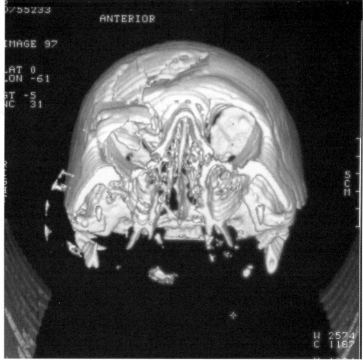

522 Fractures of the frontonaso-ethmoid complex. CT.

FRACTURES OF THE ZYGOMATIC COMPLEX

The zygomatic complex comprises the inferolateral walls of the orbit, the superolateral walls of the maxillary antrum and the zygomatic arch. Fractures may therefore involve all these structures. Reduced exposure SMV radiographs show fractures of the zygomatic arch well. In the example (**523**) there is a fracture (arrow) and lateral displacement of the left arch.

A further example (**524**) shows three fractures (arrows) of the right zygomatic arch resulting in the formation of two separate fragments, both of which have been displaced inwards towards the coronoid process of the mandible. This may result in limitation of the mouth opening.

In another example (**525** and **526**) of a fracture of the left zygomatic complex, there is inward rotation and displacement of the fragment. The fracture involves the inferolateral aspect of the floor of the orbit, with widening of the zygomaticofrontal and zygomaticotemporal sutures. There is opacity of the left maxillary antrum. The displaced fragment was elevated into its correct position and retained by stainless steel wires (**526**) at the zygomaticofrontal suture and the orbital rim. In addition, further support has been temporarily provided by ribbon gauze packed into the maxillary antrum.

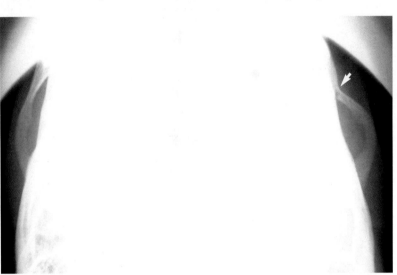

523 Fracture of the zygomatic arch. SMV.

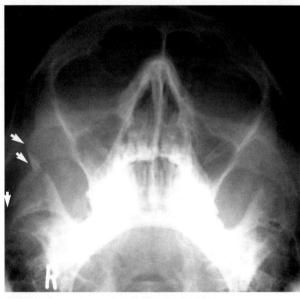

524 Fractures of the zygomatic arch. OM.

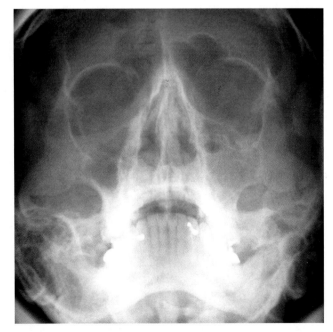

525 Fractures of the zygomatic complex. OM.

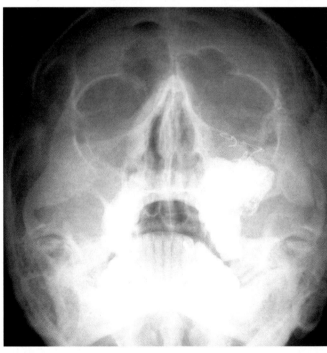

526 Treated fractures of the zygomatic complex. OM.

Another example (**527**) of a fracture of the right zygoma shows more severe inward displacement of the fragment, which appears to be in proximity to the coronoid process of the mandible. There is discontinuity of the infra-orbital margin, with a pronounced step deformity and at least one separate bone fragment lying vertically in the fracture line. The outline of the antral cavity is markedly distorted.

ORBITAL 'BLOW-OUT' FRACTURE

Direct trauma to the globe of the eye may cause transient, intra-orbital compression and result in a 'blow-out' fracture of the floor of the orbit. In the example (**528**) the infra-orbital margin remains intact but there is downward displacement of fragments of the thin bone of the orbital floor, forming a 'trapdoor' appearance (arrow). The antral cavity is radio-opaque due to haemorrhage. Note the dome-shaped, radio-opaque outline superimposed over the inferior two-thirds of the orbital cavity due to infra-orbital oedema.

Plain or computerized tomograms are helpful in determining the exact location and extent of these fractures. In the example (**529**), the defect in the continuity of the orbital floor and the soft tissues – which have herniated into the maxillary antrum forming the classical 'hanging drop' appearance – are both clearly displayed.

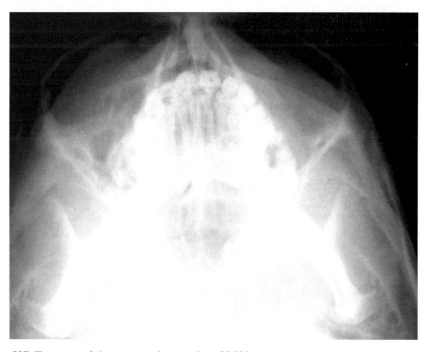

527 Fracture of the zygomatic complex. OM30.

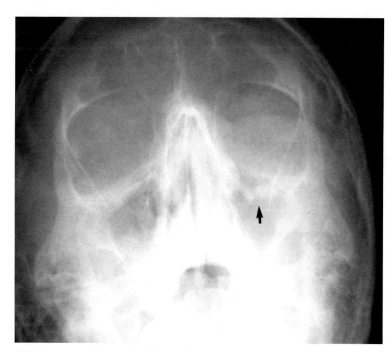

528 Fracture of the orbital floor. OM.

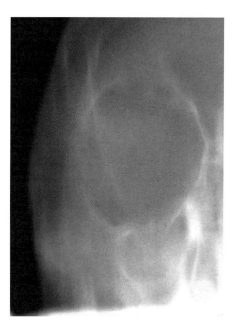

529 Fracture of the orbital floor. TG.

Tumorous conditions

Both the mandible and the maxilla may be affected by a wide range of neoplasms and other forms of tumour. In addition to masses arising from proliferation of the constituent cells of the bones, e.g. bone, cartilage and fibrous tissue, other tissues within the jaws may undergo proliferation. The most important of these is the odontogenic tissue, which gives rise to the dentition and which persists as soft-tissue residues throughout life. Tumours of odontogenic tissue may therefore arise at any age; they may also arise from other tissues in the jaw bones such as nerves, blood vessels, lymphoid and marrow tissue, and the epithelial lining of the maxillary antrum. Tumours arising within adjacent structures, such as squamous cell carcinoma of the oral mucosa, may also spread to involve the jaws. Finally, the jaw bones may also be invaded by metastases from a primary tumour in some more distant site. There is, therefore, a wide range of tumours that can affect the mandible or the maxilla. Some are more common in one jaw than the other; some are composed solely of soft tissues and others undergo mineralization to a varying degree. Some are hamartomatous or hyperplastic and, if neoplastic, they may be benign or malignant.

The use of radiographs and other imaging modalities plays a key role in diagnosis and, in particular, it may help to indicate whether a neoplasm is benign or malignant. In general terms, the boundary between an intraosseous neoplasm and the surrounding bone is well circumscribed and expansile if the tumour is benign, but poorly defined, destructive and infiltrative if it is malignant. These investigations may also reveal the full extent of a mass and whether it has spread beyond the confines of the bone into the adjacent soft tissues. Imaging techniques such as CT and MRI are of particular value in this respect. These methods also help in the identification of lymph node metastases. When a metastatic tumour is diagnosed, scintiscanning may assist in the detection of lesions in other parts of the skeleton.

Odontogenic tumours

These are a relatively uncommon group of lesions that are unique to the jaws and arise from the tissues of tooth formation. They are classified according to the tissue components that they contain and give rise to a variety of radiological appearances. They are usually benign, although malignant variants may occur.

AMELOBLASTOMA

This is the most common of the odontogenic tumours and is a benign but locally invasive epithelial neoplasm. It occurs most frequently in the molar and ramus region of the mandible in individuals in the third, fourth and fifth decades of life. The radiological appearance is variable and may be similar to that of a number of other conditions, such as dentigerous cysts and odontogenic keratocysts. Ameloblastomas are radiolucent, usually well defined and may be unilocular, loculated or multilocular; resorption of the roots of adjacent teeth is a common feature. They cause enlargement of the jaws with thinning of the cortical bone, which may become perforated. Histologically, there are two main forms, follicular and plexiform and although both may show the whole range of radiological appearances, plexiform tumours are more likely to be unilocular, whereas the follicular form tends to be multilocular.

The first example (**530**) has an appearance similar to a dentigerous cyst and is associated with the crown of a horizontally impacted, lower-right third molar in an edentulous mandible. The lesion consists of an approximately circular, radiolucent area in the lower part of the mandible, with a smaller, more oval, loculated area in the expanded edentulous ridge above. The main locule is clearly defined and contains a more radiolucent area centrally, indicating extreme thinning or perforation of a cortical plate.

Another example (**531**) is associated with a vertically placed, unerupted third molar in the left side of the body of the mandible. The radiolucent area extends from the canine region anteriorly to the mid-portion of the ascending

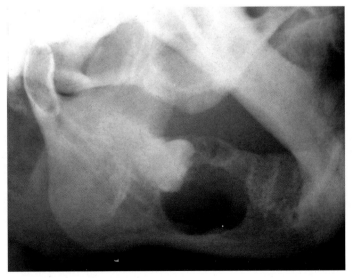

530 Ameloblastoma. OLM.

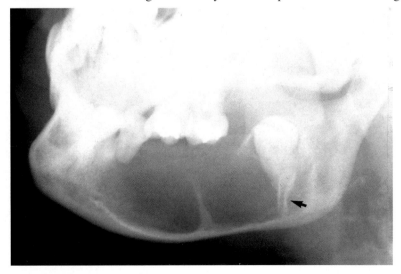

531 Ameloblastoma. OLM.

ramus posteriorly. It is basically a unilocular, well-defined lesion, less clearly outlined anteriorly, with an incomplete, vertical septum arising from the midpoint inferiorly. Another structure apparently overlying the apex of the associated third molar tooth is the image (arrow) of the body of the hyoid bone superimposed upon the lesion. There is apical resorption of $\overline{5}$ and thinning and expansion of the cortical bone buccally (arrows) (**532**).

The infiltrative pattern of growth through the bone marrow spaces, particularly of the follicular type of ameloblastoma, tends to give rise to a multilocular appearance radiologically. The next example (**533**) shows a

lesion in the left side of the mandible, extending posteriorly from $\overline{3}$ to involve the majority of the ascending ramus. It has a well-defined, scalloped margin and the cortical bone at the inferior border of the mandible is thinned, but remains intact. There is resorption of the roots of $\overline{456}$ and also of the unerupted $\overline{7}$, which has been displaced towards the base of the coronoid process. There is expansion and thinning of the cortical bone lingually and buccally (**534**) where the outline is discontinuous due to its perforation.

Another multilocular lesion (**535**) is shown, this time in the right body and ramus of the mandible, extending from $\overline{6}$ anteriorly to the base

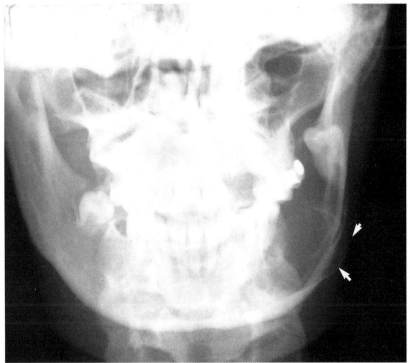

532 Ameloblastoma. PA.

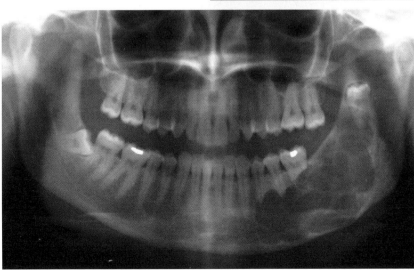

533 Ameloblastoma. DPR.

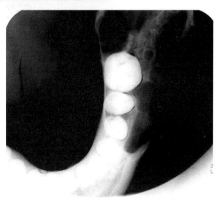

534 Ameloblastoma. LTO.

187

of the coronoid and the condylar processes posteriorly. There are numerous radio-opaque bony septa within the radiolucency, giving it a honeycombed appearance. The lesion is clearly defined peripherally with a radio-opaque lamina and there is expansion and thinning of the cortical bone inferiorly and at the anterior base of the ascending ramus. A displaced unerupted $\overline{8|}$ is present within the lesion and there is resorption of the root apices $\overline{7|}$. The honeycomb pattern is confirmed on the axial CT scans (**536, 537, 538**)

which also reveal the marked expansion of the lingual cortical plate, which is thinned and eroded. There is both buccal and lingual expansion, but the buccal cortical plate remains intact, in contrast to the perforation present at the higher plane. The dark areas of low attenuation at the anterior aspect of the lesion (**536, 537**) indicate cyst formation, which is not uncommon in these tumours.

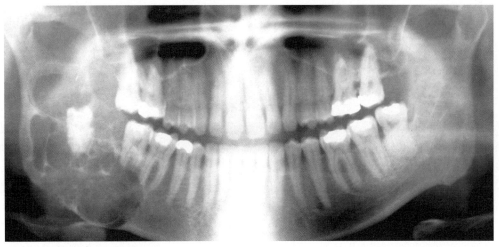

535 Ameloblastoma. DPR.

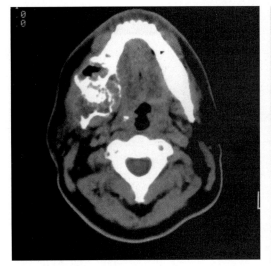

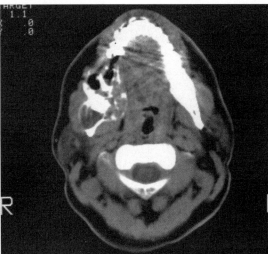

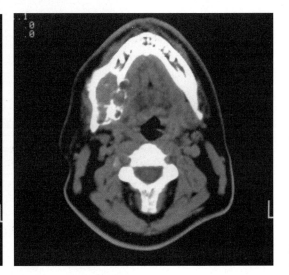

536 Ameloblastoma. CT.

537 Ameloblastoma. CT.

538 Ameloblastoma. CT.

The growth of ameloblastomas is usually slow and they may reach a considerable size before the patient seeks treatment. The next example (**539**) shows a large, predominantly unilocular, radiolucent lesion in the left ramus of the mandible with thinning and expansion of the cortical bone inferiorly, anteriorly and posteriorly. Almost the entire ramus of the mandible is radiolucent and only a small amount of radio-opaque bone remains in the region of the angle, where a bony septum curves into the tumour mass. There is expansion of the coronoid process and flattening of the sigmoid notch. $\overline{8}|$ is displaced antero-inferiorly towards the lower bor-

der of the mandible and its crown appears to project into the radiolucent defect, thus simulating a dentigerous cyst. The images of the hyoid bone and the epiglottis are superimposed upon the lesion. On the intra-oral radiograph (**540**) a dentigerous relationship between the crown of $\overline{8}|$ and the lesion is apparent once again and the thin, radio-opaque lamina on the outer aspect of the expanded ramus indicates that the cortical bone is still intact. In addition, there is expansion of the buccal and lingual (arrows) aspects of the ramus (**541**), the buccal cortical outline being indistinct.

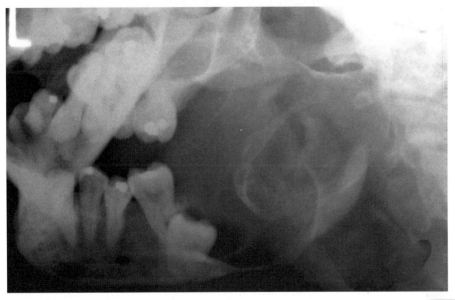

539 Ameloblastoma. OLM.

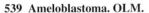

540 Ameloblastoma. P.

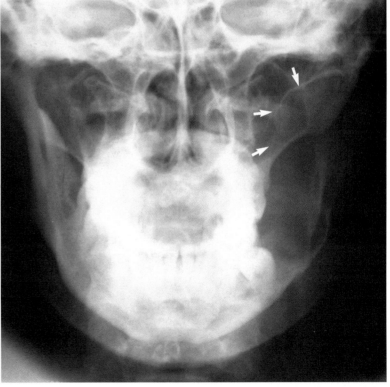

541 Ameloblastoma. PA.

PLEXIFORM UNICYSTIC AMELOBLASTOMA

In contrast to the more common forms, this type of ameloblastoma usually occurs in younger individuals and the tumour mass grows predominantly into the cyst cavity rather than invading the adjacent marrow spaces. In the example (542) showing a unilocular lesion in a 14-year-old, the radiolucent defect extends from the first molar region anteriorly and occupies the entire ramus of the right side of the mandible, apart from the condylar process. There is thinning of the cortical bone inferiorly, anteriorly and posteriorly, with expansion anteriorly, inferiorly and in the region of the sigmoid notch, which is flattened; 8| is partially formed and displaced into the coronoid process, and 7| is displaced antero-inferiorly. The radiolucent defect is superimposed upon 7| causing an appearance similar to that of a dentigerous cyst. The outline of the incompletely calcified hyoid bone is superimposed upon the lesion. The buccal position of 7| and the buccal and lingual bony expansion of the ramus are confirmed in the postero-anterior radiograph (543).

ADENOMATOID ODONTOGENIC TUMOUR

This benign, expansile, epithelial tumour characteristically arises in the anterior part of the jaws in individuals in the second and third decades of life and is often associated with the crown of an unerupted tooth. In the example (544) in an 18-year-old, the clearly defined, radiolucent lesion is associated with the mesial aspect of the unerupted 3| where the lamina dura and the follicular space are absent; it is partly surrounded by a thin, radio-opaque lamina. Not infrequently, such lesions contain a number of radio-opaque foci of dystrophic mineralization, as seen here. C| is retained, although there has been some resorption of the apex.

Another example (545) is shown in the left canine and premolar region of the mandible, this time not associated with an unerupted tooth. This lesion is circular and there is marked buccal expansion of the bone although the cortical lamina remains intact. The radio-opaque lamina demarcating the medial wall of the lesion is superimposed upon the canine and first premolar teeth, between which there is a diastema. A number of

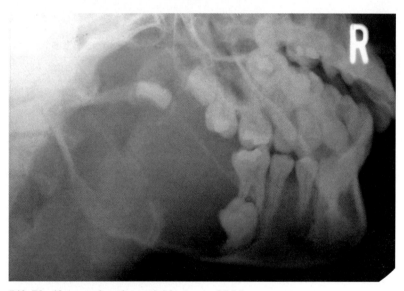

542 Plexiform unicystic ameloblastoma. OLM.

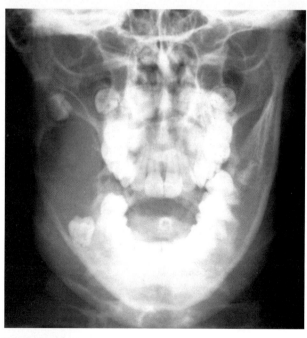

543 Plexiform unicystic ameloblastoma. PA.

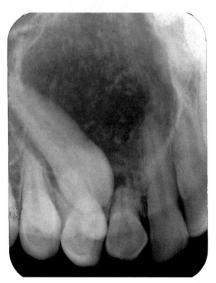

544 Adenomatoid odontogenic tumour. P.

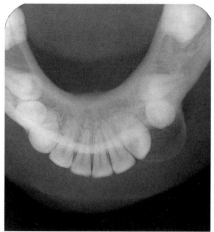

545 Adenomatoid odontogenic tumour. LTO.

radio-opaque foci of mineralization are present, characteristically towards the centre of the mass rather than at the periphery.

CALCIFYING ODONTOGENIC CYST

This lesion is essentially an expansile cystic epithelial tumour, which, in some instances, contains varying amounts of dystrophic mineralization and is occasionally associated with an odontome. Sometimes the lesion presents as a solid tumour mass (dentinogenic ghost cell tumour) and therefore has a variable radiographic appearance, which may be unilocular or multilocular in outline. In the example (**546**), there is an ovoid, clearly defined, radiolucent lesion in the right premolar region of an edentulous mandible. It is bounded by a thin, radio-opaque lamina of cortical bone except superiorly, where the alveolar bone has been eroded. Two areas of darker radiolucency within the lesion indicate that one of the cortical plates has been thinned. The smaller, round area of radiolucency (arrow) beneath the lesion is not a separate locule but the mental foramen.

Another example (**547**) shows a lesion in the left maxilla containing areas of dystrophic mineralization. Within a clearly defined, round, radiolucent area extending from |1 to |6 , numerous irregularly shaped masses of variable size and of uniformly dense radio-opacity are present, mostly in the anterior part of the lesion. The lamina dura is absent around the apices of |345 , which are blunted, indicating the presence of resorption; their roots have been displaced by the tumour, together with |1 .

The next example (**548**) shows a solid form of the lesion in which a uniformly radio-opaque mass occupies the whole of the left antrum. There appears to be erosion of all the bony walls of the antrum, an appearance similar to that of a malignant neoplasm, with expansion of the mass laterally, inferiorly and medially into the nasal cavity. The expansile, rather than invasive, nature of the lesion is shown on the CT scan (**549**) in which the walls of the antrum are shown to be intact.

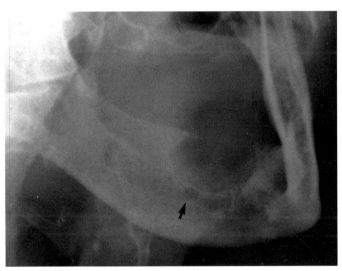

546 Calcifying odontogenic cyst. OLM.

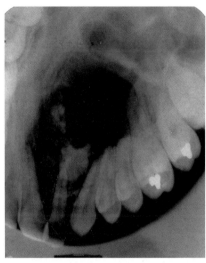

547 Calcifying odontogenic cyst. UOO.

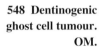
548 Dentinogenic ghost cell tumour. OM.

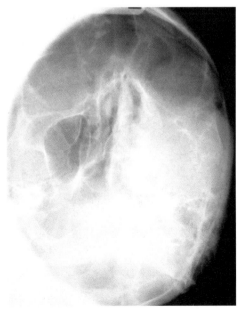

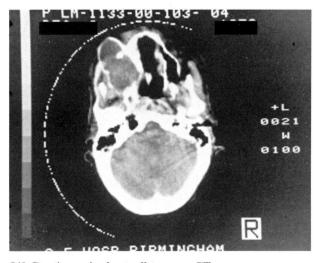

549 Dentinogenic ghost cell tumour. CT.

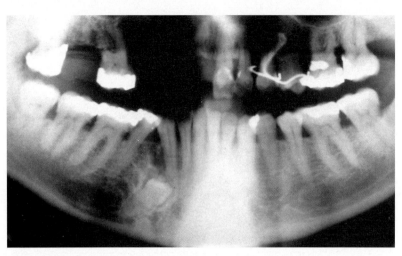

550 Calcifying epithelial odontogenic tumour (Pindborg tumour). DPR.

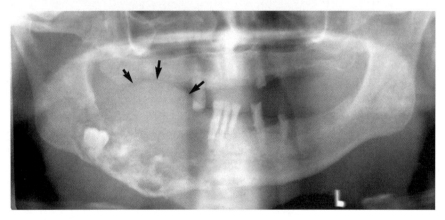

551 Calcifying epithelial odontogenic tumour (Pindborg tumour). DPR.

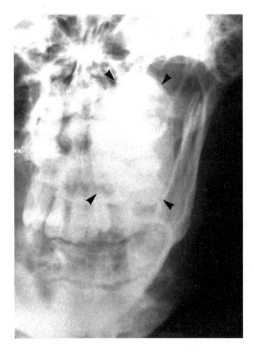

552 Cementifying fibroma. PA.

CALCIFYING EPITHELIAL ODONTOGENIC TUMOUR (PINDBORG TUMOUR)

This rare, benign, epithelial tumour undergoes mineralization to a variable extent, so that areas of radio-opacity of different shapes and sizes may sometimes be present within the predominently radiolucent lesion. It is more common in the mandible and is also sometimes associated with an unerupted tooth, as in the example (**550**) involving $\overline{4|}$. There is a loculated radiolucency lying between $\overline{5|}$ and $\overline{3|}$, the roots of which are divergent. $\overline{4|}$ is displaced inferiorly and the crown is surrounded by a normal follicular space and cortical lamina, except superiorly adjacent to the lesion.

Another example (**551**) shows a large tumour of long standing in the right side of the mandible of an elderly patient. It is mainly a radiolucent lesion with a clearly defined margin posteriorly and is poorly defined anteriorly where it has extended beyond the midline. Superiorly, there is complete destruction of the alveolar bone and a large soft tissue swelling (arrows), whereas the cortical bone of the inferior border of the mandible has, so far, simply been expanded and, in places, markedly thinned. A malformed, unerupted $\overline{8|}$ is present in the posterior part of the tumour, which contains numerous, irregular, radio-opaque structures some of which are residual bone trabeculae and others are areas of dystrophic mineralization. The cortical margins of the inferior alveolar canal, although clearly present in the ramus, are absent within the tumour.

CEMENTIFYING FIBROMA (CEMENTO-OSSIFYING FIBROMA)

This rare, benign neoplasm, which most commonly affects young adults, is composed of fibrous tissue containing a variable amount of mineralized cementum-like tissue. It is difficult histologically to distinguish from ossifying fibroma and so the term cemento-ossifying fibroma is being increasingly used. The radiographic appearance depends upon the stage of maturity of the lesion and varies from radiolucent to radio-opaque. It is encapsulated and so tends to be well defined around its periphery. In the large lesion in the left side of the maxilla (**552**) the mass is oval in outline and clearly defined (arrowheads), with uniform radio-opacity. Around the superior and lateral margins there is a distinct radiolucent capsular space and a thin, radio-opaque cortical lamina. Another example (**553**, **554**) shows a radiolucent lesion in the left side of the body of the mandible which contains much less mineralized tissue than the example in the previous radiograph. There are scattered radio-opacities particularly inferiorly and the tumour has a well defined, slightly lobulated margin. It has expanded the bone, particularly in the medial and lateral directions (**554**). The outline of the socket of the recently extracted ⌐6 is visible (**553**).

BENIGN CEMENTOBLASTOMA

This uncommon, benign neoplasm – which is composed of sheets of cementoid that are mineralized to a varying degree – typically develops on the mesial root of mandibular molars in young males. Mandibular premolars may also be involved. In the example (**555**) there is an approximately circular mass of uniform radio-opacity overlying and obscuring the mesial root ⌐6 and circumscribed by a radiolucent capsular space. Blunting of the apex of the distal root of the tooth indicates early resorption. Unusually, in this example there is some radio-opacity of the surrounding bone due to reactive osteosclerosis.

The second example (**556**) shows a larger lesion, in this instance on the distal root 6⌐, which shows evidence of resorption. The neoplasm is well circumscribed with a radiolucent capsular space and cortical lamina around most of its periphery and with a mottled radio-opaque appearance.

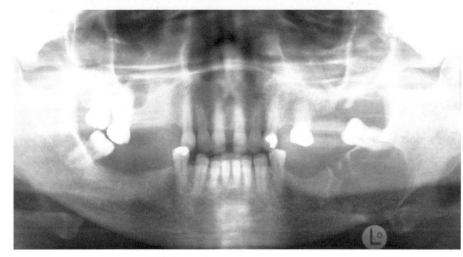

553 Cementifying fibroma. DPR.

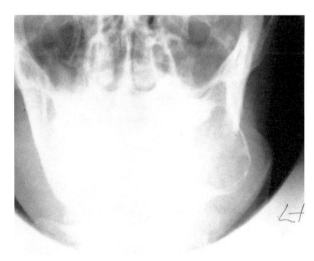

554 Cementifying fibroma. PA.

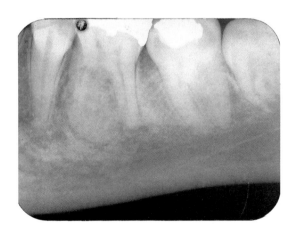

555 Benign cementoblastoma. P.

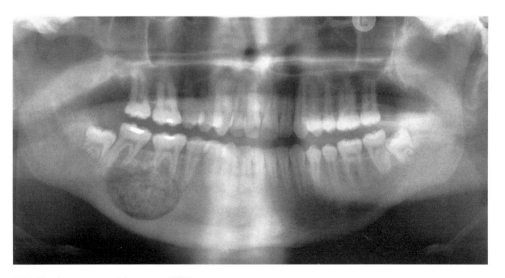

556 Benign cementoblastoma. DPR.

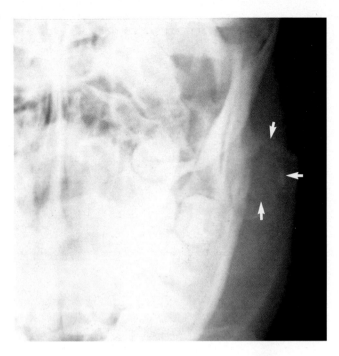

**557
Dentinoma.
PAC.**

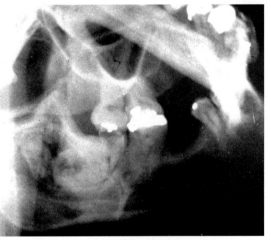

**558 Dentinoma.
OLM.**

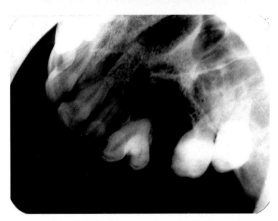

**559 Odontogenic
myxoma. UOO.**

DENTINOMA (AMELOBLASTIC FIBRODENTINOMA)

This condition arises from the abnormal proliferation of odontogenic mesenchyme, within which increasing amounts of mineralized dentine matrix are laid down. In the example (**557**) in a 16-year-old, an immature lesion has arisen in a rather unusual site on the buccal aspect of the left lower molar region. There is an approximately circular radiolucency (arrows) which contains randomly arranged radio-opacities. In the deep part of the mass superiorly, there is a triangular area of reactive, subperiosteal bone formation. Increasing amounts of mineralized dentine matrix become deposited in these lesions so that they become more radio-opaque, as in the example in an adult (**558**) where there is an ovoid lesion in the right mandibular molar region with a clearly defined margin. It is quite densely radio-opaque anteriorly although the posterior part still contains a number of areas of radiolucency.

ODONTOGENIC MYXOMA

This rare form of odontogenic tumour occurs most commonly in the second and third decades of life and is more frequent in the mandible. It does not seem to occur in bones other than the jaws. The tumour may be well or poorly defined and is typically loculated, particularly when large, giving a honeycomb appearance, as in **559**, **560** in the left side of the maxilla. This lesion, although it is well defined, lacks a peripheral cortical lamina and extends from |2 to the left tuberosity region. Numerous delicate, radio-opaque, bony septa run randomly through the lesion and there has been some displacement of the root apices |34 so that they are overlapping.

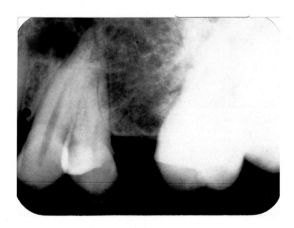

560 Odontogenic myxoma. P.

Another example (**561**) shows a large tumour in the left body and ramus of an edentulous mandible, forming a clearly defined, radiolucency with a scalloped outline. A randomly arranged reticular pattern of bone septa is seen within the defect, giving the honeycomb appearance characteristic of this condition. The cortical plate is expanded lingually and thinned on all surfaces.

Central giant cell tumour

Most central giant cell tumours are granulomas and are confined to the tooth-bearing areas of the jaws, usually anteriorly. They are most common in individuals under the age of thirty; in the early stages they arise in the alveolar bone displacing the roots of the adjacent teeth and causing bone expansion. The main radiographic features are a well defined radiolucency with loculated or multilocular outline and internal septa or trabeculations. In the example (**562**) of a lesion which arose in a nine-year-old, there is a well defined, pear-shaped homogenous radiolucency with displacement of the apices $\overline{21}$ distally and mesially respectively. The thin radio-opaque lamina dura is still present around the teeth.

As the lesions enlarge they may become less well defined (**563**) and show coarse radio-opaque trabeculations within the radiolucency, producing a honeycomb appearance. As in the previous example the roots of the adjacent teeth have been displaced, but in this case the lamina dura is missing.

Example **564** shows a much larger tumour in the anterior part of the mandible, occupying almost the entire depth of the alveolus. The radiolucency has a loculated, clearly defined margin and contains several thin, radio-opaque septa. There is displacement of the roots $\overline{11}$ distally and loss of the lamina dura around the apical halves of the roots of all four incisor teeth, the apices of which appear absorbed. Occasionally these aggressive lesions are associated with pregnancy, as was the case in this example.

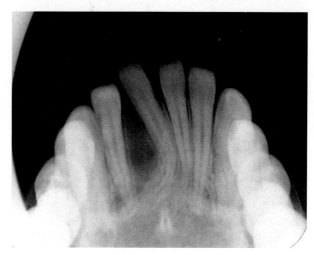

562 Central giant cell tumour. LAO.

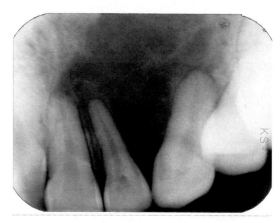

563 Central giant cell tumour. P.

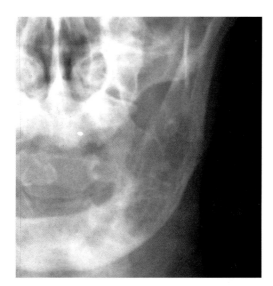

561 Odontogenic myxoma. PA.

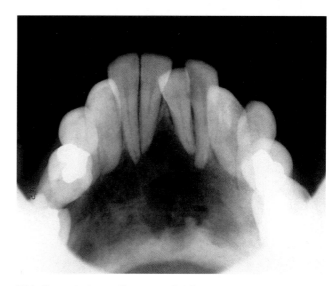

564 Central giant cell tumour. LAO.

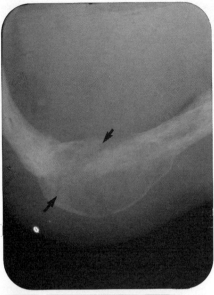

565 Central giant cell tumour. LTO.

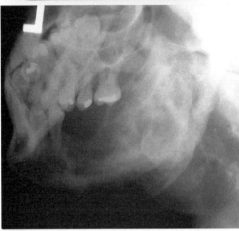

566 Central giant cell tumour. OLM.

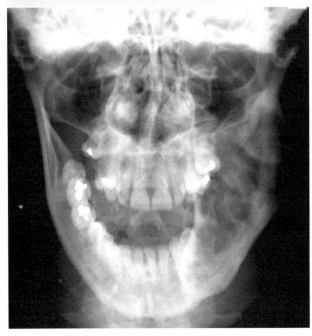

567 Central giant cell tumour. PA.

Less commonly, giant cell tumours occur in older patients and are thus sometimes seen in edentulous jaws. In **565**, in the anterior region of the mandible, there is pronounced expansion and thinning of the labial cortical bone and slight lingual expansion. A pathological fracture (arrows) has occurred running obliquely from the midline lingually to the $\overline{2|}$ region. Aggressive giant cell tumours are sometimes classified as osteoclastomas but such lesions are uncommon in the jaws.

An example (**566** and **567**) shows a large tumour occupying the ramus and body of the left side of the mandible as far forward as $\overline{|3}$. In the ramus, the tumour has extended into the coronoid process, causing expansion of the anterior border and flattening of the sigmoid notch. This expansile tumour has a clearly defined margin apart from the $\overline{|34}$ region and is essentially radiolucent, although there are numerous coarse, radio-opaque trabeculations running through it. The image of the hyoid bone is projected across the middle of the lower part of the ramus of the mandible. In addition, there is marked lingual and buccal expansion (**567**), the former projecting beyond the inferior border of the mandible.

Fibromas

OSSIFYING FIBROMA (CEMENTO-OSSIFYING FIBROMA)

This benign neoplasm is composed of fibrous tissue within which increasing amounts of bone matrix and dystrophic mineralization are deposited as the lesion matures. It is difficult histologically to distinguish from cementifying fibroma and so the term cemento-ossifying fibroma is being increasingly used (see p.192). It is essentially radiolucent in appearance but contains scattered foci of radio-opacity which may coalesce. It usually has a well defined border with a distinct cortical outline. The first example (**568**) shows an expansile, approximately circular mass (arrows) in the left side of the maxilla of a six-year-old, that has displaced the antral floor superiorly and expanded the alveolus inferiorly. $\underline{|E}$ has been displaced occlusally and distally and a large portion of the roots is missing. $\underline{|45}$ are absent and the unerupted $\underline{|3}$ has been displaced mesially and overlies the unerupted $\underline{|12}$.

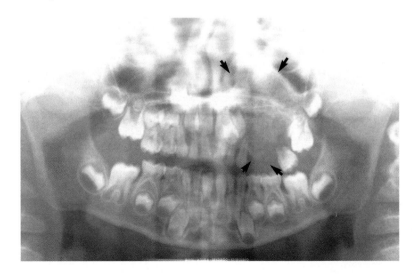

568 Ossifying fibroma. DPR.

The internal structure of the lesion is more clearly demonstrated on the intra-oral radiographs (**569**, **570**) which demonstrate randomly arranged granular radio-opacities in a radiolucent background. Somewhat atypically, this neoplasm appears to blend into the adjacent bone and is not demarcated by a clear margin. Occasionally, ossifying fibromas are very aggressive in children and may be confused with malignant neoplasms. CT may be helpful in distinguishing these entities.

Example **571** shows a large mass in the left body of the mandible which has caused expansion of the buccal and lingual cortical plates which remain intact. The mass is almost circular in outline, suggesting an expansile lesion and has encroached upon the nasopharynx, lateral pterygoid plate and lateral wall of the maxillary antrum. The lesion contains several areas of low attenuation indicative of more cellular, less mineralized areas within the tumour.

A third example (**572**, **573**) shows a more extensive lesion in an adult, which has caused expansion of the mandible buccally, lingually and inferiorly. The mass extends from the midline to the base of the coronoid process and the posterior margin is clearly defined. A thin cortical lamina persists inferiorly, but buccally and lingually this is indistinct and the buccal outline is undulating. The tumour is composed of randomly arranged, relatively coarse radio-opacities of varying density with a radiolucent background. As such lesions develop, the radio-opacities tend to become increasingly coarse and more numerous as greater amounts of mineral are deposited.

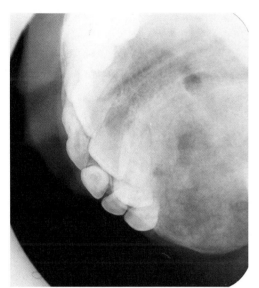

569 Ossifying fibroma. UOO.

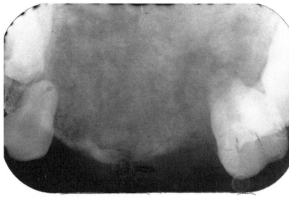

570 Ossifying fibroma. P.

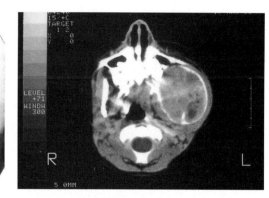

571 Aggressive ossifying fibroma. CT.

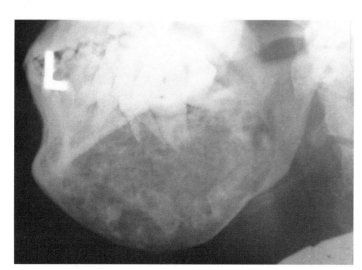
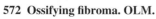

572 Ossifying fibroma. OLM.

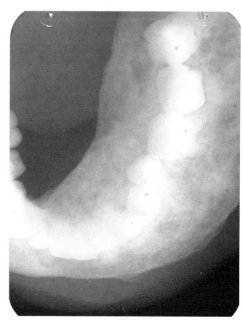

573 Ossifying fibroma. LTO.

CENTRAL FIBROMA

Rarely, a benign neoplasm of cellular fibrous tissue arises centrally within the jaws, most cases being in the mandible. The example (**574, 575**) shows a lesion occupying the ascending ramus and molar region of the right side of the mandible. It extends from the base of the coronoid process to the mesial aspect 7̄| and has a clearly defined margin with a thin, radio-opaque, cortical lamina. 8̄| has been displaced inferiorly by the tumour which is radiolucent and contains several randomly arranged, delicate, radio-opaque trabeculae and an area of more dense mineralization towards its centre. There is marked lingual expansion of the mandible, which has resulted in the projection of two apparently separate margins to the lesion superiorly on the oblique lateral film.

CHONDROMYXOID FIBROMA

This benign neoplasm which is rare in the jaws, forms a multilocular, radiolucent defect, as shown in example **576** in the third molar region of the mandible. The locules which are clearly defined contain numerous randomly arranged trabeculations. The incompletely formed third molar has been displaced towards the lower border of the mandible.

Osteoma

Osteomas are benign, slow-growing neoplasms of mature bone and are usually classified histologically into cancellous and compact types, according to the density of the bone they contain. They most commonly occur in the skull, especially in the region of the frontal and ethmoid sinuses. In the jaws the mandible is more commonly affected and the tumours are frequently peripherally placed. The radiographic appearance depends upon the histological type, but they usually have clearly defined margins. In the example of a cancellous lesion (**577**), there is an exophytic, radio-opaque mass protruding from the mental surface of the mandible. It has a regular, circumscribed boundary and is made up of randomly arranged trabeculae.

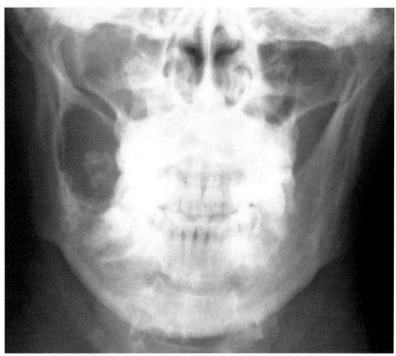

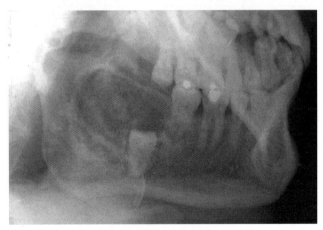

574 Central fibroma. OLM.

575 (above) Central fibroma. PA.

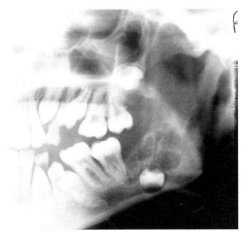

576 Chondromyxoid fibroma. DPR.

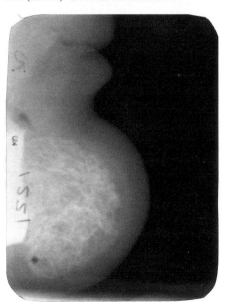

577 (left) Osteoma. S.

A CT scan (**578**) assists in determining the relationship of the mass to the bone of origin and confirms that the outer cortical plate of the mandible is intact and that the neoplasm has arisen from its periosteal surface.

Compact (ivory) osteomas are more densely radio-opaque than the cancellous type. The example (**579**) shows a compact (ivory) osteoma arising from the inferior border of an edentulous mandible. It forms an approximately circular mass of uniform radio-opacity, although the peripheral part is more granular in appearance. Being composed of dense compact bone, its radio-opacity is similar to that of the cortical bone of the mandible.

The next example (**580**) is that of a uniformly radio-opaque exophytic lesion, projecting inferiorly from the lower border of an edentulous mandible. The image of the body of the hyoid bone is superimposed upon the lower part of the mass. Note the presence of the upper denture with porcelain teeth, the anteriors being pin retained.

Gardner's syndrome

Gardner's syndrome is inherited as an autosomal dominant condition and consists of a number of abnormalities including multiple osteomas, sebaceous cysts, subcutaneous fibromas and intestinal polyps. The intestinal polyps are premalignant and may develop into carcinomas. Multiple supernumerary teeth may also be present. The osteomas of the jaws usually occur in the second decade of life as in the example (**581**) in which tumours are present in both sides of the mandible. The densely radio-opaque mass on the right is clearly defined and circumscribed by a radiolucent capsular space which is partly demarcated by a thin, radio-opaque cortical lamina, particularly posteriorly and laterally. The lesion at the left angle is less densely radio-opaque, although it also has a clearly defined margin, and is protruding laterally. A third, less radio-opaque osteoma (arrows) protrudes from the inferior border of the right side of the body of the mandible.

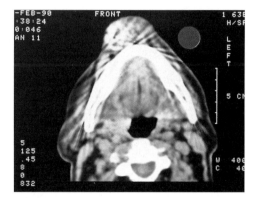

578 Osteoma. CT.

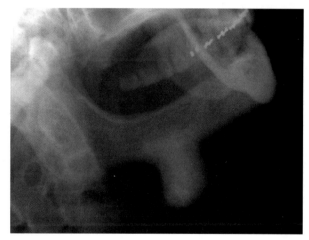

580 Osteoma. OLM.

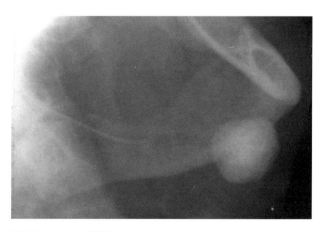

579 Osteoma. OLM.

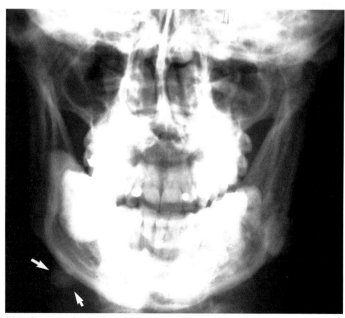

581 Gardner's syndrome. PA.

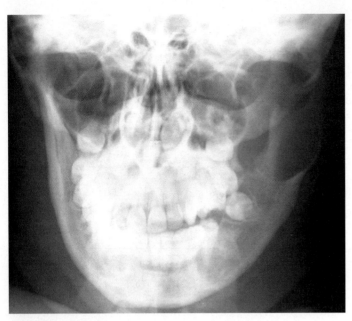

582 Central neurilemmoma. PA.

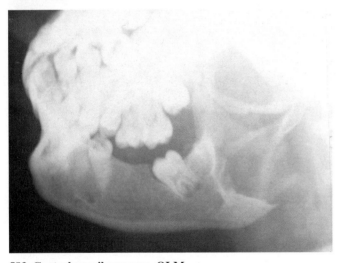

583 Central neurilemmoma. OLM.

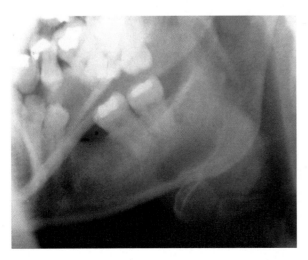

584 Central neuro-fibroma. OLM.

Neurilemmoma and neurofibroma

Benign neoplasms of nerve sheaths may arise on the intra-osseous portion of the nerves and are then described as being central in origin. They occur more commonly in the mandible than the maxilla, where they develop in association with the inferior alveolar nerve. In such cases there is a clear association between the radiolucent tumour mass and the unaffected part of the inferior alveolar canal. The first example (**582**) shows a large neurilemmoma arising in the left ramus of the mandible. It has a clearly defined outline, particularly at its inferior margin, where there is a radio-opaque lamina. The benign, expansile neoplasm has caused thinning of the cortical bone buccally, but posteriorly the bone has been mostly resorbed (**583**). Because of the position of this tumour at the posterior end of the inferior alveolar canal, the usual relationship between the two is not clearly displayed. Note that the image of the hyoid bone is superimposed upon the lesion.

The second example (**584**) shows a neurofibroma, which has arisen from the inferior alveolar nerve, in which the relationship between the two is more classically displayed. There is a clearly defined radiolucent fusiform enlargement of the inferior alveolar canal beneath the molars and in the base of the ramus of the mandible. The area is clearly defined and surrounded by a thin radio-opaque corticated margin, which is scalloped inferiorly and is continuous with the outline of the inferior alveolar canal anteriorly and posteriorly.

Bone cysts

ANEURYSMAL BONE CYST

Aneurysmal bone cysts occur occasionally in the jaws and are most common in the mandible of young adults. They may cause rapid bone expansion. The condition is widely believed to arise from cystic change within some other pre-existing pathological condition, such as an ossifying fibroma, although the evidence for the presence of such pre-existing lesions is not always clear. They contain numerous wide, irregularly shaped blood channels lying within a fibrocellular stroma containing giant cells. The radiographic features include a moderately well-defined unilocular or loculated radiolucency, frequently containing randomly arranged septa. Fluid levels may be seen in the vascular channels on CTs. In the example (**585**) there is an oval, radiolucency with a clearly defined outline surrounded by a thin, radio-opaque, cortical lamina in the left body of the mandible. There are numerous, coarse trabeculae running through the lesion and antero-inferiorly there is a lobulated area of radiolucency suggesting marked thinning or perforation of a cortical plate. The alveolar surface of the cyst is slightly expanded, but the cortex remains intact.

In the second example (**586**), the cyst has arisen in a 19-year-old, probably within an ossifying fibroma. The lesion occupies the entire left body of the mandible and contains several variably shaped areas of radio-lucency; otherwise the mass has a granular radio-opaque appearance. The inferior border of the mandible is considerably expanded forming a typi-cal 'soap bubble' pattern and there is also expansion of the alveolar crest. The unerupted |8 lies transversely in the posterior part of the cyst.

SOLITARY BONE CYST (TRAUMATIC BONE CYST; HAEMORRHAGIC BONE CYST)

Solitary bone cysts arise most commonly in the posterior region of the body of the mandible in relation to the apices of the roots of the molar teeth, in adolescent males. In this site, expansion of the bone may be only slight and the cyst has a characteristic scalloped pattern where it extends between the roots of the teeth. Occasionally such lesions occur in the ramus of the mandible, as in the example (**587**) of a ten-year-old, and, in this site, bone expansion may be more obvious. The radiograph shows a large, clearly defined radiolucency in the left ramus with marked buccal and lingual expansion of the cortical plates, both of which remain intact.

Pleomorphic salivary adenoma

In the maxilla, this benign epithelial tumour, although arising in the mucosal salivary glands, may cause destruction of the underlying bone. In **588** – an edentulous patient – there is a recurrent tumour in the left side of the maxilla which has produced a large, radiolucent defect with a clearly defined oval outline. The alveolar ridge is expanded and the radio-opaque lamina of the palatal shelf is absent on the affected side. CT is helpful in determining more fully the extent of such lesions.

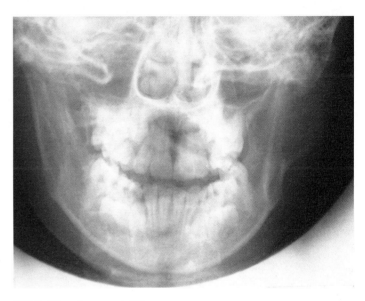

587 Solitary bone cyst. PA.

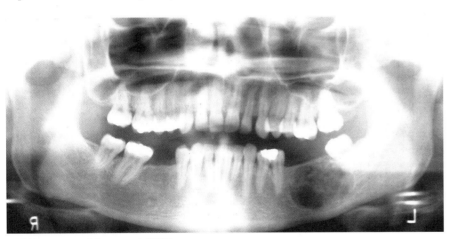

585 Aneurysmal bone cyst. DPR.

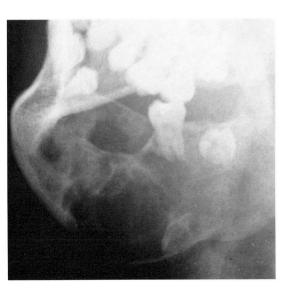

586 Aneurysmal bone cyst. OLM.

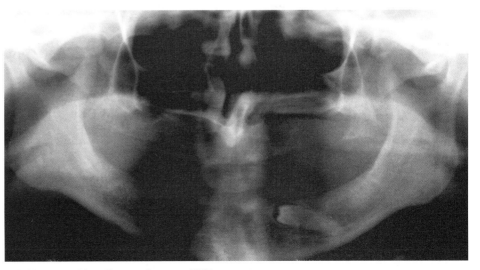

588 Pleomorphic salivary adenoma. DPR.

The axial (**589**) and coronal (**590**) scans reveal the size of the tumour and suggest that it is a benign, expansile lesion rather than an invasive one. In the planes illustrated, the slightly radio-opaque tumour (arrow) is shown expanding into the antrum and the lateral wall of the nose.

Langerhans' cell reticulosis (Histiocytosis X)

This condition is now known to arise from the abnormal proliferation of Langerhans cells and has been divided into three forms namely Letterer–Siwe disease, Hand–Schüller–Christian disease and eosinophilic granuloma, according to the clinical presentation.

Letterer–Siwe disease occurs in infants and is the most severe form. It affects both bone and soft tissues with lesions occurring throughout the body.

In Hand–Schüller–Christian disease, there are usually multiple deposits of tumour leading to a triad of symptoms of exophthalmos, diabetes insipidus due to pituitary damage and multiple bone lesions with clearly defined, punched-out margins. This form of the disease is usually diagnosed in the first two decades of life and extensive destruction of alveolar bone may result in premature loosening of the primary and/or permanent dentition. Such an example has been presented previously (see **368**). If the condition is extensive, extraction of teeth may be necessary, as in **591**, which shows two large deposits of tumour, one in the maxilla and one in the mandible. The lesions are radiolucent with clearly defined, rather lobulated margins and contain occasional incomplete septa. The cortical bone in the alveolar part of both jaws is eroded.

In adults, the tumour deposits may occur in the periapical region of the jaws, thus simulating periapical granulomas and presenting a difficulty in diagnosis. In the example (**592**), there is a radiolucent tumour deposit within the periapical and interdental tissues 1|123 . The lesion has an irregular margin, although it is clearly defined and there is loss of the lamina dura around the affected teeth.

In Hand–Schüller–Christian disease and Letterer–Siwe disease, multiple deposits of tumour are also often present in the skull. Several large, clearly defined radiolucent defects are present in the vault of the skull in the example (**593**), although the sella turcica appears normal. Erosion of the latter may be a feature of Hand–Schüller–Christian disease due to infiltration of the posterior part of the pituitary gland. Eosinophilic granulomas are a more localized, less aggressive form of the disease and are usually diagnosed in adolescents or adults. They may, however, reach a large size, as in **594** in the mandible, which extends from the lateral incisor region to the base of the ascending ramus. The lesion is clearly defined with a scalloped outline and is variably radiolucent with darker areas suggesting there has been erosion of the cortical plates. There is destruction of the alveolar bone apically around 3̄4̄ and widening of the periodontal ligament space mesially 3̄ .

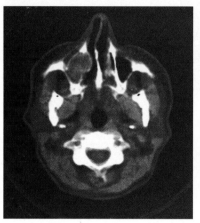

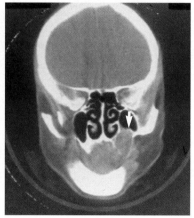

589 Pleomorphic salivary adenoma. CT.

590 Pleomorphic salivary adenoma. CT.

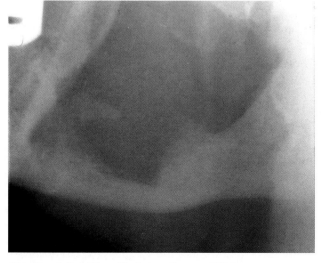

591 Hand–Schüller–Christian disease. OLM.

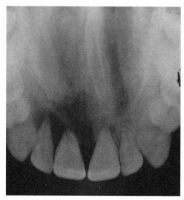

592 Hand–Schüller–Christian disease. USO.

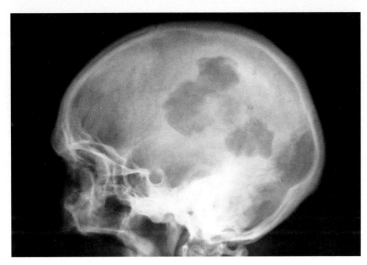

593 Hand–Schüller–Christian disease. L.

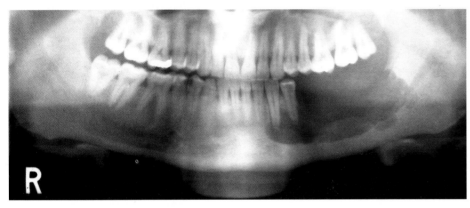

594 Eosinophilic granuloma. DPR.

Carcinomas

SQUAMOUS CELL CARCINOMA

Squamous cell carcinoma of the oral mucosa arises most commonly on the lateral margin or the ventral surface of the tongue, the floor of the mouth and the gingival and ridge mucosa, including that in the retromolar region. When it occurs in the mucosa closely related to the jaws, the underlying bone may become invaded and the infiltrating growth pattern produces poorly defined areas of radiolucency with irregular, destructive ragged margins. In the example (**595**) of a tumour which arose in the mucosa of the left retromolar region, there is invasion of the adjacent ramus of the mandible. There are irregularly shaped radio-opacities of varying size within the lesion, which are residual trabeculae of bone which have not yet been completely resorbed by the tumour. The carcinoma has spread anteriorly to ⎸7 , around which most of the alveolar bone has been destroyed and the cortical outlines of the internal and external oblique ridges of the anterior surface of the ramus are almost completely eroded – this is typical of a lesion that has grown into the mandible from the overlying tissues. A residual portion of the external oblique ridge can be seen within the lesion (arrow). Note the image of the transverse process (arrowhead) of the atlas vertebra projecting laterally beyond the maxillary molars.

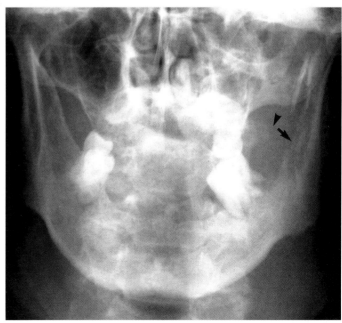

595 Squamous cell carcinoma of the retromolar mucosa with spread into the mandible. PA.

Another example (**596**) is shown, this time arising from the buccal mucosa, with invasion of the left side of the body and angle of an atrophic edentulous mandible. There is an extensive, poorly defined, variably radiolucent defect with a ragged, 'moth eaten' appearance typical of an invasive tumour. The step-like irregularity of the inferior border, together with the loss of a distinct cortical outline, is indicative of a pathological fracture. The soft tissues lying inferolaterally to the mandible are expanded due to spread of the tumour.

A further example (**597**) shows an extensive tumour invading the left side of the body of the mandible and a pathological fracture with a step deformity of the inferior border.

PRIMARY INTRA-OSSEOUS CARCINOMA

Rarely, a carcinoma arises primarily from epithelial residues in the jaw bones, usually the mandible and thus the tumour grows outwards from within the bone. In the lesion (**598**) in the body of the left side of the mandible, there is an extensive, 'moth eaten' area of radiolucency which is poorly defined and extends from the $\overline{5}$ region to the posterior border of the ramus. The 'moth eaten' appearance is characterized by numerous, randomly scattered, pinhead-sized foci of radiolucency throughout the tumour where the infiltrative pattern of bone destruction is more advanced. In the molar region, at the inferior border of the mandible, the cortical bone has been eroded and there is a more confluent radiolucent defect in the alveolar process. Much of the alveolar bone around $\overline{8}$ has been destroyed. The diffuse loss of bone has distorted the outline of the inferior alveolar canal over much of its course, although it can still be identified in the ramus and $\overline{8}$ region.

CARCINOMA ARISING IN AN ODONTOGENIC CYST

Occasionally a squamous cell carcinoma may develop in the epithelial lining of an odontogenic cyst. These tumours are usually diagnosed in elderly patients, suggesting that a cyst has been present for some conserable time before the development of the carcinoma. Such transformation has been reported in residual cysts as well as odontogenic keratocysts and the lesions are low grade carcinomas that cause slow destruction of bone. In example **599** the lesion is radiolucent and quite well circumscribed anteriorly at the site of the original cyst. The definition is less clear distally and crestally where there is evidence of infiltration. There is also a step deformity of the inferior border of the mandible due to a pathological fracture.

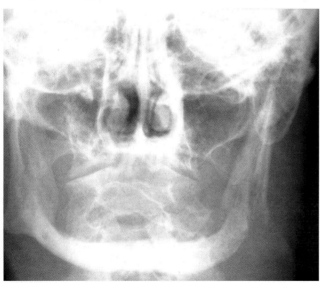

596 Squamous cell carcinoma of the buccal mucosa with spread into the mandible. PA.

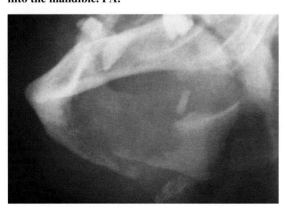

597 Squamous cell carcinoma of the floor of the mouth with extensive spread into the mandible. OLM.

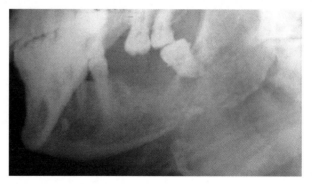

598 Primary intra-osseous carcinoma. OLM.

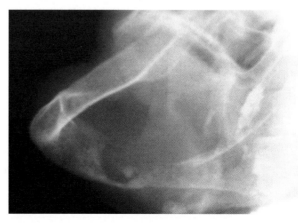

599 Squamous cell carcinoma arising in a residual cyst. OLM.

MUCO-EPIDERMOID CARCINOMA

Although approximately 45% of tumours of the minor salivary glands are malignant, there is considerable variation in the degree and pattern of local invasion and a wide range of histological types of salivary gland neoplasms is now recognized. The most commonly occurring malignant tumours are adenoid cystic carcinomas, muco-epidermoid carcinomas and polymorphous low grade adenocarcinomas. The underlying bone of the maxilla or the mandible may become involved by lesions arising from salivary glands in the adjacent mucosa. Illustration **600** shows an example of such a relatively slowly growing muco-epidermoid carcinoma which has arisen in the mucosa of the left retromolar region of the mandible, with invasion of the anterior part of the ramus, which is expanded. There is an irregularly loculated radiolucent defect and many of the locules are surrounded by radio-opaque laminae. Because of the slow rate of growth, reactive bone formation may occur and in this example there are numerous, irregular, radio-opaque trabeculae within the tumour.

BASAL CELL CARCINOMA

These neoplasms usually arise from the epithelium of the skin but occasionally they may occur on the oral mucosa, as in **601** in the right retromolar region which has invaded the underlying mandible. There is a quite well defined, radiolucent defect with a scalloped outline and loss of the radio-opaque cortical margin of the internal oblique ridge.

METASTATIC CARCINOMA

Metastatic tumours of the jaws are most likely to arise in areas where there are residues of erythropoietic marrow, for example in the molar and retromolar regions of the mandible. The most common sites for the primary lesions are the lung, breast, gastrointestinal tract and prostate. As a consequence, the metastases are more commonly adenocarcinomas rather than squamous cell carcinomas. The majority of metastatic deposits appear as single or multiple ill defined osteolytic areas. However, some lesions – notably those from the prostate gland – may demonstrate radio-opacity due to bone deposition. The first example (**602**) shows a metastatic tumour originating from a primary carcinoma of the lung, presenting as a large, radiolucency in the left ascending ramus of the mandible. The boundary is irregular, ill defined and involves the proximal part of the inferior alveolar canal.

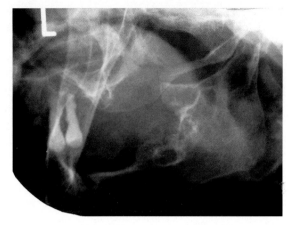

600 Muco-epidermoid carcinoma arising in the retromolar mucosa with spread into the mandible. OLM.

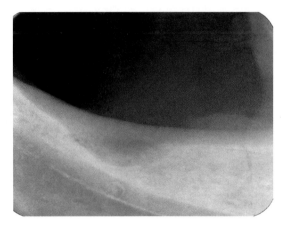

601 Basal cell carcinoma in the retromolar region with spread into the mandible. P.

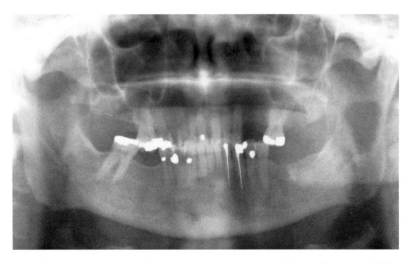

602 Metastatic carcinoma from a primary tumour arising in the lung. DPR.

Another example (**603**) is that of a metastatic carcinoma from a primary tumour in the breast, occurring in the body of the right side of the mandible. The lesion is patchy and poorly defined and extends from 8̅| region to the midline and from the alveolar crest to the inferior border. The remaining radio-opaque trabeculae within the radiolucency have become resorbed and indistinct, especially at the lower border of the mandible.

The next example (**604**) shows a metastatic carcinoma in the left side of the body of an edentulous mandible, which has arisen from a primary tumour in the prostate. There is a poorly defined, radiolucent lesion with a 'moth eaten' appearance in which numerous radio-opaque, irregularly shaped trabeculae of reactive bone are present. The latter are particularly well demonstrated (arrows) within the region of the mass that extends beyond the mandible as a radio-opaque, soft tissue swelling. Such metastases are described as osteoplastic and are a particular feature of carcinoma of the prostate.

When metastatic tumours are suspected, scintiscanning (SC) may be a useful adjunct to diagnosis and may reveal other unsuspected deposits in the skeleton. In example **605** the dark 'hot spot' at the site of the jaw metastasis is prominent, although in this case no other intra-osseous metastases are apparent. The circular hot spot in the pelvic region is due to the accumulation of radioactive material in the bladder.

Sarcomas

OSTEOGENIC SARCOMA

Osteogenic sarcomas usually arise centrally within bone and rapidly destroy the overlying cortex. Less frequently they arise from the periosteal surface of the bone (juxtacortical osteogenic sarcoma) in which situation they are less aggressive. In the jaws, osteogenic sarcomas occur more commonly in males between the ages of 20 and 40, although they may also arise as a complication of Paget's disease in older people. According to the degree of differentiation of the tumour cells, variable amounts of bone may be deposited and so the radiographic picture may vary. In the early stages a characteristic feature is widening of the periodontal ligament spaces and the inferior alveolar canal, due to infiltration of poorly mineralized tumour tissue along these anatomical pathways. In the example (**606**) there is obvious widening of the radiolucent periodontal ligament space around |34 6 .

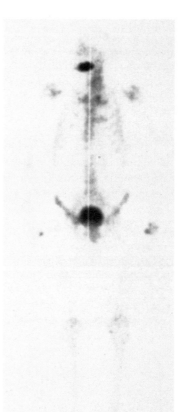

605 Metastatic carcinoma from a primary tumour arising in the prostate gland. SC.

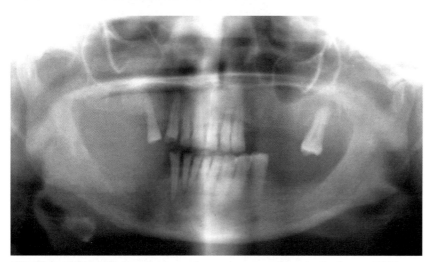

603 Metastatic carcinoma from a primary tumour arising in the breast. DPR.

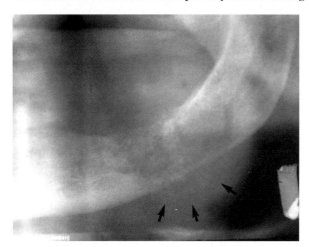

604 Metastatic carcinoma from a primary tumour arising in the prostate gland. DPR.

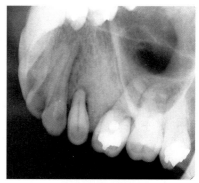

606 Osteogenic sarcoma. UOO.

The adjacent bone has an increased radio-opacity and a granular appearance, particularly between |46 and the margins are poorly defined. The DPR **607** confirms the malignant nature of the lesion as indicated by the loss of the cortical lamina outlining the antral floor between |4 and |8 . Note the fragment of root filling material in the coronal part of |3 which was placed at an early stage when the lesion was misdiagnosed as a periapical infection.

As the tumour grows beyond the confines of the cortices of the bone in which it has arisen, bone is deposited in a radial, 'sunray' pattern, visible beyond the original bony outline. In the next example (**608**), the cortical bone in the region of the angle of the mandible has been eroded and there are radiating spicules of tumour bone projecting inferiorly, giving this classic 'sunray' appearance. The image of the hyoid bone is superimposed upon the tumour and appears as a radio-opacity over the distal part of the third molar root. Note the recent extraction socket |6̄ with a small circular area of osteosclerosis apical to the distal root and a similar area close to the mesial root |7̄ , both of which are incidental findings.

The final example (**609**) shows a very large tumour involving the entire left side of the mandible. The original bony outline of the mandible is still faintly discernible; radiating from it in all directions are numerous, coarse, radio-opaque trabeculations of tumour bone which become progressively thinner towards the outer surface. The tumour is covered inferiorly by a thickened, soft tissue shadow. The trabeculations of tumour bone show some variation in width and radio-opacity according to their stage of development and the degree to which they are mineralized. The air shadow of the pharynx, larynx and trachea is displaced to the right, indicating that the tumour has spread inferomedially to involve these structures.

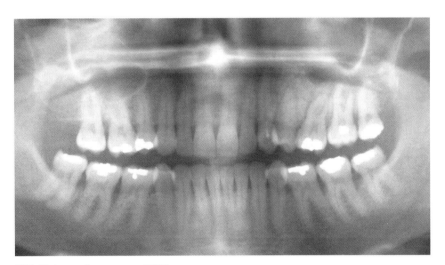

607 Osteogenic sarcoma. DPR.

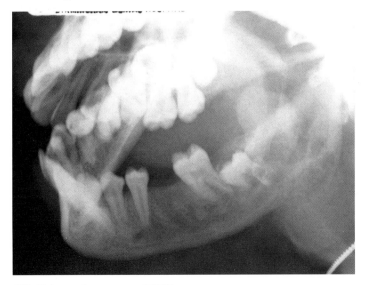

608 Osteogenic sarcoma. OLM.

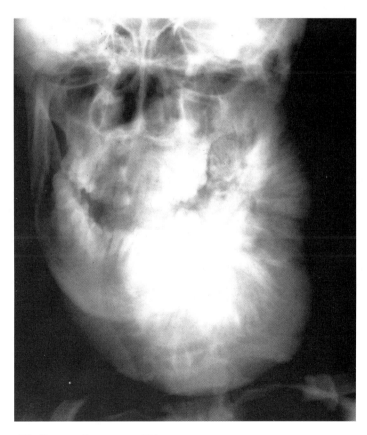

609 Osteogenic sarcoma. PA.

CHONDROSARCOMA

These are rare tumours of the jaw bones, tending to occur from the fourth decade onwards. They occur more commonly in the maxilla and may arise centrally or peripherally. The example **610** shows a poorly defined, radiolucent area with indistinct margins at the base of the right ramus of the mandible with thinning of the cortical bone at the inferior border. On the intra-oral radiograph (**611**) there is an absence of the normal trabecular bone pattern and this contrasts with the bone around the roots $\overline{6|}$. A second example (**612**) in the anterior part of the maxilla, shows an extensive lesion with poorly defined margins.

EWING'S SARCOMA

This tumour usually occurs in children or young adults and is rare in the jaws. It is a rapidly growing lesion that produces early widespread metastases. The example (**613**) shows a poorly defined mass in the left side of the body of the mandible extending from $\overline{5|}$ to $\overline{8|}$. The lesion is variably radiolucent with speckled radio-opacity and there is loss of the normal pattern of the bone trabeculae. Where the mass protrudes below the inferior border there is a faint sunray pattern caused by the formation of reactive bone. $\overline{67|}$ have been displaced superiorly and there is almost total destruction of the supporting bone around $\overline{7|}$ which is displaced posteriorly, as is the unerupted $\overline{8|}$. At a less advanced stage of these lesions, the reactive bone may show a more laminated, 'onion skin' type of reaction on the periosteal surface of the bone.

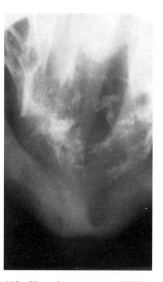

612 Chondrosarcoma. UTO.

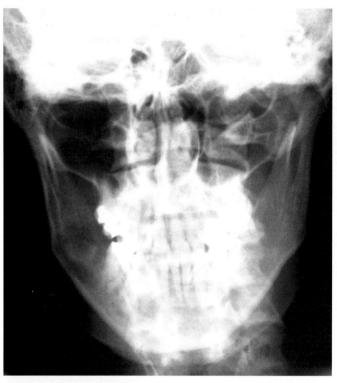

610 Chondrosarcoma. PA.

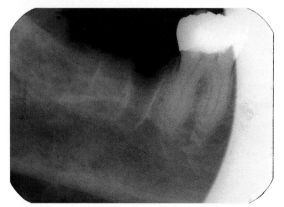

611 Chondrosarcoma. P.

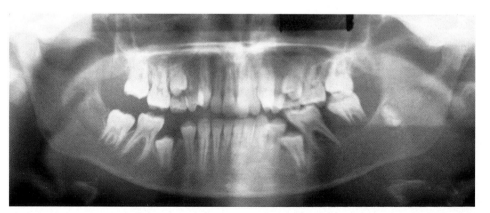

613 Ewing's sarcoma. DPR.

FIBROSARCOMA

Fibrosarcomas are also rare tumours of the jaw bones, but they occasionally arise from the intrinsic fibrous tissue of the bone or in association with the sheaths of the nerves which pass through them (neurofibrosarcoma). They tend to occur from the fourth decade onwards. The example (**614**) shows a tumour in the left molar region of the mandible which has grown into the socket |6 , a few months after the tooth had been extracted. There is a poorly defined, radiolucent area with ragged, ill defined margins except mesially, where remnants of the lamina dura of the mesial wall of the |6 socket are still present. The dome-shaped, soft tissue mass (arrows) on to which |7 was occluding is just visible above the bony defect.

The second example (**615**) shows a larger tumour of the right body and ramus of the mandible, extending from the premolar region to the base of the coronoid process. The radiolucent lesion has caused considerable bone destruction and its boundary is more clearly defined buccally than lingually, where more of the cortical bone has been eroded. Note the calcified pineal gland (arrow) projected over the middle of the frontal sinus.

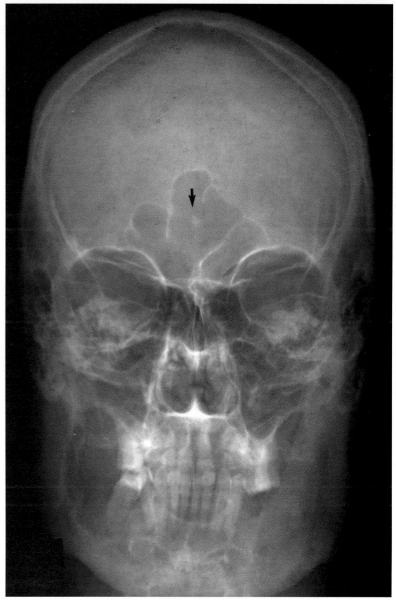

615 Fibrosarcoma. PA.

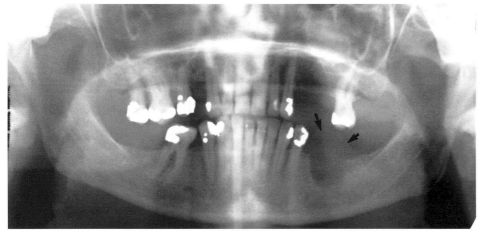

614 Fibrosarcoma. DPR.

MALIGNANT FIBROUS HISTIOCYTOMA

This is an aggressive form of sarcoma which, although more frequent in the soft tissues, may also occur in the bones. Multiple lesions are common. In **616** there is loss of the normal trabecular pattern in the right molar and premolar region of the maxilla and a diffuse radio-opacity in the lower half of the right antrum. The cortical outline of the floor of the antrum is absent. All the features suggest the presence of an infiltrating tumour. These changes are confirmed in the periapical radiograph (**617**) which also demonstrates the destruction of the lamina dura, mesially to 6⌋ .

Multiple myelomatosis

This malignant tumour of plasma cells occurs most commonly in males between 40 and 70 years of age and is characterized by the presence of multifocal osteolytic tumour deposits which may involve the jaw bones. It is, however, unusual for the jaws to be affected before other bones. In this example (**618**, **619**) there are multiple irregularly loculated, radiolucent areas of bone destruction with ill defined outlines, affecting predominantly the alveolar bone ⌐3–6 around which the lamina dura has been destroyed. Areas of bone resorption are superimposed upon the apices of the roots of these teeth, giving an appearance that may be confused with root resorption. There is, however, resorption of the apex ⌐4 as indicated by its shortened, irregularly concave outline.

In another example (**620**), in addition to lesions in the ramus of the mandible, there are skull deposits, of varying size, shape and density, most of them being clearly defined with a characteristic 'punched out' appearance.

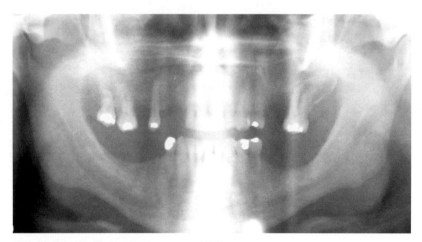

616 Malignant fibrous histiocytoma. DPR.

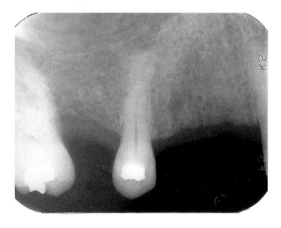

617 Malignant fibrous histiocytoma. P.

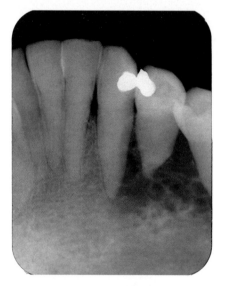

618 Multiple myelomatosis. P.

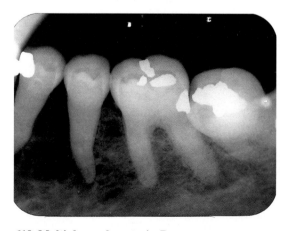

619 Multiple myelomatosis. P.

Malignant lymphoma

Extranodal lymphomas occasionally arise in and around the jaws and are usually of the non-Hodgkin's type, derived from B cells. Lymphomas that involve bone produce ill defined radiolucent destructive lesions. In the example (**621**) of a centrally arising lymphoma in the $\overline{654|}$ region, there is a poorly defined radiolucency of variable density within which the trabeculae show an abnormal pattern. The periodontal ligament space $\overline{6|}$ is irregularly widened with loss of most of the lamina dura around the distal root. Although $\overline{7|}$ was extracted only a few weeks before and the radiolucent socket persists, the lamina dura is absent and is surrounded by some osteosclerosis.

Burkitt's lymphoma

Burkitt's lymphoma is a particular form of lymphoma which is endemic in certain parts of the world, notably central Africa and New Guinea. It usually affects children between 5 and 15 years of age with multiple lesions being common in the jaws. The tumour occurs spasmodically in other parts of the world, but these cases are usually diagnosed in older individuals. The radiological appearance is that of expansion of the jaws accompanied by multiple, poorly defined radiolucent tumour masses which may affect all four quadrants. The lamina dura of affected teeth is extensively destroyed. The example (**622**) shows a large, ill defined lesion in the right side of the mandible of a 13-year-old, which is particularly radiolucent in the anterior part of the ascending ramus. There is advanced bone destruction around $\overline{5|}$ giving the appearance of exfoliation of the tooth.

Malignant melanoma

Malignant melanoma occasionally arises in the oral soft tissues where it has a predilection for the palatal mucosa. Invasion of the underlying maxilla is an early feature. In the example (**623**), the tumour has arisen in the right maxillary premolar/molar region in a patient with long-standing chronic periodontitis and there is advanced loss of alveolar bone around the standing teeth. The tumour involves the gingival mucosa; the soft tissue swelling is clearly displayed. The bone deep to the mass, particularly in relation to $5|$, exhibits increased radiolucency with an ill defined, margin and loss of surface cortical lamina due to invasion by the infiltrating tumour. $5|$ has been displaced by the lesion, and the radio-opaque lamina outlining the floor of the antrum is incomplete anteriorly, suggesting early destruction.

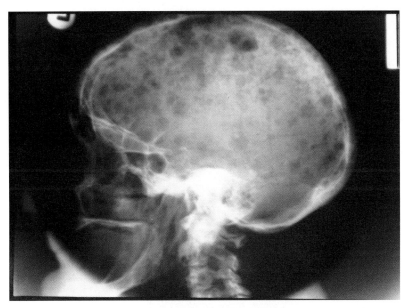

620 (above) Multiple myelomatosis. L.

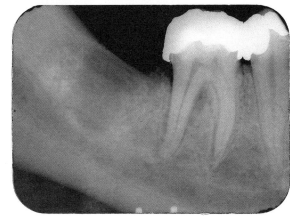

621 Malignant lymphoma. P.

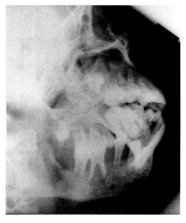

622 Burkitt's lymphoma. OLM.

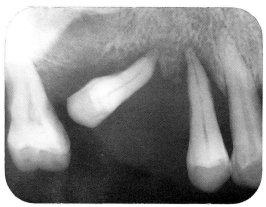

623 Malignant melanoma. P.

Malignant granuloma of the maxilla

These lesions – some of which have been shown to be a type of lymphoma – usually arise in the midline of the upper jaw. In the example (**624**) however, the condition affects the edentulous, left maxillary ridge extending from the |4 socket to the mesial aspect |7 . The bony architecture is indistinct and the lack of definition of the radio-opaque lamina of the floor of the antrum is particularly noticeable. Overall the margins of the lesion are ill defined. Bone destruction is more advanced on the edentulous ridge where, in most parts, the cortical bone has been completely destroyed and the surface is ragged and contains irregular, separate, radio-opaque fragments of incompletely resorbed bony trabeculae.

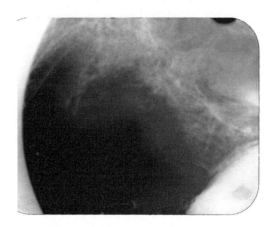

624 Malignant granuloma of the maxilla. P.

Metabolic conditions

Being part of the skeleton, the mandible and the maxilla are often involved in more generalized disorders of bone. Hence radiographic changes seen in the jaws justify the use of other types of imaging to investigate the provisional diagnosis of more widespread bone disease. Such investigation may include a radiographic survey of the whole skeleton or of selected bones. The presence of subperiosteal cortical erosions in the carpals and metacarpals would, for example, support a suspected diagnosis of hyperparathyroidism. Similarly, US and/or SC with a radioactively labelled, parathyroid-seeking chemical may assist in the diagnosis of a parathyroid adenoma. SC of the skeleton using a technetium-labelled, bone-seeking chemical may also be helpful in assessing the extent of metabolic disease of bone.

Osteoporosis

Osteoporosis is a condition in which there is a reduction in bone mass and density but the bone remains histologically normal. The condition is broadly classified into two types: primary and secondary. Primary osteoporosis is an age-related phenomenon and particularly affects post-menopausal women; secondary osteoporosis occurs as a result of accelerated bone loss (in disorders such as hyperparathyroidism) or as a complication of prolonged steroid therapy. Initially osteoporosis affects the cancellous bone and is therefore seen in those parts of the skeleton which contain relatively large proportions of this type of bone, e.g. the vertebrae. However, other bones may also be affected to a variable extent. The radiological appearances include a decrease in bone density, a reduction in the number of bone trabeculae and a thinning of the cortices. In **625** these appearances are particularly noticeable in the mandible where the cortex of the lower border is thinned and the laminae of the inferior alveolar canal are absent.

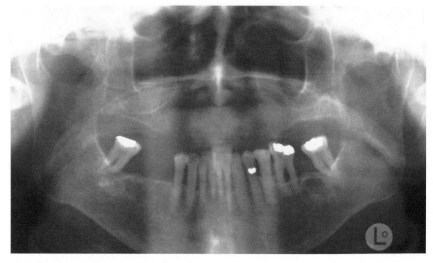

625 Osteoporosis. DPR.

Acromegaly

This condition occurs in young adults and is caused by excess secretion of growth hormone from the pituitary gland, usually due to the presence of an adenoma. Excess production of growth hormone in the young results in gigantism (where generalized growth is still possible) but in acromegaly the potential for active growth persists at only a few sites, such as the cartilage in the mandibular condyle. In the example (**626**), there is gross elongation of all parts of the mandible resulting in prognathism, prominence of the mental process and markedly obtuse angles. The pituitary fossa (sella turcica) is enlarged, with thinning of the posterior wall. In addition, there is general thickening of the diploë of the vault of the skull.

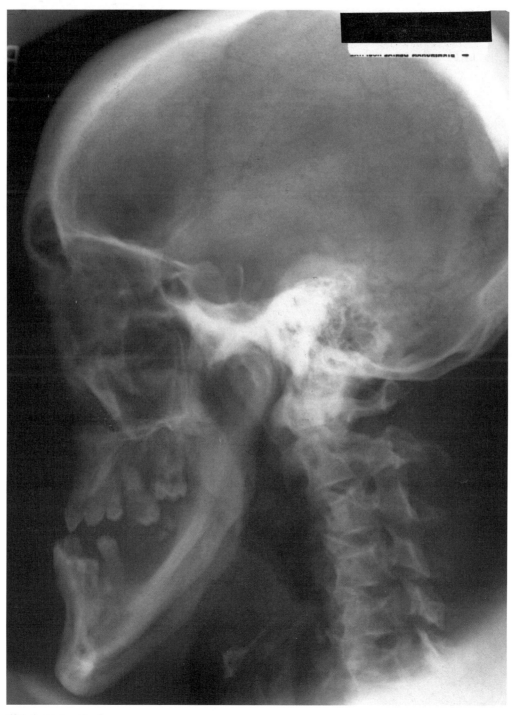

626 Acromegaly. L.

Paget's disease of bone (Osteitis deformans)

The cause of this generalized disturbance of bone metabolism is uncertain, but the condition is more common in individuals over the age of 40. In its early stages it is characterized by bone resorption, whereas in the later stages there is deposition of excessive amounts of increasingly dense bone. These progressive changes, which in the jaws are more common in the maxilla, may occur at different rates in adjacent parts of the same bone and thus a very variable radiographic appearance may be seen. Typical dental features include hypercementosis, an absence of a distinct lamina dura and focal areas of bony sclerosis in the periapical regions.

In the first example (627, 628, 629) the normal trabecular pattern of the maxilla is lost and the bone has a diffuse granular appearance. In several areas there are irregularly shaped, radio-opaque masses of varying size where bone sclerosis has occurred. The latter changes, which are particularly marked in the |34 region, contribute to the typical 'cotton wool' appearance of the condition. The expansion of the maxilla has resulted in spacing of the teeth, most of which exhibit bulbosities of the apices of their roots due to hypercementosis. The lamina dura around the roots of the teeth is obscured in many areas, as are the boundaries of the antrum and the floor of the nose in the occlusal radiograph 627. The early resorptive stage of the disease is often particularly obvious in the vault of the skull and gives rise to confluent areas of radiolucency, usually starting anteriorly. This appearance is known as osteoporosis circumscripta.

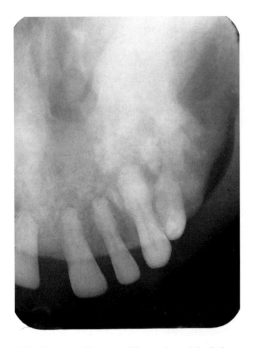

627 Paget's disease of bone (osteitis deformans). UOO.

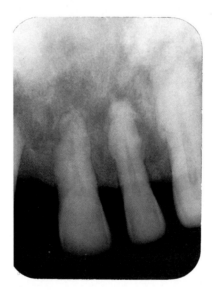

628 Paget's disease of bone (osteitis deformans). P.

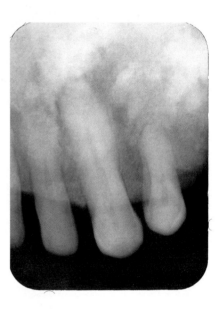

629 Paget's disease of bone (osteitis deformans). P.

In the example (**630**), the radiolucency extends across the lower part of the vault from front to back and has a scalloped superior margin. Anteriorly there is thinning of the diploë above the frontal sinus. Note the oval outline of the pinna of the ear encircling the dense radio-opaque image of the petrous part of the base of the skull. In the osteosclerotic stage, there is often involvement of the skull and the jaws.

The next example (**631**) illustrates an advanced case in an edentulous patient. The bones of the vault of the skull show patchy radio-opaci-

ties of varying size, shape and density, together with scattered, poorly defined, radiolucent areas forming the classic 'cotton wool' appearance. There is marked thickening and sclerosis of the diploë anteriorly and thinning in the basi-occipital region. Both antra are almost fully occluded by abnormal bone and there is marked enlargement and thickening of the alveolar part of the maxilla, which exhibits a more granular pattern of radio-opacity in the DPR **632**. The mandible is unaffected.

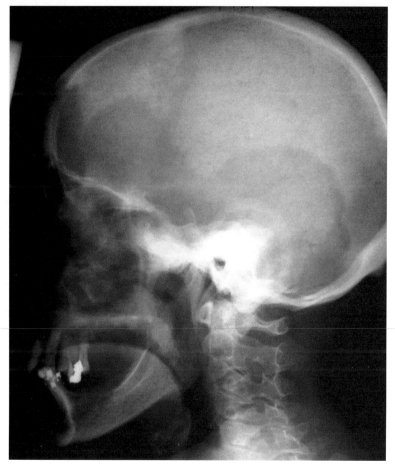

630 Paget's disease of bone (osteitis deformans). L.

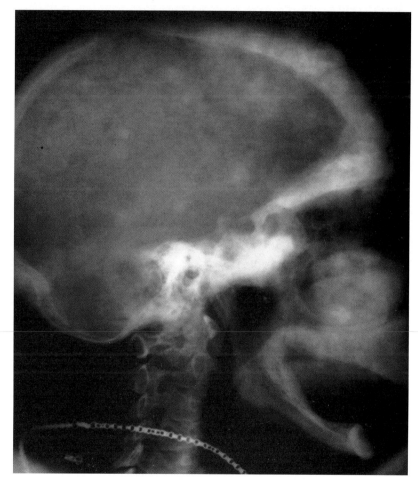

631 Paget's disease of bone (osteitis deformans). L.

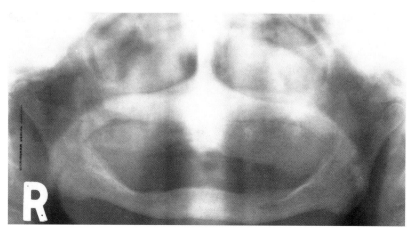

632 Paget's disease of bone (osteitis deformans). DPR

Hyperparathyroidism

This condition may be primary, due to the secretion of excess parathormone by a parathyroid adenoma, or secondary and tertiary due to various forms of renal disease. As a consequence, mineral is removed from the skeleton by bone resorption and these changes may be first detected in the jaws. The bone loss may be either focal in pattern or diffuse and, in extreme cases, may result in pathological fracture. If focal, there is a radiolucent, cyst-like defect, with a clearly defined outline which may be smooth or loculated.

In the example (633) there is a clearly defined lesion, with a loculated margin extending from $\overline{2|}$ to $\overline{|6}$ with thinning of the inferior border of the mandible and some resorption of the apices $\overline{|245}$. Although soft tissue mineralizations are common in the kidneys and the joints due to the raised levels of blood calcium, they are rare elsewhere. In this patient there are irregular, radio-opaque areas of mineralization superimposed upon the rami of the mandible, which probably represent areas of dystrophic mineralization of the soft tissues as a result of hypercalcaemia. Note the periapical osteosclerosis $\overline{|6}$ which has a large pinned amalgam restoration and the recent extraction socket $\overline{|6}$. If diffuse, the changes affect all parts of the jaws. In particular there is a generalized loss of the lamina dura with osteoporosis which is manifested as an overall radiolucency of the bone, as seen in the final example (634).

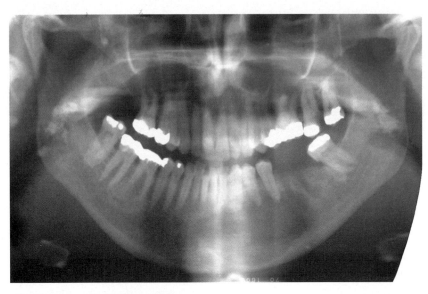

633 Hyperparathyroidism. DPR.

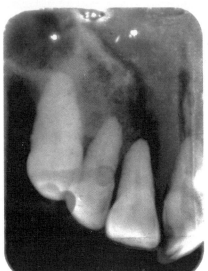
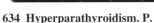
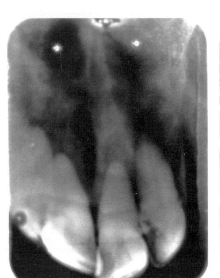
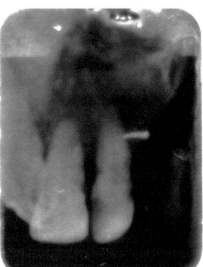

634 Hyperparathyroidism. P.

Iatrogenic conditions

Treatment of disorders of the teeth and jaws may give rise to characteristic radiographic appearances, either as a normal consequence of the treatment procedure or as an unwanted complication. The extraction of teeth, for example, is followed by a complex healing process of the socket with a characteristic sequence of radiographic changes. Radiotherapy for tumours close to the jaws may result in bone being included in the field of irradiation, with the subsequent hazard of necrosis and infection. Extraction of teeth may also lead to unwanted side affects under these circumstances.

Extraction sockets

The extraction of a tooth leaves a blood-filled socket which becomes organized over a period of several months and replaced by bone. Initially the socket is filled with woven bone, which is often relatively poorly mineralized, but subsequently with lamella bone which appears similar to that of the adjacent bone. In addition, the alveolar bone crests and lamina dura of the socket wall are progressively resorbed and remodelled, so that after a period of three to six months, there is usually no further radiological evidence of the pre-existing tooth socket.

In the first example (**635**), the sockets of the mandibular incisors and canines are shown following the recent extraction of these teeth. The lamina dura is still intact around the margins of the sockets and there is no evidence of bony repair. The crest of the interdental septum $\overline{21}$ has been fractured and is displaced slightly medially.

In the next example (**636**) showing some maxillary premolar sockets, several weeks after extraction of the teeth, the interdental septa and lamina dura are still clearly visible and there is early infilling of their apical parts with bone. The radio-opaque lamina of the antral floor runs vertically above the $\underline{5|}$ socket, and the root of the zygomatic process overlies the $\underline{65|}$ sockets.

In a further example (**637**) showing an $\overline{8}$ socket, approximately six weeks after the tooth extraction, the lamina dura outlining its original boundary is still discernible, although not clearly defined, indicating that remodelling is in progress. The socket is largely filled in with poorly mineralized reparative bone and is thus still relatively radiolucent. The rate of healing of a tooth socket is very variable and may be influenced by many factors, such as the presence of foreign material.

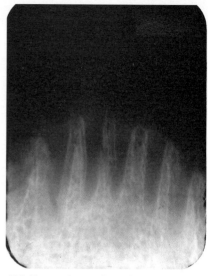

635 Extraction sockets. P.

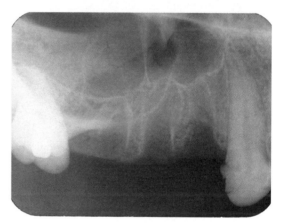

636 Extraction sockets. P.

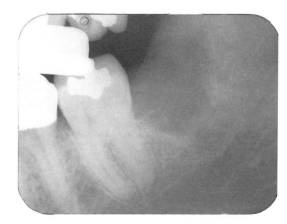

637 Extraction socket. P.

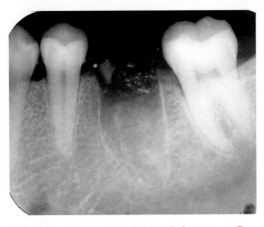

638 Extraction socket with tooth fragments. P.

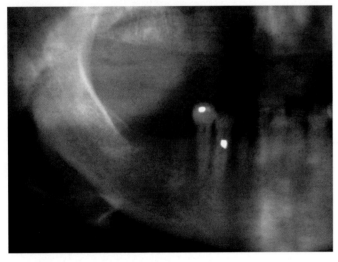

639 Extraction socket sclerosis. DPR.

In the example (**638**) showing a 6̲ socket approximately six weeks after extraction of the tooth, the apical part is healing normally and has been infilled with reparative bone, although the lamina dura is still just discernible. However, the coronal part contains several radio-opaque bodies and there is no evidence of bony repair in this area. The larger mesial body is a tooth fragment, while the numerous, fine, more dense particles are remnants of filling material.

Sometimes, the process of bone infilling is excessive and the residual socket can still be identified from sclerotic deposits of bone, which may resemble retained tooth roots. The example (**639**) shows a 5̲ socket in which the lamina dura is still just visible, but the bone within the socket is more radio-opaque than the surrounding tissue.

In the second example (**640**) both root sockets 7̅ and the distal root socket 6̅ are uniformly more densely radio-opaque than the surrounding bone, although there is no obvious presence of the lamina dura. The lack of a periodontal ligament space and root canals distinguishes these sclerotic extraction sockets from retained tooth roots. In addition, in this example, there is periapical osteosclerosis 4̅.

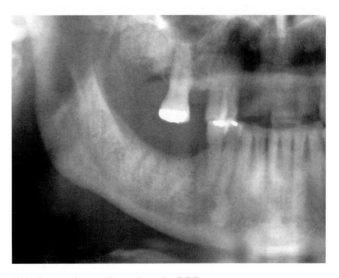

640 Extraction socket sclerosis. DPR.

Iatrogenic fracture of the mandible

The example (**641**) shows an iatrogenic fracture of the mandible, which occurred during the attempted removal of $\overline{8|}$, running from the tooth socket obliquely backwards towards the angle of the mandible. The mesial root of the tooth is retained. Note the medial displacement of the ascending ramus due to the forces of the attached muscles, the $\overline{|8}$ socket and the transversely positioned $\underline{|8}$.

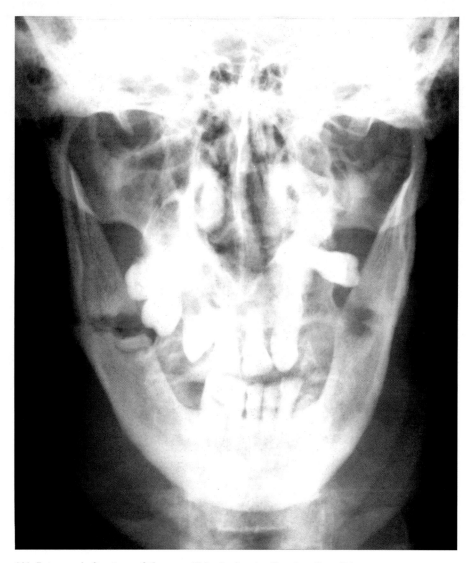

641 Iatrogenic fracture of the mandible during tooth extraction. PA.

Osteoradionecrosis

Exposure of bone to ionizing radiation may lead to localized areas of necrosis, following the development of endarteritis obliterans in the blood vessels of the irradiated bone. Because of the distribution of its blood supply, the mandible is more frequently affected, as in the example (**642, 643**) of a patient who had received radiotherapy some years previously for a squamous cell carcinoma of the floor of the mouth. There is an ill defined, irregular radiolucency of the body of the mandible extending from $\overline{6|}$ to $\overline{|6}$, reaching to the inferior border in several places. Within the affected area, the normal trabecular pattern of the bone is absent and there is a coarsely mottled appearance with some clearly defined areas of radiolucency. A large radio-opaque sequestrum (arrows) is present in the alveolar part of the incisor region.

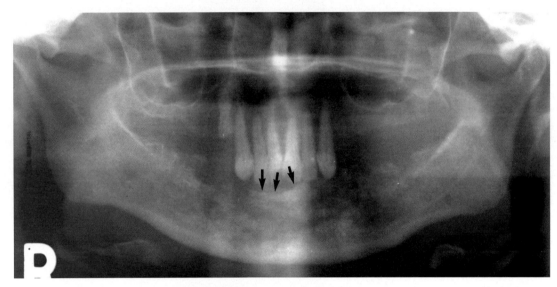

642 Osteoradionecrosis of the mandible. DPR.

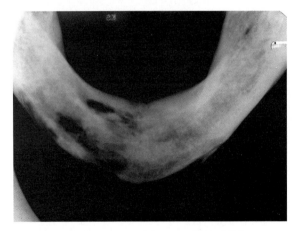

643 Osteoradionecrosis of the mandible. LTO.

7

The temporomandibular joint

Introduction

Radiography of the temporomandibular joint may be complicated by the superimposition of one joint upon the other when viewed in a lateral direction or by other anatomical structures when viewed in an anteroposterior direction. To overcome these effects it is necessary to employ oblique views or tomography. Plain radiographs display the osseous structures of the joint but provide little information about the soft tissue components such as the articular disc. Hence plain radiographs are mainly used to demonstrate disorders of the condylar neck and head and the articular surfaces. The position and form of the disc may be assessed by arthrographic techniques, MRI and to a lesser extent by CT. The latter two procedures also have the advantage of being non invasive. Dynamic studies of the disc position may be demonstrated on video fluoroscopy or with multiple view video-loop MR techniques. Occasionally radionuclide imaging of the joints is undertaken using a labelled isotope technetium 99m to assess bone activity which may be increased in hyperplastic or neoplastic conditions.

Developmental conditions

Condylar hypoplasia

Hypoplasia of the mandibular condyle is uncommon and arises as a genetically determined growth abnormality, as a consequence of trauma affecting the condylar head or as a result of disease of adjacent structures, such as the middle ear. If genetically determined, it is often part of a wider growth abnormality and may be bilateral. In **644** – an eight-year-old child – the right mandibular condyle is rudimentary but the neck is widened anteroposteriorly with a deep, V-shaped sigmoid notch. There is underdevelopment of the right side of the mandible, the ramus of which is medially positioned relative to the other side, causing facial asymmetry (**645**)

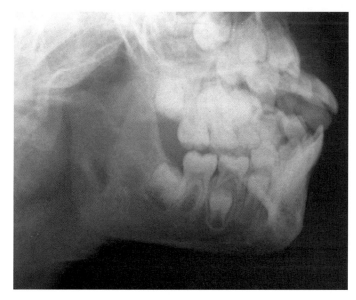

644 Condylar hypoplasia. OLM.

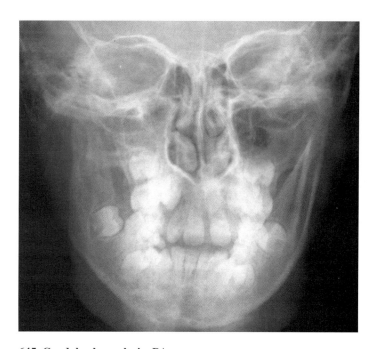

645 Condylar hypoplasia. PA.

221

Condylar hyperplasia

Hyperplasia of the mandibular condyle is also uncommon and is a consequence of overactivity in the secondary cartilage in the condylar head. It is usually diagnosed in the second and third decades of life and may occur in association with systemic diseases such as pituitary gigantism and acromegaly, when it is bilateral. More frequently however it is unilateral and not associated with other abnormalities. Excessive growth of the mandibular condyle usually results in abnormalities of the shape of the mandible on the affected side and can be divided into two basic types. In one there is enlargement and abnormality of the shape of the condylar head, often associated with distortion of the body and ramus of the mandible on the affected side and a lateral open bite. In this type there is usually little or no alteration in the position of the midline of the mandible. In the other, it is the neck of the condyle which is elongated, but the shape of the body and ramus of the mandible is relatively normal, although the midline is displaced away from the affected side.

In the first example (646), in a 15-year-old with enlargement of the head of the left mandibular condyle, the hyperplasia has caused marked bowing of the inferior border of the mandible, with a prominent, lateral open bite on the affected side and only minimal displacement of the midline of the mandible. The inferior alveolar canal (647) is positioned closer to the inferior border of the mandible on the affected side, a feature seen in this form of the condition.

In the next example (648) in an adult, there is gross enlargement of the left condyle with thickening of the condylar neck. There is no obvious asymmetry or deviation of the midline of the mandible. Another example (649) in an adult shows enlargement of the right condylar head, which projects antero-inferiorly, and downward displacement of the inferior border of the body of the mandible and hence the occlusal plane on the right.

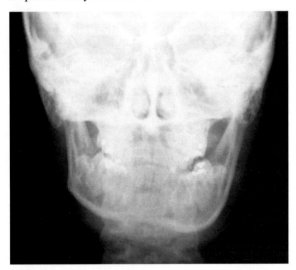

646 Condylar hyperplasia. PA.

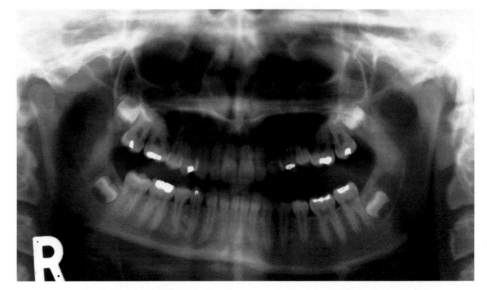

647 Condylar hyperplasia. DPR.

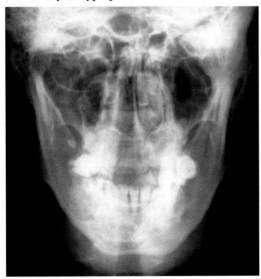

648 Condylar hyperplasia. PA.

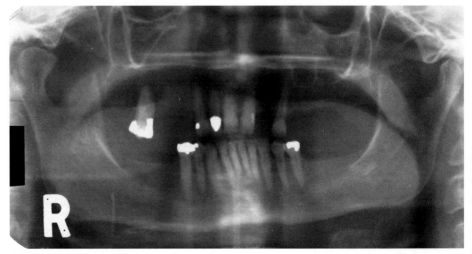

649 Condylar hyperplasia. DPR.

In the example (**650**) of the second type of condylar hyperplasia, the neck of the right condyle is elongated although the head is approximately normal in size. In this 16-year-old there is anterior displacement of the body of the mandible and a shift of the midline away from the affected side. All the mandibular teeth remain in occlusion, but their anterior displacement has resulted in 7̲| being out of occlusion and over erupted. There is no obvious bowing of the inferior border of the mandible.

Conventional radiographs do not allow any conclusions to be drawn about the level of osteoblastic activity in the affected condyle, particularly when the head remains relatively normal in size. Scintiscanning is useful under these circumstances – as in example **651** – where there is a zone of increased uptake of the radioisotope within the affected side (arrow). A further example (**652**) of marked elongation of the mandibular condyle illustrates how tomography in a lateral position is useful to demonstrate the extent of the change.

Inflammatory conditions and their sequelae

Rheumatoid arthritis

Although rheumatoid arthritis is a relatively common disease typically affecting the joints of the hands and feet in females of middle age and above, the temporomandibular joints alone are only rarely involved. When they do become affected it is usually in patients with established disease in other joints. The joint surfaces are replaced by granulation tissue which progressively erodes the underlying bone. The main radiographic features are flattening and erosion of the condylar heads. In the example (**653**) in a 40-year-old, a transcranial view of the right temporomandibular joint shows an irregular, oval radiolucency in the condylar head and narrowing of the joint space.

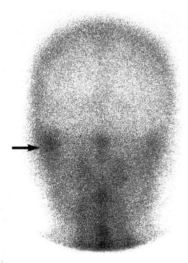

650 Condylar hyperplasia. DPR.

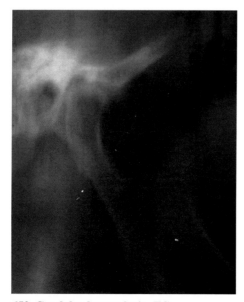

651 Condylar hyperplasia. SC.

652 Condylar hyperplasia. TG.

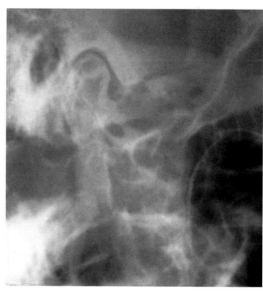

653 Rheumatoid arthritis. TMJ.

223

Juvenile rheumatoid arthritis (Still's disease)

In the juvenile form of rheumatoid arthritis there is a polyarthritis which involves both small and large joints, particularly those with the most active metabolism. The disease is usually diagnosed by the age of 15 and the temporomandibular joints are frequently involved. Once again this usually occurs in patients with established disease in other joints. The changes are often more florid than in the adult form and may progress to marked reactive bone formation and joint ankylosis. As the disease occurs during the phase of general body growth, abnormalities in the development of the mandible are a common sequel. In the example (**654**) showing advanced disease of the right temporomandibular joint, there is gross enlargement of the head of the condyle, particularly in its anterior aspect, with partial obliteration of the sigmoid notch due to reactive bone formation. The ramus and the body of the mandible on the affected side are both underdeveloped with displacement of the midline to the right. Marked antegonial notching of the inferior border of the mandible and elongation of the coronoid process (arrows) are both present, due to masseter and temporalis muscle activity attempting to overcome the restriction in joint movement. The gross enlargement of the condylar head and the shift of the midline are both clearly displayed on the postero-anterior radiograph **655**. In addition to the obvious enlargement and the abnormal shape of the condylar head, the transcranial (**656**) and tomographic (**657**) views demonstrate the marked irregularity of the articular surfaces of the condylar head and glenoid fossa, and osteosclerosis in both the mandible and temporal bone adjacent to the joint. Although there is marked limitation of joint movement, there is no radiographic evidence of bony ankylosis.

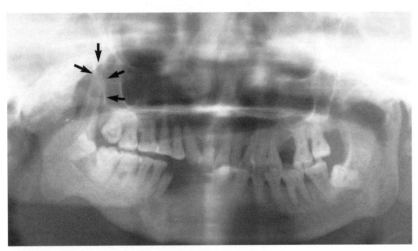

654 Juvenile rheumatoid arthritis (Still's disease). DPR.

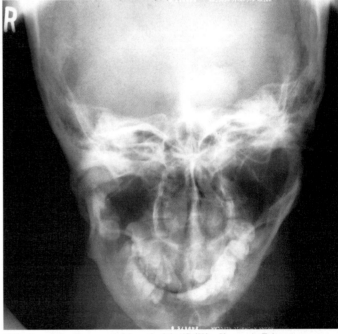

655 Juvenile rheumatoid arthritis (Still's disease). PA.

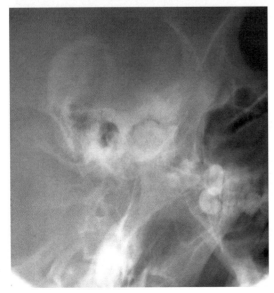

656 Juvenile rheumatoid arthritis (Still's disease). TMJ.

657 Juvenile rheumatoid arthritis (Still's disease). TG.

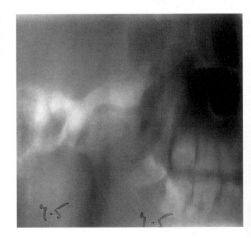

In the second example (**658**) ankylosis has occurred, with bony continuity between the head of the condyle and the articular eminence and wall of the glenoid fossa, together with obliteration of the joint space on this aspect. Elsewhere, the condylar head is bloated in shaped and the joint space is reduced in width.

Ankylosis

Infections of the middle ear or other adjacent structures in childhood sometimes result in temporomandibular joint ankylosis. This is usually unilateral and leads to subsequent growth abnormalities of the affected side of the mandible. Ankylosis may also be a consequence of trauma or, more rarely, a complication of rheumatoid arthritis (as in **658**), in which case it may be bilateral. The example (**659**) of the right temporomandibular joint of an adult shows bony ankylosis resulting from osteomyelitis and destruction of the cartilaginous growth centre of the condyle in childhood. This has resulted in impaired growth of the mandible and there is also osseous continuity between the condyle and the temporal bone, with absence of a joint cavity. In addition, there is elongation of the coronoid process and prominent antegonial notching of the inferior border of the mandible due to the pull of the temporalis and masseter muscles respectively. The deep, V-shaped sigmoid notch, with the inferior alveolar canal opening into it, is also a result of the limited development of the mandible. Fibrous tissue may form within or around the joint space as in the example (**660**). There is apparent ankylosis of the right mandibular

658 Juvenile rheumatoid arthritis (Still's disease). TMJ.

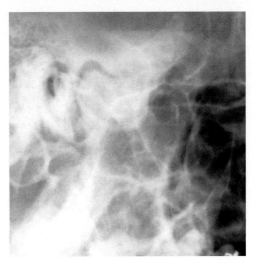

condyle to the temporal bone following osteomyelitis at the age of 12 and destruction of the condylar head. The right side of the mandible is underdeveloped and there is deviation of the midline to the affected side. The glenoid fossa has been obliterated by sclerotic bone (**661**) and an irregular radiolucent zone of fibrous tissue separates the condylar stump from the sclerosed fossa. There is also sclerosis of the deformed condyle and bony margin of the sigmoid notch, with pronounced underdevelopment of the mental process.

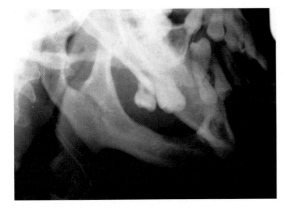

659 Ankylosis. OLM.

661 Ankylosis. TG.

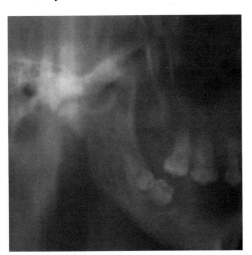

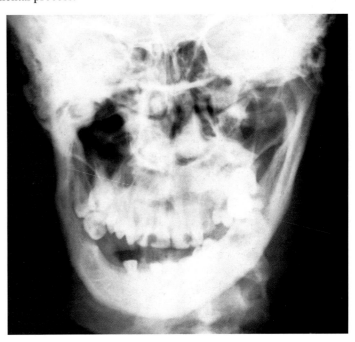

660 Ankylosis. PA.

Another example (**662**) shows deformity of the left side of the mandible that has arisen from osteomyelitis in childhood. The disease process involved most of the body and ramus of the mandible, both of which are smaller than normal, and there is also deformity of the angle. The walls of the inferior alveolar canal are poorly defined. The condyle has undergone extensive destruction (**663**) but there is still some anterior movement during mouth opening (**664**) suggesting a more fibrous form of ankylosis. There has been compensatory hyperplasia of the left coronoid process which exhibits some cortical sclerosis due to the traction of the attached muscle.

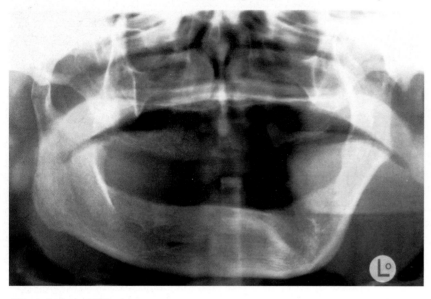

662 Ankylosis. DPR.

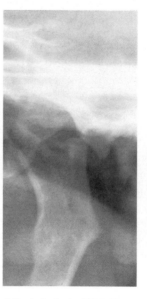 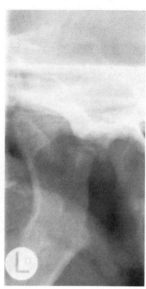

663 Ankylosis. DPR(J).   **664 Ankylosis. DPR(J).**

Traumatic conditions

Dislocation of the mandibular condyle

When the mandibular condyle translates excessively over the articular eminence it remains within the confines of the capsule of the temporomandibular joint but may be unable to return to the normal rest position. This situation may occur unilaterally or bilaterally and may arise as a result of trauma, particularly if the mouth is open at the moment of impact. It may also occur if fibromuscular joint tone is reduced as in elderly or medicated individuals. It is important to appreciate that the extent of condylar head movement during normal mouth opening varies greatly, so that an apparently dislocated condyle in one patient may be a quite normal appearance in another. In some individuals the condylar head may simply subluxate out of the glenoid fossa and then return to its normal position when the mouth is closed.

In example **665**, with true bilateral dislocation of the mandibular condyles, there is a wide open bite with inability to close the mouth. This is confirmed by the ovoid radiolucent outline in the midline, between the two dental arches, caused by the patient's inability to seal the lips. The position of the heads of the condyles are anterior to the articular eminence on both sides as clearly demonstrated by the TMJ(Z) **666**.

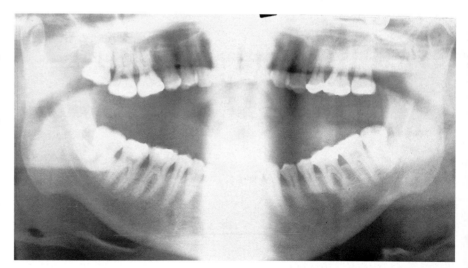

665 Dislocation of the mandibular condyle. DPR (Z).

Another example (**667**) of dislocation of the mandibular condyle is illustrated in a transcranial view of the temporomandibular joint. The head of the condyle (arrow) lies anterior to the articular eminence with the patient's mouth in the closed position, the glenoid fossa being empty.

Fracture of the mandibular condyle

Traumatic fractures of the mandibular condyle usually occur at the point of greatest weakness, i.e the neck, and hence the line of fracture is most commonly outside the joint capsule. Such fractures may give rise to displacement of the condylar head fragment due to traction from the attached lateral pterygoid muscle. Much less commonly the fracture is intracapsular and in this case there is little or no displacement of the condylar head; the fracture line is often difficult to identify on radiographs. Condylar fractures may be unilateral or bilateral (see Chapter 6) and may occur alone or in association with fractures of other parts of the mandible. In the case of bilateral fractures there may be some alteration of the occlusion, such as an anterior open bite. Despite the displacement of the condylar head fragment, there is often little interference in normal function and the injury may be unrecognized clinically. If this happens in a child, abnormal development of the mandible on the affected side may result. In the radiograph (**668**), there is a bifid left mandibular condyle. This condition may arise developmentally or, as in this example, as a consequence of trauma during childhood. The lateral half of the condylar head has been displaced and lies (arrow) just anterior to the remainder of the condyle (**669**). The body and ramus of the left side of the mandible are underdeveloped and there is deviation of the midline to the left on opening (**668**).

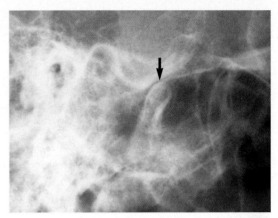

667 Dislocation of the mandibular condyle. TMJ.

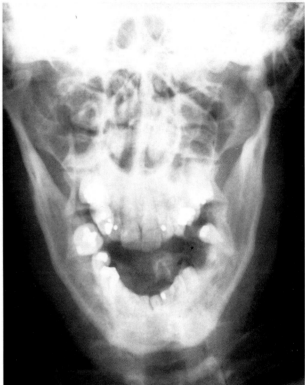

668 Bifid mandibular condyle following trauma. PAC.

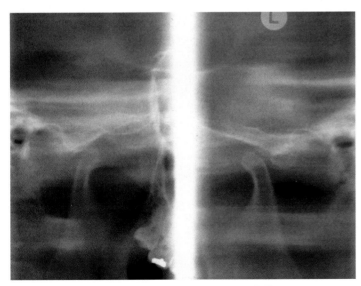

666 Dislocation of the mandibular condyle. TMJ(Z).

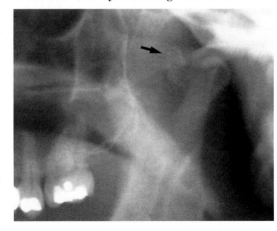

669 Fracture of the mandibular condyle. DPR.

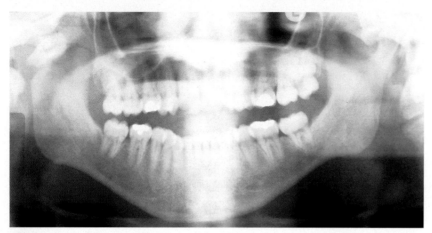

670 Fracture of the mandibular condyle. DPR.

In the next example (**670**), there is a fracture at the base of the right condylar neck with anterior displacement of the bone fragment by muscle traction. In another view (**671**) taken at approximately 90° to the previous one, it is clear that the displacement is also medial, confirming the direction of pull of the lateral pterygoid muscle.

A further example (**672**) shows a fracture of the neck of the left mandibular condyle with marked displacement of the condylar head fragment medially.

Finally, (**673**) a fracture of the head of the left mandibular condyle is demonstrated on a slightly rotated postero-anterior view. The radiolucent fracture line runs inferomedially from the articular surface (arrows) and is intracapsular, with no displacement of the fragment.

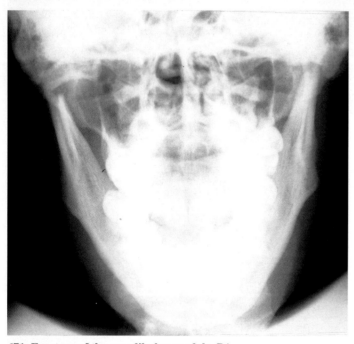

671 Fracture of the mandibular condyle. PA.

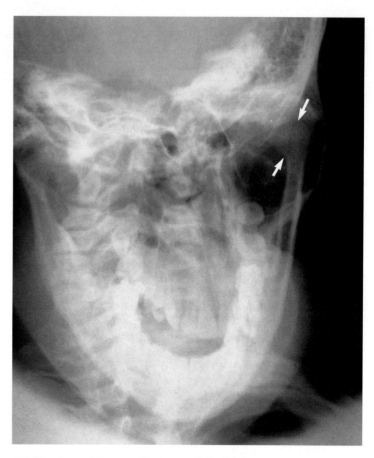

673 Fracture of the mandibular condyle. PAC.

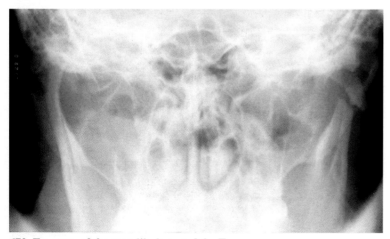

672 Fracture of the mandibular condyle. T.

Regressive conditions

Osteo-arthrosis

Facial pain associated with altered function of the temporomandibular joint and its supporting fibromuscular components is quite common, particularly in young adult females. The symptoms may be unilateral or bilateral, although when bilateral one side may be affected before the other. The condition, often known as the myofascial pain dysfunction syndrome, has a complex aetiology but in the majority of these patients no osseous abnormality of the temporomandibular joints can be detected on plain radiographs. When radiolographical features are observed they are believed to be associated with progressive degenerative changes in the articulating surfaces of the joint. These give rise to bone erosions with replacement by fibrous tissue and damage to and displacement of the intra-articular disc. This form of osteo-arthrosis is often associated with signs and symptoms of joint dysfunction such as clicking, crepitus, deviation of the jaw on opening and localized pain. The earliest radiographic features are areas of erosion which involve the articular surfaces and are usually first seen on the lateral aspect of the joint. Subsequent changes include bony sclerosis, the development of cystic radiolucencies (Ely's cysts) beneath the condylar surface, osteophyte formation predominantly on the anterior aspect of the condyle and flattening of the condylar head and articular eminence. These features are demonstrated below.

On the standard transcranial radiograph (**674**), illustrating an early stage of the disease, the outline of the anterior aspect of the head of the left condyle is poorly defined suggesting that degenerative changes are present, although there is a normal cortical outline on the posterior aspect. Also, there is apparent narrowing of the joint space anteriorly.

Tomography is often helpful both to confirm these changes and to determine the extent of the disease. At the level of the tomograph illustrated (**675**), an irregular, radiolucent crater is clearly visible, indicating erosion of the articular surface of the condyle (arrow). Osteo-arthrosis is often bilateral, and the right joint is also affected (**676**), with the changes being more advanced; the erosion involves most of the articular surface anteriorly resulting in flattening.

Sometimes the areas of subchondral erosion can reach considerable size forming clearly visible, cyst-like radiolucencies (Ely's cysts) in the head of the condyle (**677**). In this example, there is also some sclerosis in the temporal bone around the joint.

675 Osteo-arthrosis. TG.

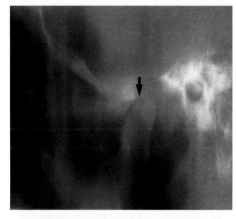

677 Osteo-arthrosis. TG.

674 Osteo-arthrosis. TMJ.

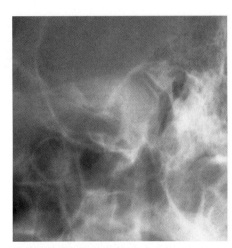

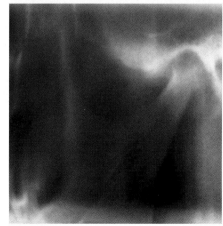

676 Osteo-arthrosis. TG.

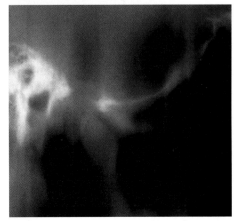

The destructive changes may lead to alteration in the shape of the condylar head with flattening of the articular surface as illustrated in **678**.

Both joints are affected, that on the right showing more advanced changes and with slight osteosclerosis. On the left side, there is still some erosion of the anterior part of the condylar head where the outline of the surface is indistinct, whereas on the right characteristic 'lipping' of the bone surface is seen anteriorly due to compensatory bone remodelling. This change is confirmed in the tomogram **679**.

The process of bone remodelling may produce quite marked, bony protruberances at the margins of the condylar head, forming 'beak-like' structures, as shown in both condyles in **680**. In addition, the tomogram **681** shows that the outlines of the glenoid fossa and the condylar head are indistinct and that there is mild bone sclerosis in both.

Less commonly the site of erosion is predominantly on the anterior aspect of the condylar head. In **682**, the condition is again bilateral, with a clearly defined, irregularly shaped radiolucency and a nodular bony protruberance on the anterior aspect of each condylar head.

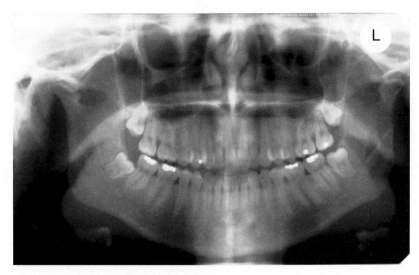

678 Osteo-arthrosis. DPR.

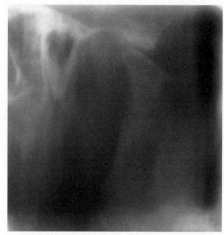

679 Osteo-arthrosis. TG.

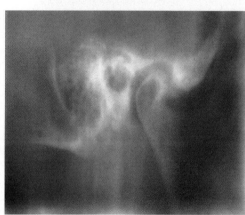

681 Osteo-arthrosis. TG.

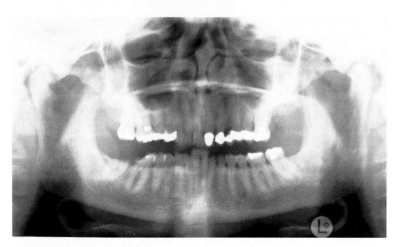

680 Osteo-arthrosis. DPR.

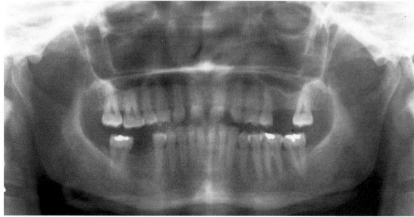

682 Osteo-arthrosis. DPR.

The tomograms (**683**, **684**) confirm the presence and the extent of these lesions and indicate that the articular surfaces are also involved, with radiolucent erosions on both sides.

The next example (**685**, **686**, **687a,b**) of bilateral osteo-arthrosis show a series of computerized tomograms. On the left side (**685**) there is early destruction of the cortex of the lateral pole of the condylar head (arrow) with reactive sclerosis of the underlying bone and also a small erosion of the articular surface of the glenoid fossa (arrowhead). On the right side (**686**) the changes are much more advanced with irregularity of the outline of the lateral two-thirds of the head of the condyle which is expanded and

exhibits extensive sclerosis. The outline of the glenoid fossa is also irregular and there is bridging between it and the condylar head anteromedially (arrow). It is difficult to obtain direct views of the temporomandibular joint in the sagittal plane but these can be obtained by reformatting contiguous axial tomograms. In the example (**687a,b**), a sagittal view of the previous illustration has been constructed through the joint in the anteroposterior plane, indicated by the white line. Here the joint space is markedly reduced in size and there is irregularity of the bone surface and sclerosis of the condylar head.

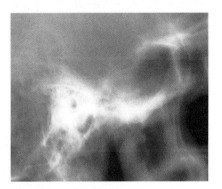

683 Osteo-arthrosis. TG.

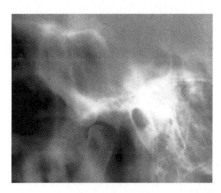

684 Osteo-arthrosis. TG.

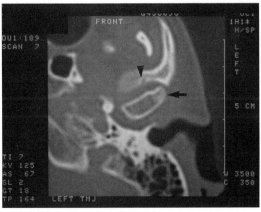

685 Osteo-arthrosis. CT.

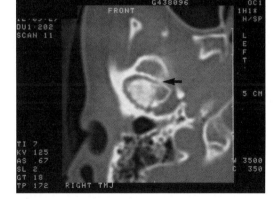

686 Osteo-arthrosis. CT.

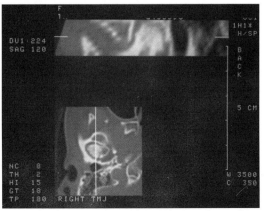

687a (left), b (right) Osteo-arthrosis. CT.
A: coronoid process;
B: root of zygoma;
C: external auditory meatus;
D: mastoid air cells.

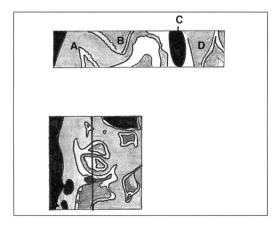

Temporomandibular joint disc abnormalities

In some patients with myofascial pain who have temporomandibular joint dysfunction, there may be evidence of displacement of the articular disc. Such displacement is usually a consequence of laxity of the capsular ligament together with spasm of the associated muscle and is almost always in an anterior or anteromedial direction. Two basic types can be identified: firstly, those with anterior displacement in which disc reduction to an approximately normal position occurs on opening; and secondly, those in which reduction does not occur. Arthrography may be used to demonstrate the displacement.

ANTERIOR DISPLACEMENT OF THE DISC WITH REDUCTION
The example (**688a,b**) of the first type, with the jaw in the closed position, shows that the anterior displacement of the disc is accompanied by enlargement of the anterior compartment of the inferior joint space, and that the cranial surface is concave due to the presence of the disc. On the mouth opening, the disc moves posteriorly, relative to the head of the condyle, from its anteriorly displaced position so temporarily assuming a more normal relationship. This movement may be accompanied by an audible click. During this stage (**689a,b**) the distribution of a radio-opaque medium is similar to that in a normal joint in the closed position, with more medium occupying the posterior compartment. On completion of opening (**690a,b**) the arthrogram assumes a normal appearance, with most of the radio-opaque medium occupying the posterior compartment.

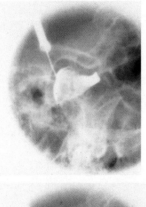
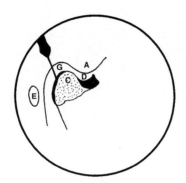

688 a,b Anterior displacement of the temporomandibular joint disc with reduction. A(J).
A: articular eminence;
C: mandibular condyle;
D: articular disc:
E: external auditory meatus;
G: glenoid fossa.

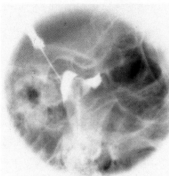
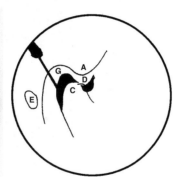

689 a, b Anterior displacement of the temporomandibular joint disc with reduction. A(J).
A: articular eminence;
C: mandibular condyle;
D: articular disc;
E: external auditory meatus;
G: glenoid fossa.

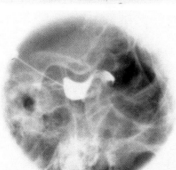
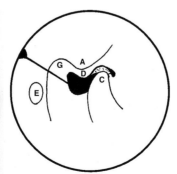

690 a, b Anterior displacement of the temporomandibular joint disc with reduction. A(J).
A: articular eminence;
C: mandibular condyle;
D: articular disc;
E: external auditory meatus;
G: glenoid fossa.

MRI may also be used to demonstrate the position of the disc, as in **691a,b; 692a,b**. The articular disc has a relatively low signal intensity and is shown to lie anteriorly to the condylar head with the mouth closed (**691**). On full opening (**692**), the disc has reduced and is situated over the condylar head in a normal relationship. Disc displacement usually occurs in an anteromedial direction. To demonstrate the medial displacement, it is necessary to undertake scans in a coronal plane, as in **693**.

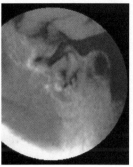 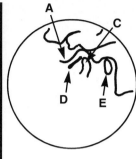 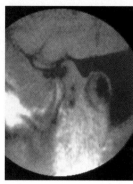 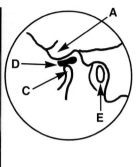 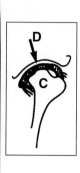

691 a,b Anterior displacement of the temporo-mandibular joint disc with reduction. MRI.
A: articular eminence;
C: mandibular condyle;
D: articular disc;
E: external auditory meatus.

692 a,b Anterior displacement of the temporo-mandibular joint disc with reduction. MRI.
A: articular eminence;
C: mandibular condyle;
D: articular disc;
E: external auditory meatus.

693 a,b Anteromedial displacement of the temporomandibular joint disc with reduction. MRI.
C: mandibular condyle;
D: articular disc.

ANTERIOR DISPLACEMENT OF THE DISC WITHOUT REDUCTION

In the example (**694a,b**) of the second type in which reduction does not occur on opening, the anterior displacement of the disc with the mouth closed is again clearly displayed by arthrography. The anterior compartment of the inferior joint space is again larger than the posterior one and its concave cranial surface reveals the outline of the inferior surface of the displaced disc. On the mouth opening, the disc remains displaced anteriorly so that even on full opening the distribution of medium is similar to that in the closed position (**695a,b**). The anteriorly displaced disc may lead to mechanical interference to the anterior movement of the head of the condyle, so that there is limitation of opening of the mouth, as here.

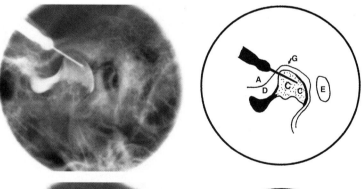

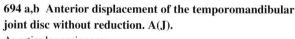

694 a,b Anterior displacement of the temporomandibular joint disc without reduction. A(J).
A: articular eminence;
C: mandibular condyle;
D: articular disc;
E: external auditory meatus;
G: glenoid fossa.

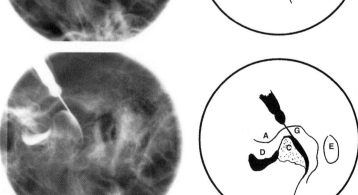

695 a,b Anterior displacement of the temporomandibular joint disc without reduction. A(J).
A: articular eminence;
C: mandibular condyle;
D: articular disc;
E: external auditory meatus;
G: glenoid fossa.

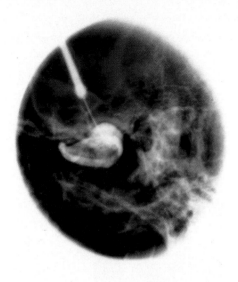

696 Perforation of the temporo-mandibular joint disc. A(J).

PERFORATION OF THE DISC

Sometimes, particularly when there is chronic displacement of the disc, perforation results, so that when a contrast medium is injected into the inferior space of the joint cavity, it spreads into the superior space as well. In **696**, the radio-opaque medium, in addition to capping the condylar head, has mushroomed into the superior joint space. Such an appearance may also be created in the absence of a perforation if the medium is inadvertently injected directly into the superior space.

Tumorous conditions

Synovial osteochondromatosis

This condition, of unknown pathogenesis, may occasionally affect the temporomandibular joint. It is characterized by the presence of numerous, predominantly cartilaginous nodules, which arise from the articular surface and intrude into the joint cavity where they may become detached and lie free. Such nodules are often too small or not sufficiently mineralized to be detected radiographically. The condition is usually accompanied by swelling of the joints and occurs most often in the elderly. In example **697**, the articular surface of the left condyle appears to be notched and to have a continuous layer of cortical bone. Several radio-opaque bodies (arrow) are present above and anterior to the condylar head occupying part of the widened joint space. These findings are confirmed on the tomogram (**698**). Occasionally, the intra-articular bodies (arrow) reach considerable size, when they are then more easily seen (**699**).

Fibrosarcoma

Malignant tumours are rare in the region of the mandiblar condyle. In the example (**700**) of a fibrosarcoma which has arisen in the neck of the left condyle there is a poorly defined radiolucency between the coronoid process (arrow) and the base of the head of condyle. The condylar head (arrowheads) is smooth and apparently unaffected. The neck of the mandible is widened with loss of the distinct cortical margins and there are scattered radiopacities within the lesion, which are remnants of the original bone.

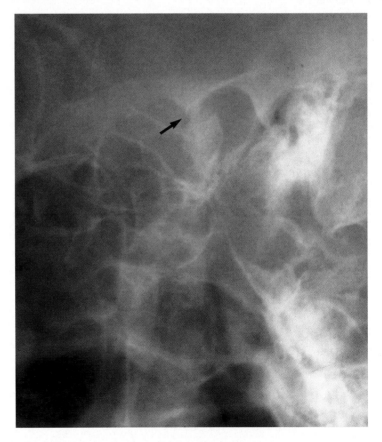

697 Synovial osteochondromatosis. TMJ.

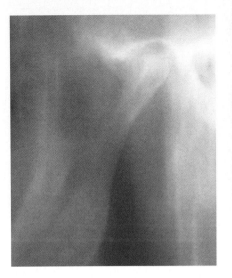

698 Synovial osteochondromatosis. TG.

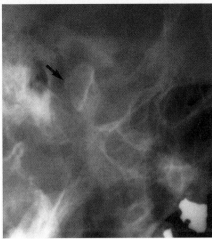

699 Synovial osteochondromatosis. TMJ.

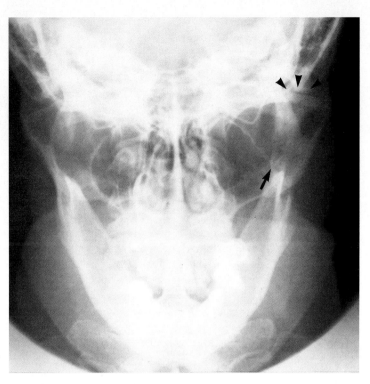

700 Fibroscarcoma. PAC.

Metastatic carcinoma

Occasionally a tumour metastasis from a primary lesion elsewhere in the body may develop in the condylar head. The example (701) shows a metastatic deposit of adenocarcinoma from a primary tumour of the colon. Compared with the normal side, the cortical outline of the right condyle is missing, particularly on the medial side (arrows), and the condyle itself has an irregularly radiolucent, 'moth eaten' appearance.

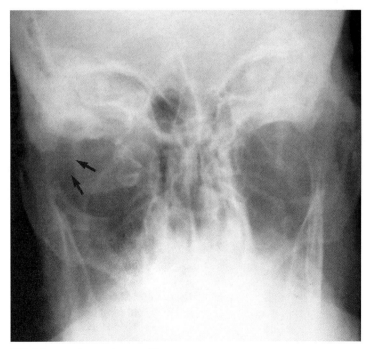

701 Metastatic carcinoma. T.

8

The maxillary antrum

Introduction

The maxillary antrum is a mucous membrane lined air sinus which is triangular in shape with its base forming the lateral wall of the nose, where there is an opening (ostium) into the middle meatus. There is one antrum on each side of the maxilla and together with the ethmoid, sphenoid and frontal sinuses, they form the paranasal sinuses. The maxillary antrum is the largest of these, occupying much of the body of the maxilla in the adult. The floor of the maxillary antrum is closely related to the apices of the posterior teeth, for the most part being separated by just a thin lamina of bone. Thus diseases arising within the antrum may be confused with those of dental origin and, conversely, dental diseases, such as infections, may spread to involve the antrum. Although intra-oral radiographs image the antral floor, extra-oral radiographs are needed to display the whole of the maxillary antrum. The occipitomental and DPRs are particularly useful for imaging the maxillary sinus, because they are largely free of super-imposition from other anatomical structures and demonstrate both sides for comparison. The occipitomental radiograph may be used as an initial screening view, after which further imaging investigations may be performed as necessary.

Microbial conditions and their sequelae

Maxillary sinusitis

Antral infections are most commonly a complication of respiratory tract infections (such as the common cold) and may be either unilateral or bilateral. However, sinusitis may also be of dental origin, for example, as a consequence of a root that has been displaced into the antrum or an oro-antral communication. In such cases the sinusitis is usually unilateral. The main radiological features of acute infection are mucosal thickening and the presence of fluid within the antral cavity due to the presence of inflammatory exudate or pus. The fluid fills the lower half of the antrum up to the level of the ostium, leaving a radiolucent shadow above it. If the ostium becomes blocked then the antrum fills completely with fluid resulting in total radio-opacity of the antral cavity. In chronic, recurrent or allergic conditions a more generalized thickening of the antral lining may be present, either with a smooth surface which contours the outline of the bony walls or with a more lobulated margin. Maxillary sinusitis may be confined to the maxillary antrum or involve other air sinuses particularly the ethmoid.

The first example (**702**, **703**) shows a patient with bilateral acute sinusitis. The fluid nature of the exudate in the antrum can be confirmed by examining the patient initially in the erect position and repeating the procedure either in the prone position or with the head tilted laterally, so inducing a change in position of the fluid level. In the first radiograph (**702**) taken in the upright position, mucosal thickening and a fluid level are present in both antra with only a small radiolucent air space persisting. The change in position of the patient through 90° to the prone position (**703**) has resulted in complete radio-opacity of both antra and loss of any fluid level which would now be in the same plane as the film. Note that the nasal mucosa also appears thickened, with opacity of the nasal cavity, particularly on the erect film; however the frontal sinuses appear to be unaffected.

In acute exacerbations of chronic disease, the radiographic features of both conditions are often present. In the next example (**704**) of bilateral maxillary sinusitis there is an empyema or collection of pus on the right side, where a distinct, horizontal fluid level is present. The radio-opaque fluid occupies most of the antral cavity and only a small air space remains superiorly. In the left antrum, there is gross thickening of the soft tissue which forms a radio-opaque contour to the cavity and is dome-shaped inferiorly, suggesting the present of a polyp.

In chronic sinusitis of either infective or allergic origin, the soft tissue lining of both antra becomes markedly thickened forming a radio-opaque contour which follows their bony outline, as shown in **705**. As a consequence, the radiolucent air shadows within them are greatly reduced in size, but no fluid levels are present. On both sides, the foramen ovale (arrows) is clearly displayed, superimposed upon the inferior medial corner of the antrum.

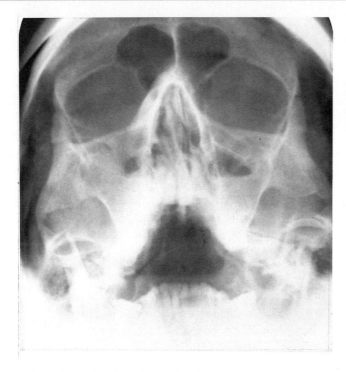

702 Acute bilateral maxillary sinusitis. OM.

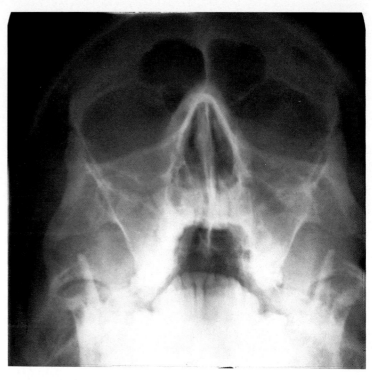

703 Acute bilateral maxillary sinusitis. OM.

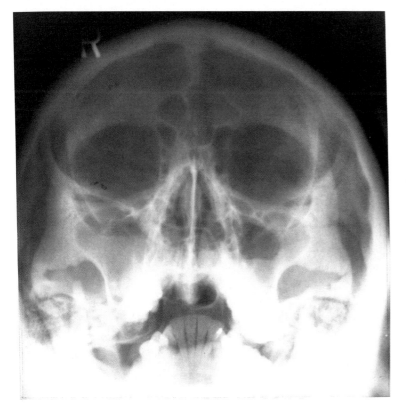

704 Acute bilateral maxillary sinusitis. OM.

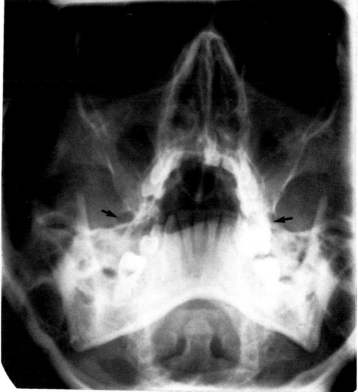

705 Chronic bilateral maxillary sinusitis. OM.

The next example (**706**) shows a unilateral sinusitis of the left antrum, with radio-opacity of most of the cavity and no obvious fluid level. Such an appearance is due to gross thickening of the lining, so that the cavity has become almost completely occluded with pus; any residual air has been displaced. Note (as an incidental finding) the presence of a clearly defined, radio-opaque mass with a smooth outline in the region of the base of the right frontal sinus. The lateral view (**707**) however suggests that the mass, which is an osteoma, is present in the anterior ethmoid air sinuses.

Unilateral sinusitis may be due to dental causes, as in example **708** – an oro-antral fistula resulting from the extraction of an upper molar tooth. The left antrum is radio-opaque towards the base and the radio-opacity is bounded by a clearly defined horizontal margin which is menisciform, indicative of a fluid level. All the other sinuses appear normal.

Antral polyp

Localized polypoid hyperplasia of the antral mucosa, in response to persistent sources of irritation, is not uncommon and is usually symptomless. The radiograph (**709**), which was taken to confirm the presence of a small root fragment distal to ⌊5 , also revealed a lesion in the floor of the antrum. The radio-opaque lamina outlining the antral floor dips inferiorly between ⌊57 , above which there is a smooth, dome-shaped, radio-opaque swelling projecting into the antral cavity with no intervening bony margin. This appearance is typical of an antral polyp.

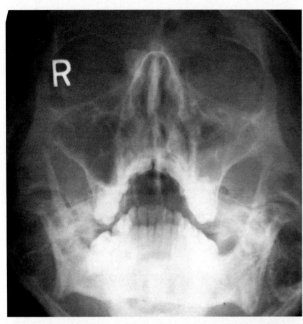

706 Chronic unilateral maxillary sinusitis. OM.

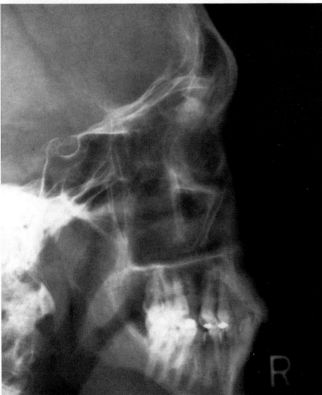

707 Chronic unilateral maxillary sinusitis. L.

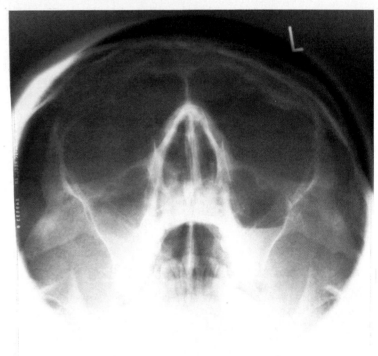

708 Acute unilateral maxillary sinusitis. OM.

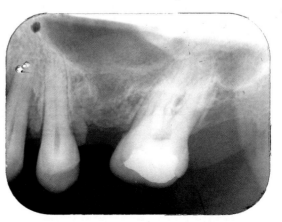

709 Antral polyp. P.

Mucous cyst

Mucous cysts probably arise as a consequence of inflammation or hyperplasia of the mucosal lining, particularly affecting the antral floor. They occur commonly and are found most frequently in the third decade of life, usually as an incidental radiographic finding. Occasionally they are found in air sinuses other than the maxillary antrum. In the example (**710**) there is a large, dome-shaped, radio-opaque lesion occupying the lower part of the right antrum. It has a smooth surface and is not separated from the antral cavity by a bony margin. The rest of the antrum appears to be normal. Note, however, the abnormally shaped, hypoplastic right mandibular condyle.

Antrolith

Antroliths form by the deposition of mineral upon the surface of a suitable nidus, which may be degenerate or infected tissue, or a foreign body. In the example (**711**, **712**), a radio-opaque antrolith (arrow) of irregular outline is present in the left maxillary antrum, in close relationship to the medial wall. The antral cavity is also radio-opaque and its bony outline is indistinct, particularly on the lateral aspect, indicating the presence of chronic sinusitis. There is a small root fragment in the alveolus in the $\underline{7}$ region.

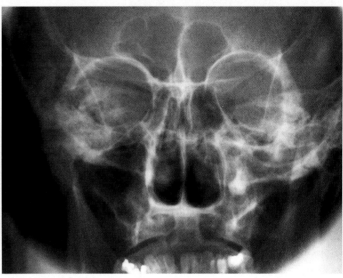

712 Antrolith. PA.

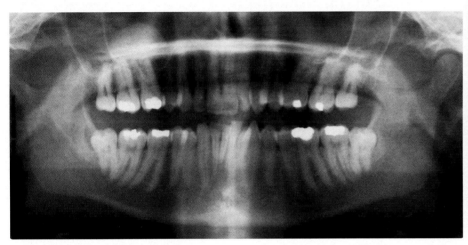

710 Mucous cyst. DPR.

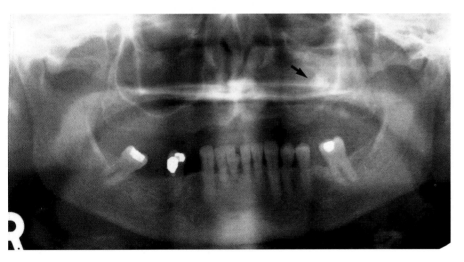

711 Antrolith. DPR.

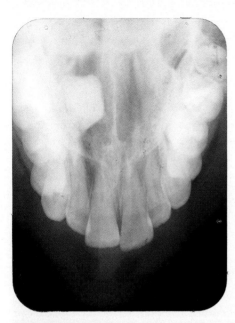

713 Rhinolith. USO.

Rhinolith

Rhinoliths arise in a similar manner to antroliths, except that they form in the nasal rather than the antral cavity. In the example (**713**) there is an irregularly shaped, radio-opaque mass in the floor of the right nasal cavity. The centre of the mass is more dense than the periphery and this pattern, together with the absence of a surrounding cortical lamina and follicular space, excludes the possibility of this being an unerupted tooth, an odontome or an osteoma. The position of the rhinolith in the nasal cavity is confirmed on the postero-anterior film (**714**).

Tumorous conditions

Tumours may involve the maxillary antrum either by arising in the tissues lining the antral cavity or by spread from lesions in adjacent tissues. In the former situation they are most commonly epithelial in origin but other types of neoplasm occur occasionally. In the latter situation, a wide variety of tumours may spread to involve the antrum and examples of these are illustrated in other chapters. In addition to plain radiographs, CT and MRI are valuable in demonstrating the extent of such lesions more accurately, particulary if they have extended widely and have metastasized to the regional lymph nodes.

Squamous cell carcinoma

The most common form of malignant tumour to affect the maxillary antrum is squamous cell carcinoma which arises from the lining epithelium. It rarely occurs in individuals under the age of 40 and as much of the tumour growth is into the antral cavity in the early stages, the mass is often of considerable size by the time it is diagnosed. The tumour produces opacity within the antrum and may also cause infection, resulting in further changes in the antral lining. When the floor of the antrum is involved, the patient may present with dental symptoms such as the inability to wear an upper denture or the presence of loose teeth.

In the example (**715**) of an early lesion in the right antrum, the slightly radio-opaque tumour mass occupies the inferior and lateral aspects of the antral cavity, with destruction of the bony walls and extension laterally into the soft tissues. The radiolucent antral air shadow is much reduced in size, although the bony infra-orbital margin and the infra-orbital foramen remain intact.

In the example (**716**), there is a more advanced lesion involving the left side of the maxilla. The alveolar process has largely been destroyed and the soft tissue mass extends inferiorly into the mouth. The inferior, medial, lateral and superior walls of the antrum have been destroyed. A further view (**717**) confirms these findings and shows that the tumour mass is also protruding into the nasal cavity. The infra-orbital foramen remains intact. There is an overlying soft tissue swelling, the margins of which run obliquely downwards across the orbit from its medial aspect. Alveolar destruction is well displayed on intra-oral radiographs as in **718** which shows the characteristic, radiolucent 'moth eaten' pattern.

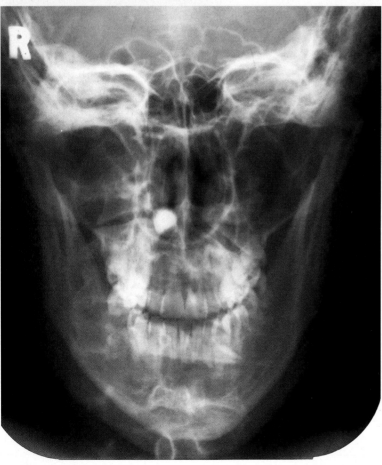

714 Rhinolith. PA.

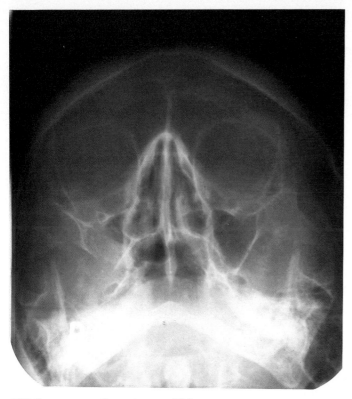

715 Squamous cell carcinoma. OM.

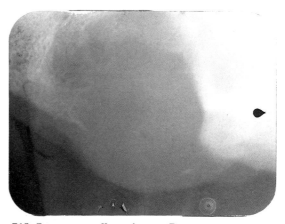

716 Squamous cell carcinoma. DPR.

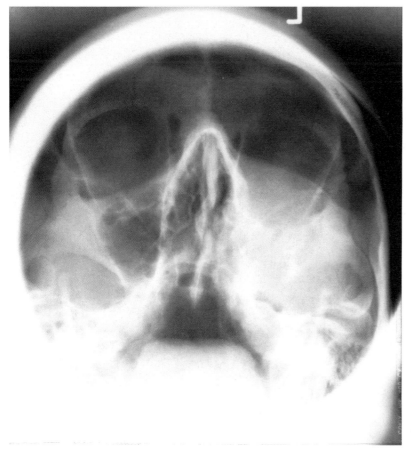

717 Squamous cell carcinoma. OM.

718 Squamous cell carcinoma. P.

In another example (**719**), of a more advanced neoplasm, there is almost complete destruction of the medial, inferior and lateral walls of the left antrum. The slightly radio-opaque tumour mass has extended into the nose (arrowhead), the mouth (arrow) and the infratemporal fossa. There is thinning of the medial wall of the antrum and also evidence of bone destruction of the lateral wall. The outline of the infra-orbital foramen is indistinct. The intra-oral radiographs (**720, 721**) show an irregular pattern of bone destruction with patchy areas of radiolucency separated by irregularly arranged bone remnants. There is apical resorption |34 and the periapical areas of increased radiolucency caused by the tumour could be misinterpreted as periapical granulomas. The soft tissue outline overlying the alveolus can just be determined. The greater radio-opacity of the bone on the right of the radiograph (**721**) is due to superimposition of the shadow of the zygomatic arch, which remains intact.

Another example (**722–725**) shows an extensive neoplasm in the right maxillary antrum which has resulted in generalized opacity with loss of the bony outline.

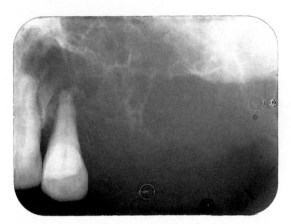

721 Squamous cell carcinoma. P.

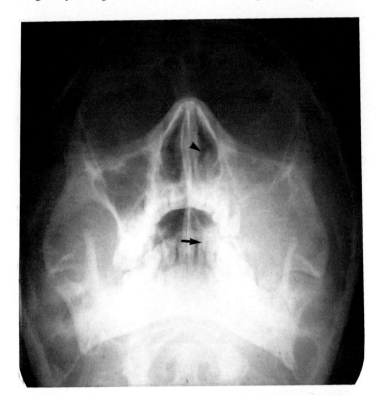

719 Squamous cell carcinoma. OM.

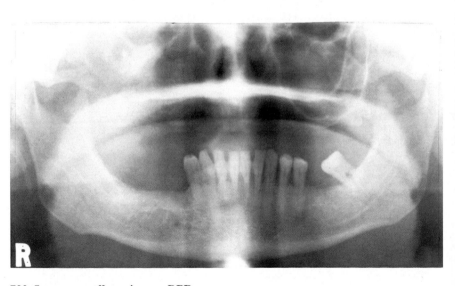

722 Squamous cell carcinoma. DPR.

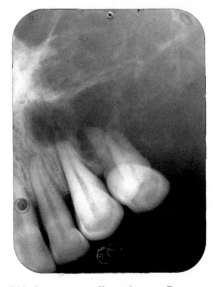

720 Squamous cell carcinoma. P.

The overall extent of the lesion is more clearly displayed in the occipitomental radiograph (**723**) which shows that although the medial wall of the antrum remains intact, the roof, lateral wall and floor have all been destroyed. The tumour mass has also extended posterolaterally into the infratemporal fossa and has caused destruction of the zygomatic arch (arrow). There is swelling of the infra-orbital soft tissues resulting in a horizontal zone of radio-opacity superimposed upon the lower half of the right orbit. The neoplasm is well displayed on the CTs which show destruction of the anterior wall of the antrum and the invasion into the pterygoid plates posteriorly (**724**). A further tomographic slice at the level of the condylar head of the mandible (**725**) confirms the destruction of the posterolateral wall of the antrum with spread of the tumour into the infratemporal fossa and the nasal cavity.

In another example (**726**) of an extensive neoplasm, again arising in the right antrum, the walls of the antrum have been completely destroyed. The mass has spread into the infratemporal fossa, the lower part of the orbit and both sides of the nasal cavity. The nasal septum has been partially destroyed and displaced to the left and the lateral wall of the nose on the left is partially eroded.

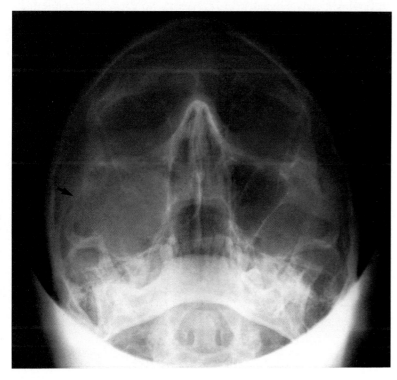

723 Squamous cell carcinoma. OM.

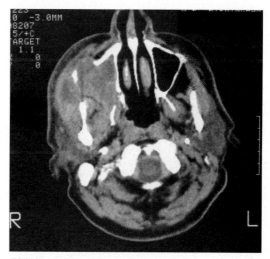

724 Squamous cell carcinoma. CT.

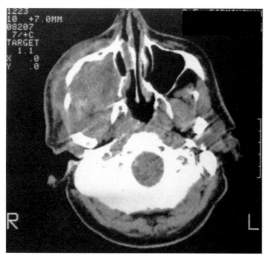

725 Squamous cell carcinoma. CT.

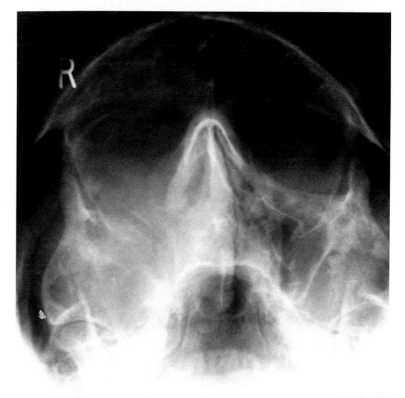

726 Squamous cell carcinoma. OM.

Spindle cell sarcoma

Sarcomas are rare in the antrum but when they occur they usually appear on radiographs as poorly defined areas of destruction of the bony walls. The example (**727–729**) shows an undifferentiated sarcoma which has caused a radiolucent defect in the right maxillary alveolar process, extending upwards into the antrum. Inferiorly, the bone of the edentulous ridge has been completely destroyed and anteriorly the bone margin is indistinct, with an irregular pattern of destruction. Swelling of the overlying soft tissues is also evident. The involvement of the antrum is confirmed by the lack of continuity (arrows) of the cortical lamina of the antral floor (**728**) and the destruction of the lateral wall (**729**).

Malignant lymphoma

Extranodal malignant lymphomas rarely arise in the maxillary antrum and are usually of the B cell type. In the example (**730**), a tumour of the follicular, centre cell type totally occupies the left antrum, which is opaque. The neoplasm has destroyed the lateral wall and the underlying edentulous alveolar ridge. The superior margin of the antrum is poorly defined medially, suggesting that it too is involved. The tumour mass has caused swelling of the alveolus occlusally and palatally (arrows). In addition, the right antrum is radio-opaque inferiorly with a clearly defined menisciform upper boundary indicating the presence of fluid. The DPR (**731**) shows that the cortical outline of the floor and posterior wall of the left antrum is missing.

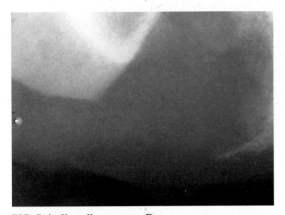

727 Spindle cell sarcoma. P.

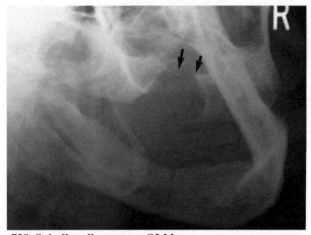

728 Spindle cell sarcoma. OLM.

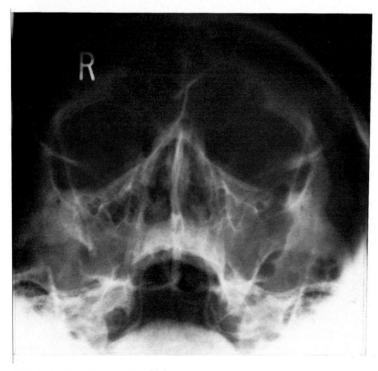

729 Spindle cell sarcoma. OM.

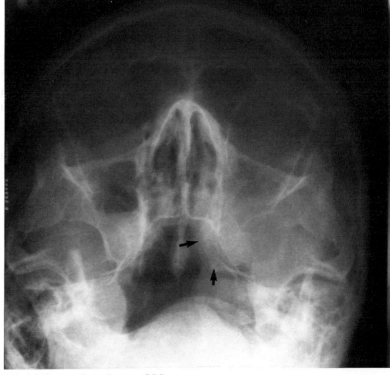

730 Malignant lymphoma. OM.

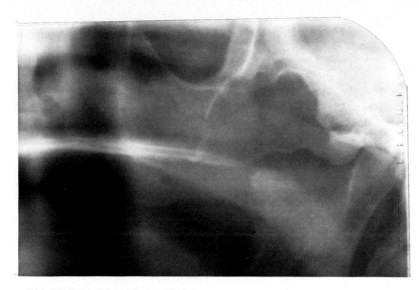

731 Malignant lymphoma. DPR.

Iatrogenic conditions

Oro-antral fistula

An oro-antral fistula may arise as a complication of tooth extraction in the maxilla when a communication between the oral and antral cavities fails to heal. Antral infection may supervene. In the example (**732**) the fistula developed after the extraction of 6|. The radio-opaque lamina outlining the antral floor runs postero-inferiorly over the apices of the roots 54| almost to the crest of the edentulous ridge but is missing over the radiolucent tooth socket 6|. It becomes continuous again posteriorly above the root 7|.

Displaced tooth roots

Tooth root fragments, most commonly those of maxillary molars or premolars, may be displaced into the antral cavity during an attempted extraction. In the example (**733**), a root fragment has been displaced into the antral cavity during the extraction of 6|. The root is inverted, with the fractured surface facing superiorly. There is a distinct root canal but the root is not surrounded by a lamina dura or a periodontal ligament space. A smaller root fragment is still present in the distal tooth socket and the cortical lamina of the antral floor above the socket is breached. Note that the antral floor dips down around the apices of the roots 54|.

Another example (**734**), following extraction of 6|, shows that the palatal root has been displaced into the antrum, lying on its floor posterior to 7|. Again the root is inverted with an obvious root canal but no surrounding lamina dura. This radiograph has been taken from a more posterior position than usual, with the X-ray tube angled anteriorly, so that the palatal root 7| is projected away from the buccal roots, which are foreshortened. Images of the zygomatic arch, pterygoid plate, pterygoid hamulus and coronoid process of the mandible are also present.

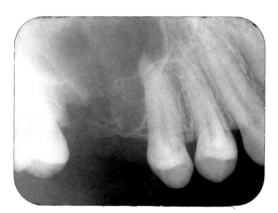

732 Oro-antral fistula. P.

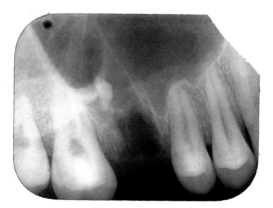

733 Displaced tooth root. P.

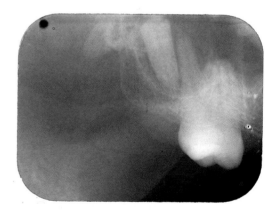

734 Displaced tooth root. P.

The next example (**735**) shows a root fragment viewed 'end on' and the root canal can just be determined, although there is no surrounding lamina dura. A second smaller root fragment is present in the alveolus distal to 4|. The thin, radio-opaque lamina of the lateral part of the floor of the nose runs obliquely across the upper part of the illustration.

The radiograph **736** shows a palatal root 7| which has been displaced into the antral cavity, lying horizontally above the roots 6|. Again, the root canal and the absence of lamina dura should be noted, together with the cortical lamina of the floor of the antrum extending down around the roots 65|. The outline of 7| socket is indistinct and is partly obscured by superimposition of the root of the zygomatic arch.

The next example (**737, 738**) shows a palatal root |6 which has been displaced into the antrum and is tilted distally at 45° close to the apex of its socket. The lamina dura outlining the socket is partly superimposed upon the root and is closely related to the antrum, which dips down almost to the crest of the edentulous ridge mesial to it. The lateral limit of the antral floor is displayed as a thin lamina running across the middle of the socket. An occlusal radiograph (**738**) includes a greater part of the antrum and may be more useful in demonstrating a root fragment that has been displaced away from the tooth socket.

In the last example (**739, 740**), the root fragment is retained high up on the medial wall of the right antrum, possibly occluding the ostium. As a consequence, drainage has been impeded and the antrum is infected and radio-opaque. The other sinuses are normal, confirming that unilateral maxillary sinusitis frequently has a local cause.

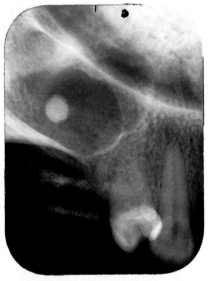

735 Displaced tooth root. P.

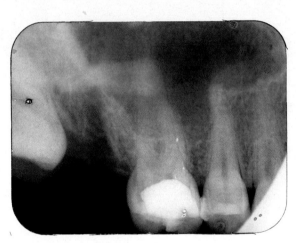

736 Displaced tooth root. P.

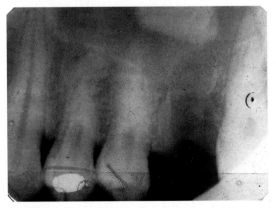

737 Displaced tooth root. P.

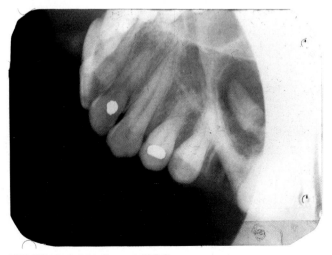

738 Displaced tooth root. UOO.

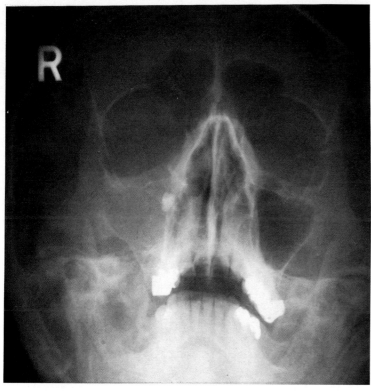

739 Displaced tooth root. OM.

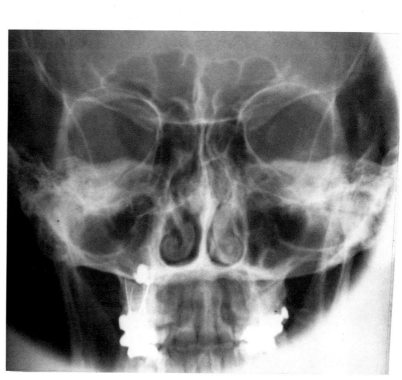

740 Displaced tooth root. L.

Foreign body

Foreign bodies may be inadvertently introduced into the maxillary antrum during dental or surgical treatment. The first example (**741**) shows a mass of radio-opaque root filling cement accidentally introduced into the antral cavity during endodontic treatment of 5|. This tooth is root filled and has a radiolucent periapical lesion, probably a granuloma, through which a trail of filling material passes up to the antral mass. The lamina dura is absent periapically but a thin cortical lamina surrounds the periapical lesion and blends with that outlining the floor of the antrum. The position of the material within the antrum is confirmed in the extra-oral radiograph (**742**) which also shows no evidence of antral infection. Note the prominent inferior nasal conchae bilaterally.

741 Foreign body. P.

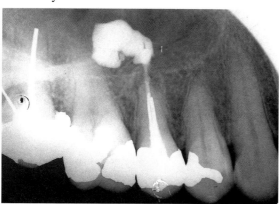

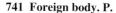

742 Foreign body. PA.

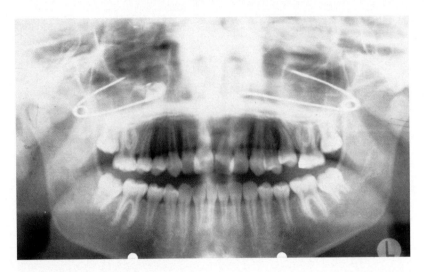

743 Foreign body. DPR.

Foreign bodies may also be introduced into body cavities by patients themselves. Such foreign bodies may have a variety of shapes and forms, sometimes rather bizarre, as in the example (**743**) of a patient who had introduced a safety pin into the right nostril several years previously. The pin is lying in the inferior meatus and has a radiographic double image. The second image (on the left) is magnified in an anteroposterior direction and is incomplete.

Postoperative maxillary cyst (surgical ciliated cyst)

Cysts sometimes arise in the maxilla at the site of a previous operation involving the antral cavity, usually a Cadwell–Luc procedure, but also following maxillary osteotomies or apicectomy. The cyst is thought to arise from the proliferation of epithelial residues that become entrapped in the wound. These cysts, postoperative maxillary cysts, may be quite destructive and result in considerable bone loss, giving, however, an appearance resembling an antral carcinoma. In the example (**744**) there is a clearly defined, approximately circular radiolucency with a radio-opaque cortical lamina between ⁀75‾. The roots of both teeth have been displaced and the lesion appeared at first sight to be a residual cyst. The diagnosis was confirmed by the history of a previous operation and the histology. In small lesions the bony outline of the adjacent antrum remains clearly visible, but as the cysts enlarge and cause erosion of the antral wall, the outline becomes less well defined.

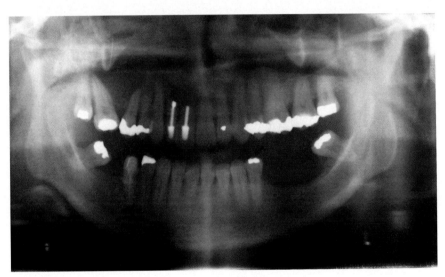

744 Postoperative maxillary cyst (surgical ciliated cyst). DPR.

9

The salivary glands

Introduction

Technological advances have allowed a wide range of investigative procedures to be applied to the imaging of the major salivary glands, the type of modality being determined by the nature of the disorder or complaint. Plain radiographs are used when an obstruction of a duct is suspected, to help in confirming its presence and in determining the size and number of any calculi. If plain radiographs fail to demonstrate a duct calculus, sialography is indicated. The contrast agent demonstrates the architecture of the duct system, the site of the obstruction and any alteration to the ductal tree arising from it. Sialography can also be used to investigate chronic recurrent sialadenitis, autoimmune sialadenitis, sialadenosis and traumatic injury to the gland. CT assists in identifying the location and the type of lesion present (e.g. solid or cystic) and whether the adjacent tissues and lymph nodes are affected. The parotid gland usually has a lower attenuation number than that of the surrounding tissues, depending upon the amount of fat present within the gland. The greater the fat content of the gland, the better the tumour is demonstrated. However, when the suspected tumour and the adjacent glandular tissues are of similar attenuation values, CT combined with sialography may be helpful in differentiating normal salivary gland tissue from the tumour mass.

The use of diagnostic ultrasound is valuable in the investigation of parotid or submandibular gland enlargement and the technique is also useful in the detection of sialoliths, which are echogenic with acoustic shadowing. Cystic lesions appear hypoechoic, usually with well defined margins, whereas solid tumours may show well or poorly defined hypoechoic areas with internal shadowing. MRI provides good contrast between different types of soft tissues and is therefore particularly suitable for imaging glandular and periglandular masses. It is also helpful in determining the relationship of a parotid tumour to the main branches of the facial nerve. The investigations so far described demonstrate any variations in the anatomical form of the salivary glands. However, functional information can be obtained using radionuclide imaging – the isotope most commonly used is technetium pertechnetate (^{99m}Tc), which releases gamma rays as it decays. Technetium, like iodine, is secreted by the intercalated ducts, the rate of accumulation of radioactivity being measured quantitatively against time. This technique also demonstrates whether the secretory activity of the gland is uniform or localized. It is useful in assessing salivary gland function in patients with chronic sialadenitis, autoimmune sialadenitis, sialadenosis (sialosis) or in some forms of salivary gland tumour.

Inflammatory conditions and associated abnormalities

Sialolithiasis

Salivary calculi (stones; sialoliths) are calcific deposits that form within the ductal system of salivary glands. They cause partial obstruction to the salivary flow, particularly at times of increased salivation, and consequently may result in salivary gland swelling and pain at meal times. Continued obstruction leads to chronic sialadenitis, which is accompanied by acinar atrophy and fibrosis with progressive loss of secretory tissue. Salivary calculi occur more commonly in the submandibular than the parotid ducts, and may be single or multiple, rounded or fusiform and show variation in radiodensity dependent upon the ratio of the inorganic to organic matter within them. Poorly mineralized calculi are difficult to demonstrate radiographically but may become more obvious if reduced exposure techniques are employed. Small calculi will also be difficult to detect, particularly if their image is obscured by superimposition upon that of the teeth or the jaws. Conversely, those that are larger and more densely mineralized, if superimposed upon the tooth bearing part of the jaws, may be misinterpreted as foci of sclerotic bone or tooth roots.

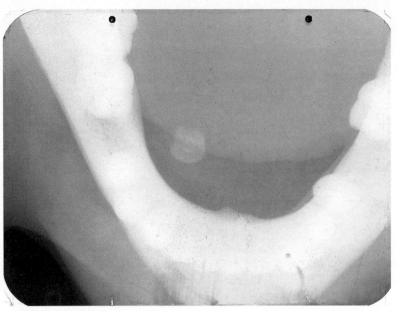

745 Submandibular duct calculus. LTO.

Submandibular duct calculus

Salivary calculi may be situated at any point along the ducts. In submandibular glands, for descriptive convenience, they are identified at the duct orifice, within its intra-oral segment, at the bend where the duct passes around the posterior aspect of the mylohyoid muscle and within the body of the gland. Since salivary calculi are formed by the deposition of successive layers of mineral upon a central nidus, they can appear as a series of concentric layers that are alternately radio-opaque and radiolucent. In the first example (**745**) there is an approximately circular calculus, which shows this concentric structure in the anterior part of the duct of the right submandibular salivary gland. The calculus is relatively poorly mineralized; to make it more visible the film was deliberately underexposed. As a consequence, the outline of the tongue, which runs across the calculus, is also demonstrated clearly.

More than one calculus in the same duct is not uncommon (**746**) but the number in the duct of the left submandibular gland in this example is somewhat unusual. One of them is clearly circular in outline with concentric laminations, whereas the others are more irregularly shaped. The genial tubercles (arrow) are displayed clearly and should not be misdiagnosed as a salivary calculus. Sometimes a calculus may become very large, as in the example (**747**) in an edentulous patient where there is a sizeable elongated,

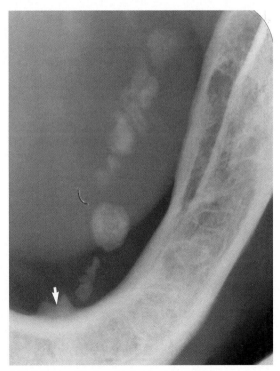

746 Submandibular duct calculus. LTO.

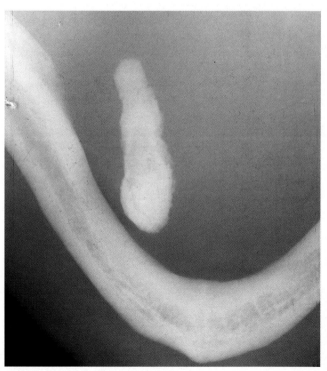

747 Submandibular duct calculus. LTO.

radio-opaque calculus in the duct of the right submandibular salivary gland. The calculus is wider anteriorly, at its probable site of origin, and tapers posteriorly. It is of variable radiodensity and has an irregular outline.

Calculi do not always cause symptoms and so may only be detected coincidentally on radiographs taken for other purposes. In the example (**748**) of a radiograph taken for the assessment of wisdom teeth, multiple calculi were found in the left submandibular duct. Their images are superimposed upon the periapical region $\overline{|4567}$ and are magnified and slightly blurred as the calculi lie outside the focal trough. The image of a duct calculus at the posterior border of the mylohyoid muscle may, on a dental panoramic radiograph, overlie the posterior part of the body of the mandible and resemble an area of osteosclerosis. In the example (**749**), the outline of the calculus is irregular and the image lies beneath the apices $\overline{8|}$.

In the body of the submandibular gland, as in the duct, calculi can reach a considerable size. The large calculus shown in **750** lies within the substance of the right submandibular salivary gland and is laminated concentrically. Its image is projected across the inferior border of the mandible and that of the body of the hyoid bone is seen below.

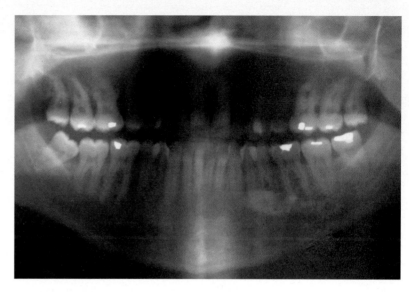

748 Submandibular duct calculus. DPR.

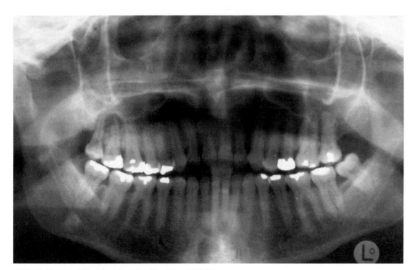

749 Submandibular duct calculus. DPR.

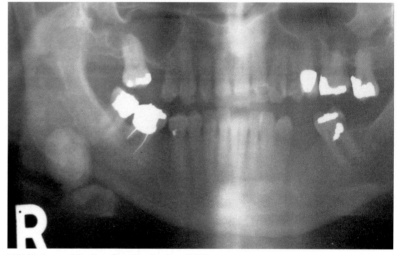

750 Submandibular gland calculus. DPR.

Another example – **751** – shows extensive mineralization of the left submandibular gland involving both the superficial and deep parts. The deep groove on the anterior aspect of the radio-opaque mass, representing the posterior border of the mylohyoid muscle, forms the boundary between the two parts of the gland. This patient was originally radiographed because of a painful ⌐7 socket (**752**) and the mass was discovered as an incidental finding.

The duct of the submandibular gland may be obstructed by mucus plugs or calculi that are poorly mineralized and hence minimally radio-opaque. This is the case in approximately 20% of submandibular calculi. When a suspected obstruction is not apparent on plain radiographs, sialography is indicated.

In the first example (**753**) of a sialogram of a submandibular gland, there is gross dilatation of the main duct and the intraglandular part of the duct system due to obstruction at the duct orifice by a non-radio-opaque calculus. The oval radiolucency within the dilated duct is not a calculus but an air bubble, which, with the patient in the upright position, has risen to the surface of the contrast medium. The looped outline of the cannula, which has been inserted into the duct, is seen clearly and the duct orifice appears to be relatively posterior in position due to retrusion of the tongue, the outline of which is also clearly visible. A second example (**754**) shows a radiolucent calculus (arrow) at the junction of the main duct and the gland. The duct outline is displayed clearly with the sharp downward

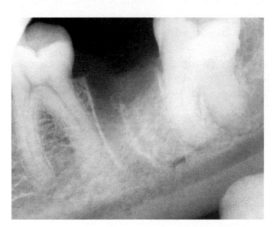

752 Submandibular gland calculus. P.

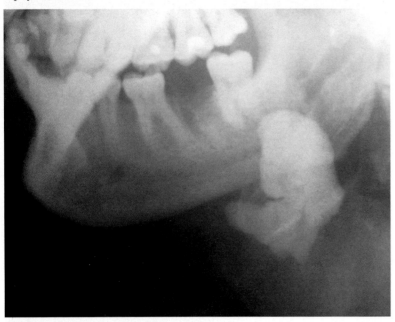

751 Submandibular gland calculus. OLM.

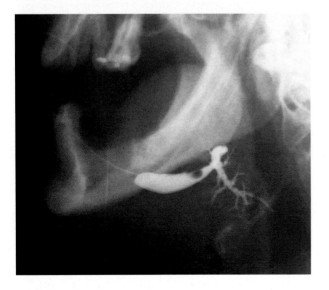

753 Submandibular duct calculus. SL(L).

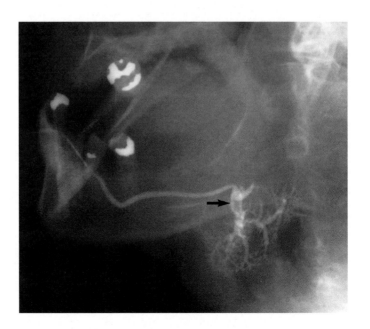

754 Submandibular duct calculus. SL(OLM).

angulation as the duct passes around the posterior border of the mylohyoid muscle. The ducts within the gland distal to the calculus are dilated but normal in distribution. In the clearance view – **755** – taken five minutes after removal of the cannula, the duct between the orifice and the calculus is now empty, but the water-based contrast medium is still present in the ducts of the gland beyond the obstruction.

Persistent partial obstruction of a salivary gland may lead to progressive atrophy of the secretory components. Although in **756** there is an obvious calculus of variable radio-opacity on the plain radiograph, a sialogram was also performed. **757** shows that proximal to the calculus the duct is normal, but distally there has been a marked reduction in the normal duct architecture. Anteromedially and disto-inferiorly the medium has diffused into the degenerative gland tissue, forming an almost homogenous radio-opacity. Loss of secretory activity can be demonstrated on a scintiscan following the injection of ^{99m}Tc. The scan **758** from a patient with sialolithiasis

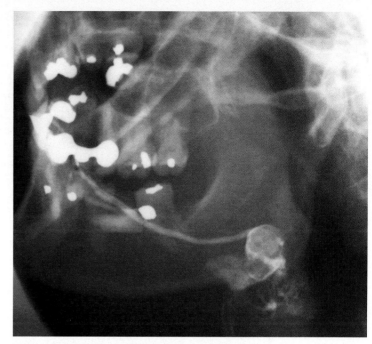

757 Submandibular gland calculus. SL(OLM).

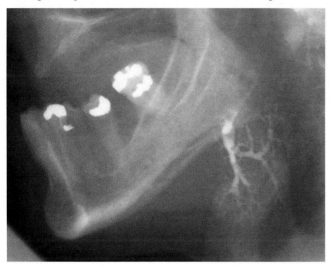

755 Submandibular duct calculus. SL(L).

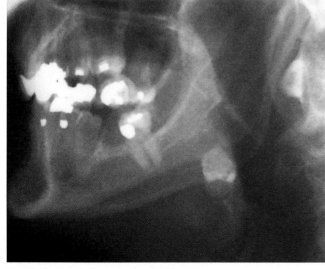

756 Submandibular gland calculus. L.

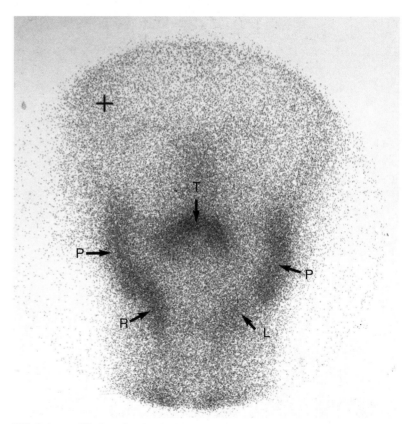

758 Submandibular gland calculus (anterior). SC. P: parotid glands; R: right submandibular gland; L: left submandibular gland; T: palatal and lingual glands.

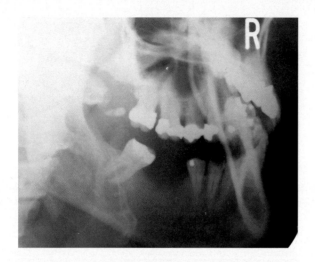

759 Parotid duct calculus. OLM.

affecting the left submandibular gland demonstrates the normal uptake of isotope in both parotid glands (P), the right submandibular gland (R) and the accessory salivary glands of the palate and tongue (T), but greatly reduced uptake in the left submandibular gland (L).

PAROTID DUCT CALCULUS

Calculi are less common in the parotid gland and tend to be smaller and generally less radio-opaque. When they form close to the ampulla of the main duct, their image may be superimposed upon that of the upper molar teeth, as in **759** where a radio-opaque oval calculus can be seen just distal to 7| . A useful technique to demonstrate parotid calculi in the region of the ampulla is to place an intra-oral film in the vestibule, hence avoiding any superimposition (**760**). Since parotid calculi are often poorly mineralized, a better image may be obtained by underexposure of the film, as in **761**. Here the calculus is demonstrated close to the mucosal surface of the air-filled, radiolucent cheek vestibule. When a suspected calculus is not demonstrated on a plain radiograph, a sialogram may be helpful, as in **762** where there is partial obstruction of the duct orifice. The main duct is dilated with a segmental outline and contains two radiolucent calculi (arrows) as shown by the oval, radiolucent filling defects. The next parotid sialogram (**763**) shows

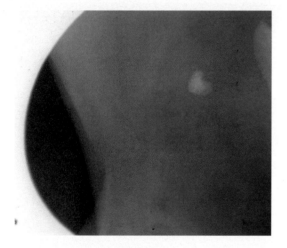

760 Parotid duct calculus. S.

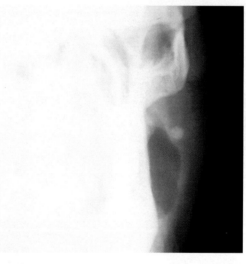

761 Parotid duct calculus. RPA.

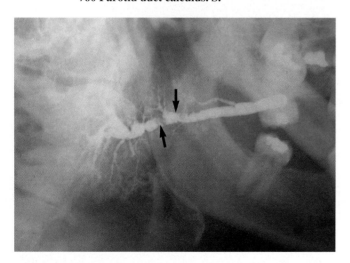

762 Parotid duct calculus. SL(OLM).

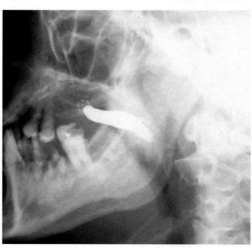

763 Parotid duct calculus. SL(L).

marked dilatation of the duct due to the presence of a radiolucent calculus at the ampulla. The calculus is outlined by a halo of contrast medium but insufficient medium has been introduced to fill all the branches of the grossly dilated duct system. A further example (**764**) shows a radiolucent calculus in the midportion of the main duct, where there is an interruption in the continuity of the column of contrast medium. The anterior portion of the duct is of normal diameter and shows the characteristic hook shape where the duct penetrates the buccinator muscle. The ducts posterior to the obstruction are dilated but retain their branching pattern. There is also discontinuity of the medium (arrow) in the first inferior branch of the duct system, which may be due to the presence of a second, smaller radiolucent calculus.

Salivary duct stricture

Calculi may promote a chronic inflammatory response in the wall of the duct, leading to fibrosis, which even if the calculus is shed or removed, may progress to a stricture. The first sialogram (**765**) shows a radiolucent calculus (arrow) in the parotid duct with dilatation distal to the partial obstruction. The calculus was subsequently passed but the patient continued to complain of symptoms and a second sialogram (**766**) revealed a stricture of the duct at the previous site of the calculus. The stricture (arrow) is demonstrated by the narrowing of the outline of the contrast medium at this point. Narrowing may also occur without any previous evidence of calculus formation, as in **767** where there is an obvious stricture of the main part of the duct with gross dilatation distal to the point of narrowing.

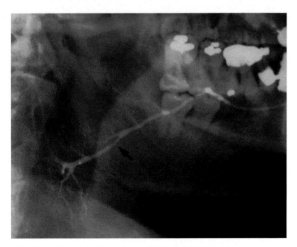

764 Parotid duct calculus. SL(L).

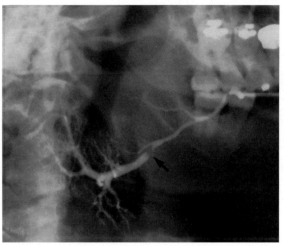

765 Parotid duct calculus. SL(OLM).

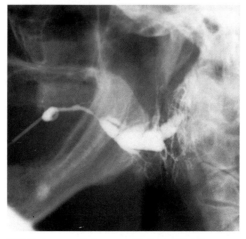

766 Stricture of the parotid duct. SL(OLM).

767 Stricture of the parotid duct. SL(L).

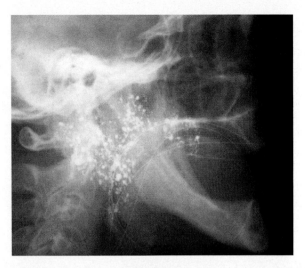

768 Sjögren's syndrome. SL(L).

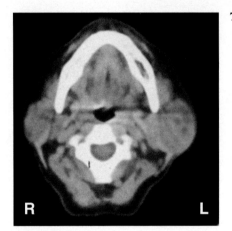

769 Sjögren's syndrome. CT.

Autoimmune sialadenitis (Sjögren's syndrome)

Sjögren's syndrome, which is believed to be a form of autoimmune disease, is characterized by progressive destruction of the acinar tissue of salivary and other exocrine glands, with progressive reduction in secretory activity. The salivary and lacrimal glands are principally affected giving rise to xerostomia and xerophthalmia (keratoconjunctivitis sicca) respectively. The destructive process may affect the glands alone (primary Sjögren's syndrome) or be associated with some other form of autoimmune disease (secondary Sjögren's syndrome) such as rheumatoid arthritis. The syndrome most commonly affects middle-aged and elderly females, although younger patients can be affected. The destruction of the acinar tissue is accompanied by progressive, lymphocytic infiltration and often enlargement of the salivary glands, in particular the parotid glands. The chronic inflammatory changes result in damage to and weakening of the walls of the finer ducts. As a result, contrast medium may leak out of the ducts during sialography to produce a characteristic, but not necessarily pathognomonic, appearance. In example **768** – of a parotid sialogram – the main ducts and many of the smaller ducts are not well demonstrated and many of them end in fine globular dilatations. Elsewhere in the gland, there are larger, apparently discrete foci of the contrast medium, probably a consequence of extravasation into the glandular tissue through the weakened duct walls. The accessory lobule of the gland also shows similar changes. Enlargement of the parotid glands may be demonstrated in computerized tomograms, as in **769** where enlargement of both glands, more advanced on the left side, is clearly shown. Such an examination is also of value in the investigation of lymphomas, which may arise in the salivary glands of patients with Sjögren's syndrome.

Chronic sialadenitis

Chronic inflammation in the major salivary glands, not associated with calculi, occurs most often in the parotid gland. Characteristically there are recurrent episodes of glandular swelling and infection. Recurrent parotitis may be divided into two types, the one affecting children and the other adults. In the first type, the condition commences in infancy or early childhood as acute swelling, which is usually unilateral, although both glands may be abnormal with intermittent swelling. In such cases sialography demonstrates diffuse sialectasia, which involves the whole gland. The adult type may be a progression of the childhood form or may arise spontaneously later in life and in addition to sialectasia, sialography will reveal ductal changes.

In the first example (**770**) in a seven-year-old, the sialogram shows narrowing of both the primary and in particular the secondary ducts, with the characteristic 'snowstorm' distribution of punctate areas of contrast medium (sialectasia) within the parenchyma of the gland. This appearance probably arises from damage to the ductal walls, which allows contrast medium to escape and gather in the periductular tissues. In the second

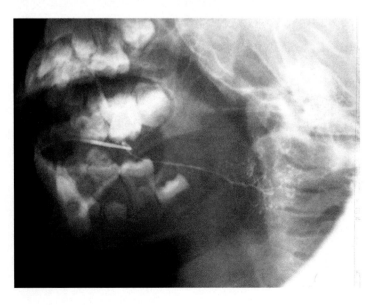

770 Recurrent parotitis. SL(OLM).

example (**771**) in a slightly younger patient, the changes are similar but more pronounced and also involve the accessory lobe of the gland.

In adults, the sialographic appearances are more varied and include changes in the structure of both the ducts and the glandular parenchyma. In the first example (**772**) the main duct is narrower than normal and there is almost complete loss of the architecture of the secondary ducts in the main lobe of the gland and to a lesser extent in the accessory lobe. A characteristic, punctate sialectasia is present in the parenchyma of the gland. Confirmation of damage to the smaller ducts and acini is obtained from a second radiograph – **773** – taken some thirty minutes later. This clearance radiograph, taken after the cannula has been withdrawn, shows that the ducts are now empty, but contrast medium is still present in the areas of sialectasia probably due to extravasation. In the next parotid sialogram (**774**) the proximal part of the main duct is dilated, suggesting partial obstruction in this region of the gland. In addition, some of the minor ducts are dilated with terminal globular dilatations characteristic of sialectasia; the overall radio-opacity of the duct system is greater than normal.

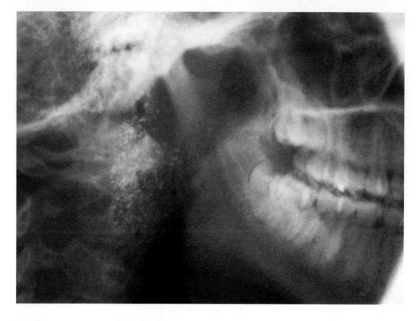

773 Recurrent parotitis. SL(L).

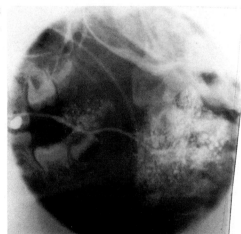

771 Recurrent parotitis. SL(OLM)).

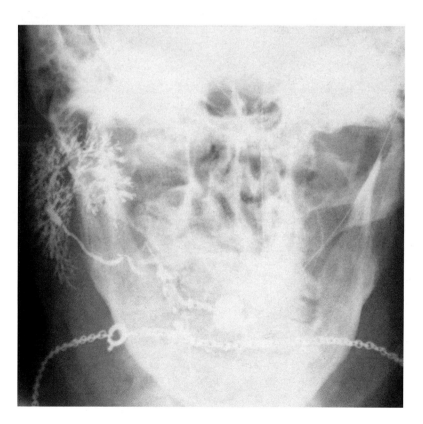

774 Recurrent parotitis. SL(PA).

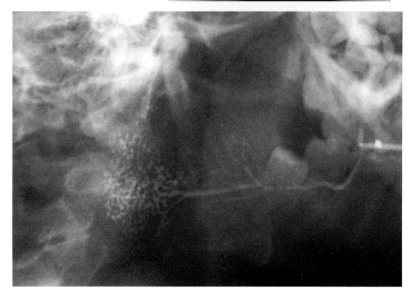

772 Recurrent parotitis. SL(OLM).

In the next example (**775**), the main duct appears normal although the number of secondary ducts is fewer than would be expected. There are several relatively large focal collections of contrast medium throughout the gland, a pattern of destruction that has been referred to as 'cavitary' sialectasia.

A possible long-term consequence of recurrent sialadenitis is progressive reduction in secretory activity. The uptake of ^{99m}Tc, measured by scintigraphy, gives an indication of the secretory activity of salivary glands. A record of the pattern of uptake of the radioactive isotope relative to time, as a time/activity uptake curve, shows the activity of the secretory acini and the subsequent discharge of secretory components after stimulation of the gland with a sialogogue. In **776**, of a patient with a long history of recurrent parotitis affecting the left parotid gland, the scintigraph shows that the rate of uptake of ^{99m}Tc on the left is less than that on the right. The first two scintigraphs also show normal accumulation of ^{99m}Tc in the submandibular salivary glands, the oropharyngeal salivary glands and the thyroid gland. Following stimulation with a sialogogue, saliva containing the radionuclide has been secreted from the salivary glands and has accumulated in the oropharynx as seen in the last two scintigraphs.

A further example of the use of scintigraphy is demonstrated in the next patient where there was uncertainty about possible remnants of the left submandibular salivary gland following previous surgery. The complete absence of secretory tissue in this site is, however, clearly displayed in the cumulative scintigraph (**777**). The uptake curves show a normal pattern of uptake of the parotid glands and in the right submandibular

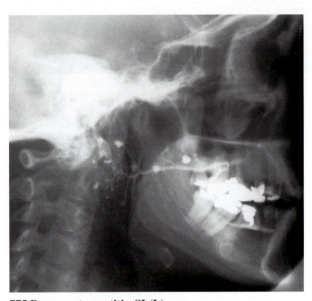

775 Recurrent parotitis. SL(L).

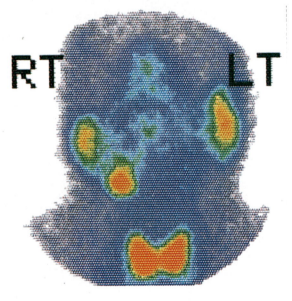

776 Recurrent parotitis. TASC.

777 Absent submandibular gland. SC.

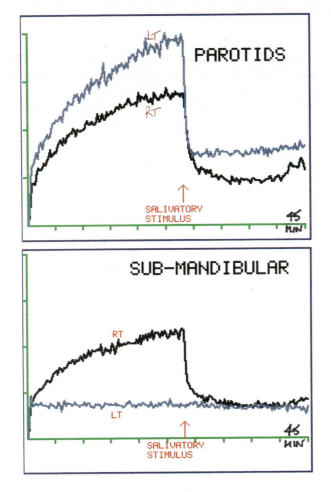

778 Absent submandibular gland TASC. Top: parotids; bottom: submandibular.

779 Absent submandibular gland. SC. 2.5 minute frames.

salivary gland (**778**) but no uptake in the region of the left submandibular salivary gland. After stimulation with a sialogogue, the emptying of the remaining major salivary glands is normal. This sequence of events is also seen in the sequential series of scintigraphs (**779**) recorded at two-and-a-half minute intervals.

Chronic sialadenitis that is not associated with calculi or autoimmune disease is less common in the submandibular gland. In **780**, the sialogram shows a stricture (arrow) of the middle part of the main duct and sialectasia in both the sublingual and submandibular glands. The normal architecture of the smaller, secondary ducts is less distinct.

780 Chronic submandibular sialadenitis. SL(OLM).

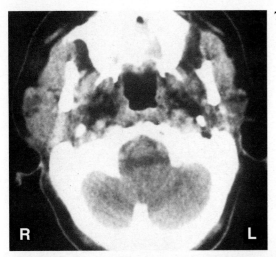

781 Parotid abscess. CT.

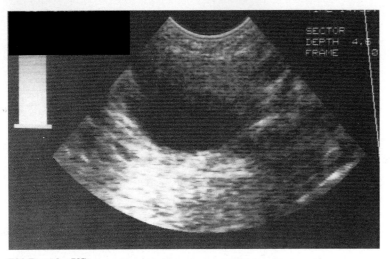

782 Ranula. US.

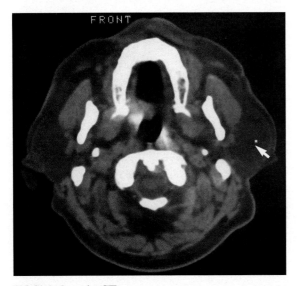

783 Sialadenosis. CT.

Parotid abscess

This is shown in **781**. A parotid abscess may arise as a result of ascending infection via the parotid duct in patients who are debilitated and/or dehydrated, including those with Sjögren's syndrome. Often the diagnosis is obvious, but in some cases the condition becomes chronic and indistinguishable clinically from other causes of unilateral parotid enlargement. US and CT may be helpful in obtaining a more accurate diagnosis. In this example, a computerized axial tomogram demonstrates a lobulated area of low attenuation in the right parotid gland. Measurement of the attenuation number (Hounsfield number) would indicate that the swelling contains fluid.

Traumatic conditions

Ranula

This is shown in **782**. Mucous extravasation cysts may be due to trauma that has damaged the ducts and allowed the escape of salivary secretion into the adjacent tissues. This phenomenon occurs most commonly in the minor salivary glands of the lower lip. Less commonly the ducts of the sublingual gland are affected resulting in a swelling in the floor of the mouth, commonly known as a ranula. On occasions the swelling may extend along fascial planes into the neck and is then known as a plunging ranula. US may be helpful in identifying ranulas by demonstrating their cystic nature. In this example, there is a well-localized, homogenous, echo-poor area with posterior enhancement, shown by the clearly echo-bright area in the lower part of the illustration. This combination of features is characteristic of a fluid-filled, cystic lesion.

Metabolic conditions

Sialadenosis (Sialosis)

This is shown in **783**. Sialadenosis is a non-inflammatory, non-neoplastic enlargement of the salivary glands. It is associated with chronic liver disease, particularly in alcoholics, and in malnutrition and hormonal disorders such as diabetes. It presents as a bilateral, painless enlargement of the parotid glands, although other glands may also be affected. The glands become enlarged, due predominantly to an increase in the size of each individual secretory cell. Although the duct architecture remains normal, as the condition progresses there is fatty infiltration of the parenchyma. In this example there is enlargement of both parotid glands, which are of low attenuation. The application of an electronic pencil (arrow) provides the attenuation or Hounsfield number of the tissue components. Here the value is -71, which indicates that there is a high fat content of the gland. Although the gland is of low density, there is a random patchwork of denser areas scattered throughout it.

Tumorous conditions

Salivary gland neoplasms arise most commonly in the parotid glands, where the majority – 80% – are benign. In other salivary glands, a greater proportion are malignant but the overall occurrence of neoplasms is much less frequent. In addition to tumours of glandular epithelium, neoplasms of stromal and interstitial tissues, e.g. lymphomas, may also occur. In the case of the major salivary glands, imaging techniques are helpful in the diagnosis of neoplasia and the determination of the site and size of tumours. Sialography may reveal the presence of more substantial space-occupying lesions that have displaced the normal duct architecture of the gland. CT, US and MRI are more reliable for the identification of smaller tumours.

Pleomorphic salivary adenoma

Pleomorphic salivary adenomas are benign, expansile neoplasms with localized, peripheral areas of growth, resulting in a lobular outline. They occur most commonly in the superficial lobe of the parotid gland, but may also occur in the deep part, as well as in the accessory lobe. In **784** there is a tumour mass occupying most of the upper two-thirds of the parotid gland. The main duct has been displaced inferiorly and the architecture of the minor ducts of the lower aspect of the gland remains normal with the typical branching pattern. However, above and posterior to the main duct, the minor ducts are fewer in number and exhibit a curvilinear shape as they are distorted around the tumour. In the superior aspect of the gland, the minor ducts are dilated (arrows) due to tumour compression. In the second illustration – **785** – the neoplasm lies in the accessory lobe of the parotid gland and has displaced the main duct inferiorly, resulting in downward curvature of the anterior part of the duct. The main duct is dilated proximally to the mass, due to partial obstruction by the tumour, but there is no obvious abnormality of the finer branches of the duct system. The posterior and inferior margins of the tumour are outlined by a thin, radio-opaque line (arrowheads) of contrast medium extravasated from the distorted acini at the periphery of the mass. (Note the image of the surface of the dorsum of the tongue outlined by globules of the contrast medium, which have escaped into the mouth.)

CT often demonstrates tumours more clearly because the parotid gland contains a significant proportion of fat, particularly in more elderly people, which has a low attenuation value. In **786** there is a slightly lobulated mass in the anterolateral aspect of the left parotid gland. It lies close to, but is separated from, the masseter muscle. The mass contrasts well with the lower attenuation of the gland, having a similar density to that of the adjacent muscle. [Note the major blood vessels (arrow) in the deeper aspect of the right parotid gland.]

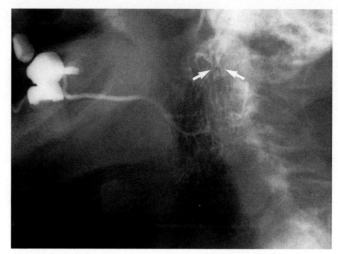

784 Pleomorphic salivary adenoma. SL(OLM).

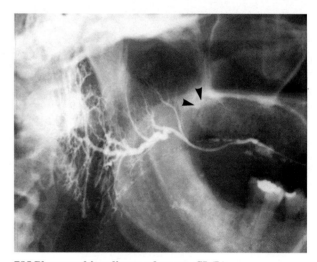

785 Pleomorphic salivary adenoma. SL(L).

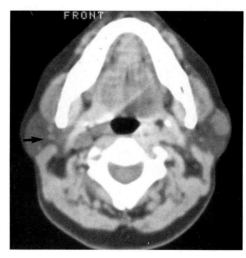

786 Pleomorphic salivary adenoma. CT.

Another example – **787** – shows a tumour in the left parotid gland. It is well circumscribed, has a slightly lobulated surface (particularly on its superficial aspect) and lies within the gland, surrounded by normal tissue of low attenuation. The external carotid artery lies posteromedial to the ramus of the mandible, close to the tumour. When the parotid glands contain relatively little adipose tissue, the attenuation values of the glandular tissue and the neoplasm may be similar. Under these circumstances, a combination of sialography and CT may prove to be a useful investigation. In the example of this technique – **788** – the neoplasm in the left parotid gland has been outlined by the radio-opaque medium.

A US scan of a representative field of a parotid tumour in another patient – **789** – shows a mass that, although less echogenic than the surrounding normal tissues, contains numerous echoes, indicating that it is largely solid in nature. The superficial boundary of the mass and the adjacent normal glandular tissue, which is echo-bright, shows that the tumour is lobulated. The dark, echo-free areas on each side of the mass are acoustic shadows caused by adjacent bony structures. The approximate dimensions of such masses may be determined by the use of electronic calipers as illustrated in **790**, which shows the two-dimensional extent of the lesion.

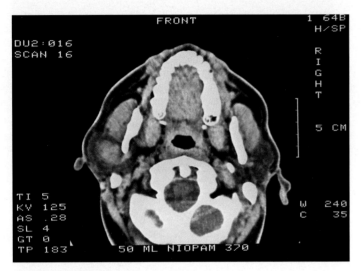

787 Pleomorphic salivary adenoma. CT.

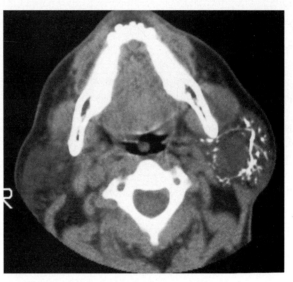

788 Pleomorphic salivary adenoma. CT(SL).

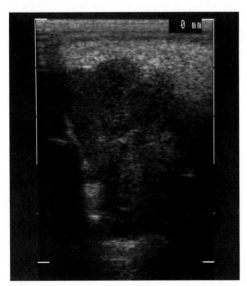

789 Pleomorphic salivary adenoma. US.

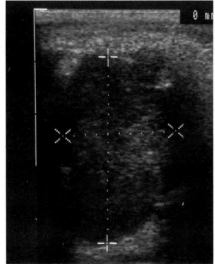

790 Pleomorphic salivary adenoma. US.

Adenocarcinoma

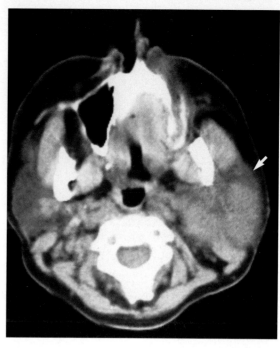

This is shown in **791**. Malignant tumours usually have an indistinct border on computerized tomograms although this is not always the case. In this example of an adenocarcinoma in the left parotid gland, the infiltrative nature of the lesion is clearly shown. The tumour occupies both the deep and the superficial parts of the gland; most of its periphery is ill defined. The mass is infiltrating posteriorly into the adjacent muscle, superficially into the subcutaneous fat and medially into the pharyngeal wall. Anterolaterally, some normal glandular tissue (arrow) of low attenuation persists between the tumour mass and the masseter muscle. The major vessels within the gland appear to have been infiltrated by tumour.

10

The soft tissues

Introduction

Imaging of the soft tissues was at one time traditionally limited to the detection of radio-opaque objects, such as foreign bodies or areas of dystrophic mineralization and to the use of contrast agents to demonstrate lesions such as vascular malformations or soft tissue cysts. However, more recent techniques have made it possible to image the soft tissues specifically (US) and to improve the contrast of individual soft tissue structures (CT; MRI). These techniques are now used to demonstrate a wide variety of solid and cystic lesions involving the soft tissues.

Dystrophic mineralization

Although dystrophic mineralization may occur in any persistent, chronic inflammation of soft tissues, it is most commonly found in tuberculous lymph nodes often as a coincidental finding. In the example (**792**), several mineralized lymph nodes are present in the upper and middle parts of the deep cervical chain on the right side of the neck. The nodes have a uniform radio-opacity but are of variable size and shape and have an irregular outline. They are seen to lie just below the angle of the mandible, along the course of the internal jugular vein. Their position distinguishes them from salivary calculi (see **745–765**).

The image of such radio-opaque masses may be superimposed upon that of other structures giving rise to unusual radiographic appearances which may lead to incorrect diagnoses. The next example (**793, 794**) shows the image of a large, mineralized lymph node at the upper end of the right, deep cervical chain which has been projected on to the second molar.

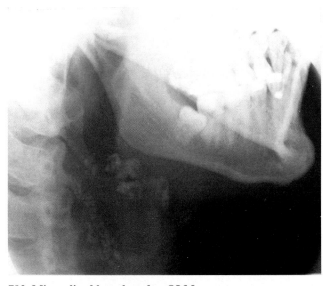

792 Mineralized lymph nodes. OLM.

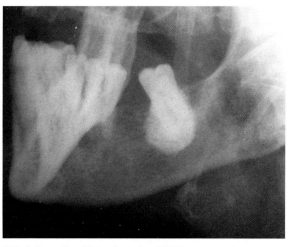

793 Mineralized lymph node. OLM.

The first impression may be that of an area of osteosclerosis or a cementoblastoma. However, closer examination confirms the absence of any radiolucent capsule or radio-opaque lamina and that the pear-shaped mass overlies part of the crown of the tooth. The true position of this lesion is confirmed on the lateral radiograph (**794**) which shows that it lies posterior to the angle of the mandible.

Less commonly, dystrophic mineralizations develop within chronically inflamed tonsils. In the example (**795**), several discrete, faintly radio-opaque foci of calcification (arrows) are present in the tonsil. Such foci, or tonsiliths, may vary considerably in shape and size. In some rare metabolic conditions, dystrophic mineralization in the soft tissues may be more generalized. For example, in calcinosis (**796**), deposition of foci of dystrophic mineralization commonly occurs within the dermis and occasionally within the oral mucosa. In this illustration, numerous rounded radio-opaque deposits are present within the soft tissues of the chin.

Vascular lesions

Vascular lesions of the soft tissues are not normally apparent on conventional radiographs, although some cavernous haemangiomas may be seen on CTs. In addition, foci of dystrophic mineralization (phleboliths) sometimes occur within dilated venous channels or haemangiomas and so may be seen on conventional radiographs. Phleboliths form by deposition of successive concentric layers of mineral around a focus of degenerative tissue or thrombus and so are roughly circular in outline but exhibit considerable variation in size. They are not densely radio-opaque and some have radiolucent centres. In the large vascular lesion (**797**) of the left side of the face, there are numerous phleboliths which are mostly superimposed over the ramus of the mandible. For the further investigation of vascular malformations, Doppler ultrasound, MRI or angiography may be used.

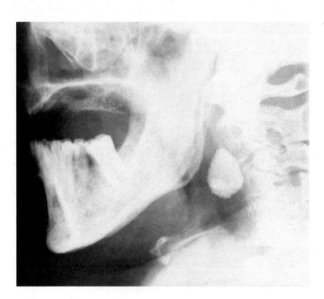

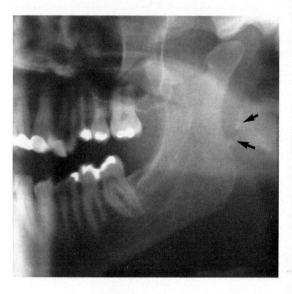

794 Mineralized lymph node. L.

795 Tonsilith. DPR.

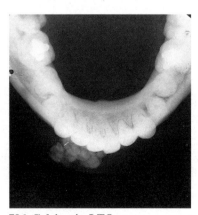

796 Calcinosis. LTO.

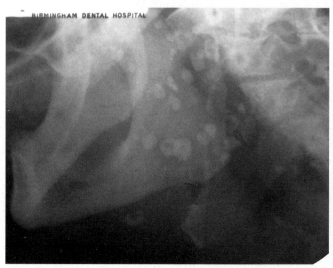

797 Cavernous haemangioma with phleboliths. OLM.

The next example (**798**) shows a traumatic aneurysm arising from the facial artery. The lesion is well demonstrated on the carotid angiogram in which radio-opaque medium has been injected into the external carotid artery. The facial artery loops downwards over the posterior part of the ramus of the mandible towards the lower border, from where a complex mass of tortuous vessels is seen overlying the body of the mandible. Also clearly displayed are the maxillary artery, running obliquely upwards and forwards to the posterior border of the maxilla from the neck of the condyle, and the superficial temporal artery with its branches extending throughout the temporal region.

The last example (**799**) shows an MRI of a recurrent cavernous haemangioma in the right cheek. This T1-weighted image demonstrates a well circumscribed, fusiform mass (arrow) lying deep to the subcutaneous fat and within the muscles overlying the maxilla. The level of the scan is indicated by the line on the topogram.

Tumorous conditions

A wide variety of epithelial and connective tissue tumours may arise in the head and neck. Various imaging techniques are invaluable in the determination of the full extent of such masses and may often indicate their benign or malignant nature. In addition to the main tumour mass, the involvement of lymph nodes may also be revealed in malignant epithelial tumours and lymphomas, so helping in the staging of these lesions.

Squamous cell carcinoma

Intra-oral squamous cell carcinoma occurs most commonly on the lateral margins of the tongue and in the floor of the mouth; incidence increases with age. When the lesions are restricted to the soft tissues, conventional radiographs are of limited assistance but CT and in particular MRI may reveal the extent of the tumour more fully. The example (**800** and **801**) of an MRI scan shows a T1-weighted image following the intravenous administration of gadolinium with an area of high signal intensity in the anterior third of the tongue, suggestive of a tumour mass. The presence of the lesion is more clearly shown in the second illustration (**801**), which shows a shortened T1-weighted image of the same patient, in which the signal from the fat tissue has been suppressed. The slice is at a different level from the previous figure and also shows the presence of an enhanced lymph node (arrow) suggesting metastatic spread.

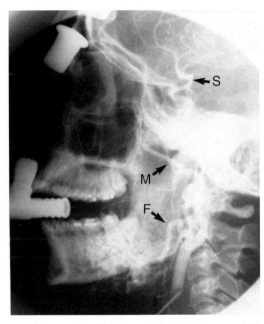

798 Traumatic aneurysm of the facial artery. AN.
F: facial artery; M: maxillary artery; S: superficial temporal artery.

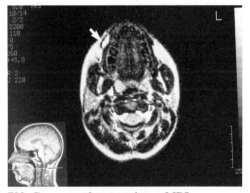

799 Cavernous haemangioma. MRI.

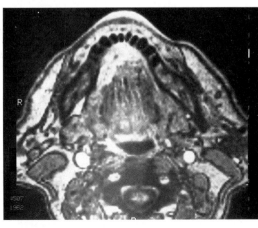

800 Squamous cell carcinoma – floor of tongue. MRI.

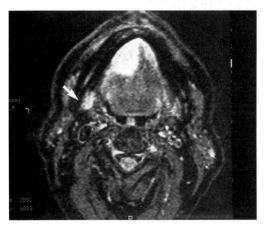

801 Squamous cell carcinoma – tongue. MRI.

Another example (**802**, **803**) shows a large carcinoma which has arisen in the left side of the floor of the mouth and has spread into the mandible. The two illustrations show how such lesions are more clearly demonstrated in T1-weighted images following enhancement with gadolinium (**803**).

Nasopharyngeal carcinoma

The example (**804**, **805**, **806**) shows a large nasopharyngeal carcinoma (arrows) in the posterosuperior part of the nasophaynx. This is visible on the plain radiograph (**804**) but the extent of the lesion is more completely displayed by CT. In the tomogram (**805**) there is a mass (cross) in the right nasopharynx extending across the midline. The tomogram at a lower level (**806**) shows an enlarged lymph node (cross) in the posterior triangle of the neck. There is also a large, approximately circular area of low attenuation, just anterior to the node, due to the presence of a haematoma, which arose following surgical investigation.

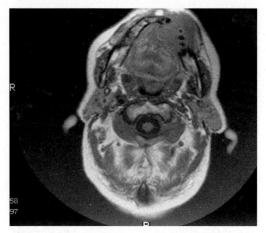

802 Squamous cell carcinoma – floor of mouth. MRI.

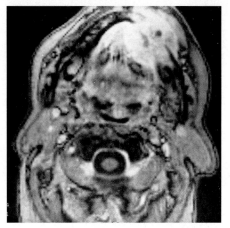

803 Squamous cell carcinoma – floor of mouth. MRI.

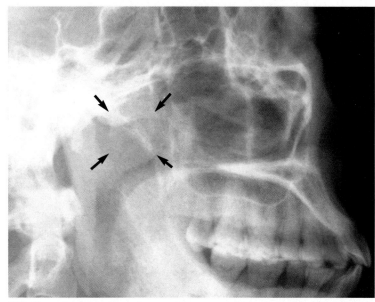

804 Nasopharyngeal carcinoma. L.

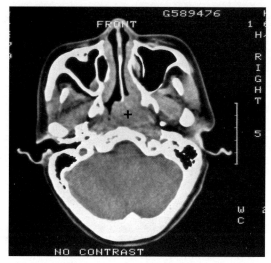

805 Nasopharyngeal carcinoma. CT.

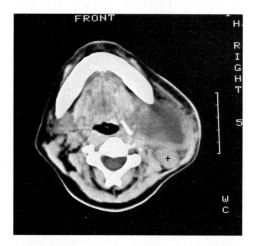

806 Nasopharyngeal carcinoma – lymph node metastasis. CT.

Lymphangioma (cystic hygroma)

Developmental abnormalities of lymphatic vessels may arise superficially in the head and neck and most commonly affect the tongue or the lips. When more deeply placed, they usually occur in the soft tissues of the neck. Cystic hygromas are most commonly diagnosed in the first decade of life and may cause considerable distortion of the tissues. Occasionally they may be found in adults. The example (**807**) shows a well-defined oval mass of low attentuation in the left submandibular space overlying the submandibular salivary gland (cross). The cystic nature of the lesion is demonstrated by the US scan (**808**) which shows an echo-free area with deeper acoustic enhancement, typical of a fluid-filled lesion. Note the echo-free linear areas indicating the presence of blood vessels adjacent to the lesion.

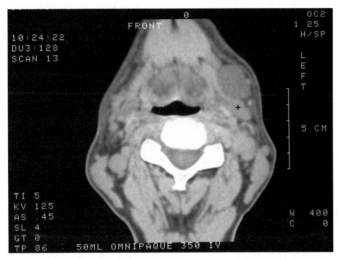

807 Lymphangioma (cystic hygroma). CT.

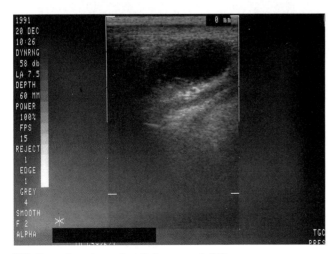

808 Lymphangioma (cystic hygroma). US.

Carotid body tumour

This rare tumour of the chromaffin system is often very vascular and may attain a large size, reaching to the base of the skull, prior to diagnosis. In the example (**809**, **810**), the MRI scans taken following injection of gadolinium show a large lobulated tumour occupying the left infratemporal and pterygopalatine fossae and extending medially into the posterior nasal air space. There are areas of irregular signal loss within the lesion, probably representing foci of necrosis or maybe a consequence of the vascularity of the tumour. The tumour has encroached upon the posterior wall of the maxillary antrum, which is reduced in size.

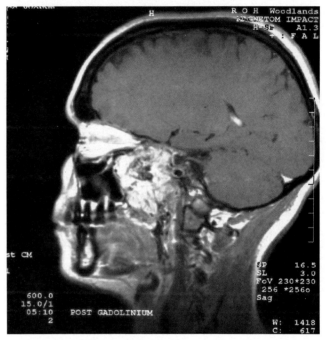

809 Carotid body tumour. MRI.

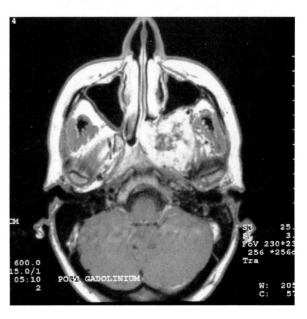

810 Carotid body tumour. MRI.

The vascular nature of this tumour can be demonstrated by angiography. The example (**811**) shows a digital subtraction angiogram following injection of contrast medium into the external carotid artery. The tortuous artery is clearly shown feeding the richly vascular tumour mass. This lesion was treated by embolization; a conventional angiogram (**812**) taken two months later demonstrates almost complete resolution of the lesion.

Foreign bodies – traumatic

Tooth fragments

Traumatic injuries to teeth, particularly the incisors, may result in tooth fragments becoming embedded in the soft tissues, most frequently those of the lips. Radiographic examination is essential in such traumatic incidents, particulary when the clinical examination fails to identify all the tooth fragments. In the example (**813**) there are fragments of the crowns of fractured maxillary incisors embedded within the lower lip. At least three pieces are present, one of which can be identified as the fragment from an oblique fracture through the crown of a central incisor. A second radiograph (**814**) of the same patient emphasizes the need for more than one view and shows a significant difference in the anteroposterior position of the fragments. This radiograph also demonstrates the swelling of the lower lip. The next example (**815**) is that of an upper lip, within which at least four tooth fragments, showing different degrees of radio-opacity, are embedded. Once again the swelling of the lip is apparent.

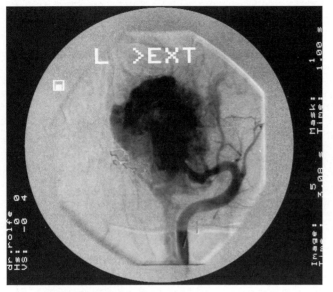

811 Carotid body tumour. AN.

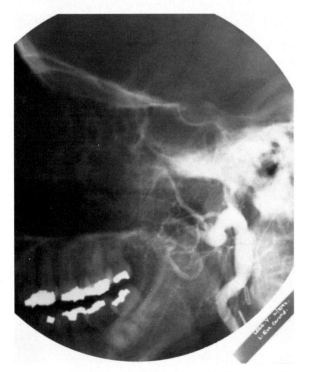

812 Carotid body tumour following embolization. AN.

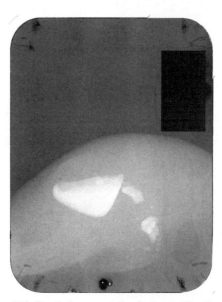

813 Tooth fragments in the lower lip. S.

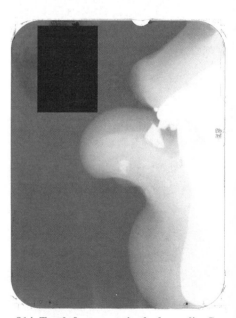

814 Tooth fragments in the lower lip. S.

Glass

In traumatic incidents such as road traffic accidents, in addition to fragments of tooth tissue, particles of glass, plastic or metal from the vehicle, and of grit from the road surface, may also become embedded in the facial tissues. The first example (**816**) shows fragments of windscreen glass embedded in the lower lip. The fragments are only slightly radio-opaque and the largest has an irregular, angular outline. Some smaller fragments lie posterolaterally.

In the second example (**817**), a fragment of windscreen glass embedded within the soft tissues of the cheek, has been displayed more clearly by underexposure of the film and by the slight rotation of the head and inflation of the cheek.

Missiles

In firearm injuries the projected missile may pass through the tissues, or become impacted within them or upon the bony structures of the facial skeleton. In the first example (**818**), there is a foreign body apparently lying against the right ramus of the mandible in the region of the sigmoid notch. The dense radio-opacity and the distinct outline of the foreign body indicate its metallic nature and the shape is characteristic of that of an airgun pellet. A postero-anterior radiograph (not shown) confirmed its position just medial to the ramus, again reinforcing the value of two differently

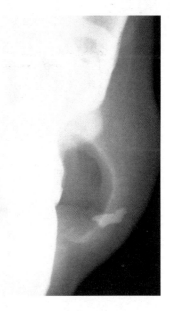

817 Glass. RPA.

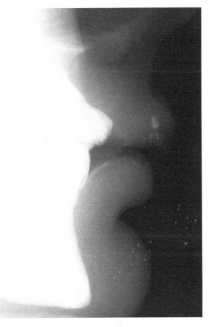

815 Tooth fragments in the upper lip. S.

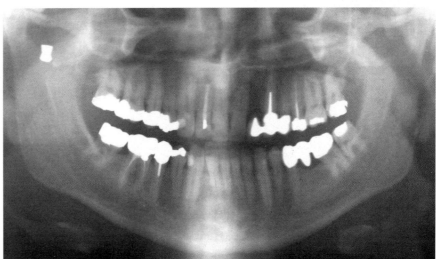

818 Airgun pellet. DPR.

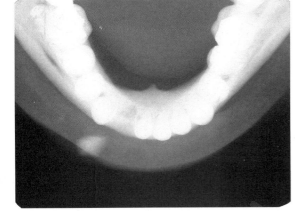

816 Glass. LTO.

angled views. The airgun pellet in the next example (**819**) is flattened against the lateral surface of the body of the mandible in the $\overline{6|}$ region. The radio-opaque foreign body is ovoid in shape and indistinct in outline due to the distortion on impact with the bone. Its position lateral to the mandible and the gross distortion is confirmed on the occlusal radiograph (**820**).

With gunshot wounds it is more likely that a collection of metallic debris, due to fragmentation of the missile rather than distinct bullets or pellets, will be seen on radiographs. In the example (**821**) in a patient who was shot with a handgun, the low velocity bullet has entered the right cheek and after fragmenting against the edentulous ridge of the maxilla, the larger fragments have settled in the tongue. A number of fragments have exited through the left side of the neck and the track is clearly outlined by a number of small, radio-opaque fragments.

The next example (**822**) is also that of a patient who was assaulted and shot with a low velocity handgun, in this case through the left cheek. There are fractures (arrows) at the right angle, left body and midline of the mandible, which have been temporarily immobilized by a loop wire around the lower incisors. The fracture in the midline is not clearly visible on this radiograph. Numerous irregular, radio-opaque fragments are retained in the missile track and are superimposed upon the left ramus of the mandible. With extensive injuries of this nature the airway may be compromised and an endotracheal tube has been inserted via the mouth and a pack placed in the oropharynx. Both the tube and the pack can be identified by their radio-opaque markers and a radio-opaque artery clip is also present.

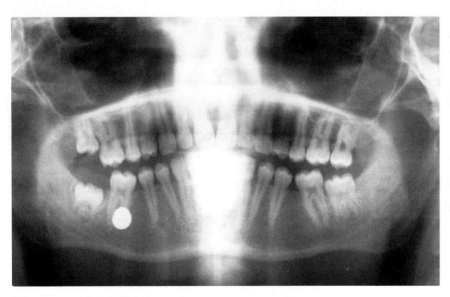

819 Airgun pellet. DPR.

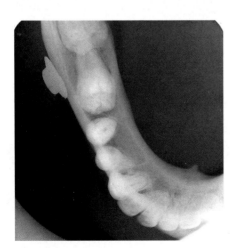

820 Airgun pellet. LTO.

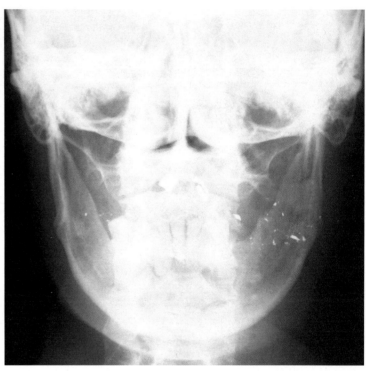

821 Low velocity bullet wound. PA.

The next example (**823**) shows a close range shotgun injury to the face. Many of the pellets have been distorted by the force of the impact and others have fragmented as indicated by the smaller radio-opaque particles. There are multiple fractures of the underlying facial skeleton particularly on the left, but these are not clearly displayed on the radiograph.

Silica

In various occupations, particularly those of polishers and grinders, small particles of radio-opaque material may become impacted into the lips and the peri-oral skin. In the example (**824**) in a machine polisher, there are multiple small particles of silica within the skin of the lower lip and chin. The particles are faintly radio-opaque, of variable size and approximately circular in outline; some have radiolucent centres. The outline of the everted vermillion part of the lip is projected beyond the main soft tissue contour. A similar radiographic appearance has been described in the condition of multiple miliary osteoma of the skin (osteoma cutis). Note that the crestal part of the edentulous alveolus is projected anterior to the inferior border of the mandible, which has a more dense cortical outline.

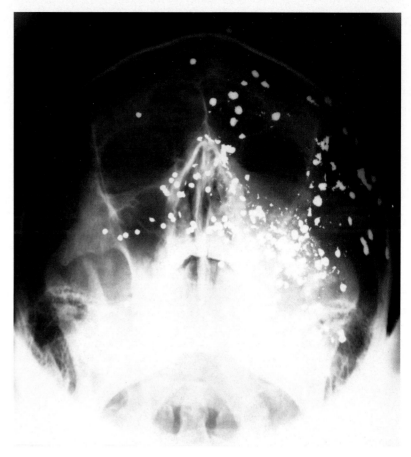

823 Gunshot wound. OM.

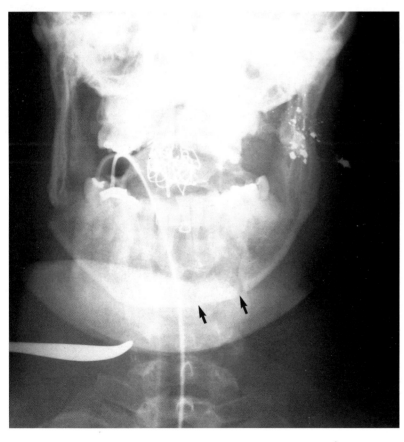

822 Low velocity bullet wound. PA.

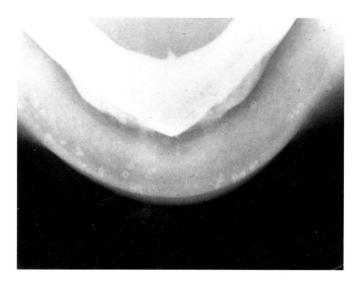

824 Silica. LTO.

Foreign bodies – iatrogenic

A wide range of foreign bodies may find their way into the oral soft tissues during dental procedures. These include not only particles of filling and impression material, but also items such as fragments of broken needles used for the injection of local anaesthetics. The latter is now a rare occurrence with the use of disposable needles.

Restorative materials

Particles of amalgam may enter the oral mucosa where they are slowly eroded to produce an amalgam tattoo. In the example (**825**) of a tattoo on the gingival mucosa, there are numerous, approximatelycircular, densely radio-opaque particles superimposed predominantly over the interdental crest $\overline{54|}$ and partly over $5|$ cervically. The density of the radio-opacity indicates the metallic nature of the material. In the next example (**826, 827**), radio-opaque rubber base impression material has been introduced into the lingual soft tissues. Two views, approximately at right angles, have been taken to provide sufficient information about the size, shape and position of the foreign body.

Local anaesthetic needles

The fracture of needles, sometimes into more than one fragment, was particularly associated with inferior alveolar nerve block anaesthesia. In the example (**828**), part of a needle which fractured during administration of a right inferior alveolar nerve block has been retained in the pterygomandibular space. Its position medial to the ramus of the mandible is

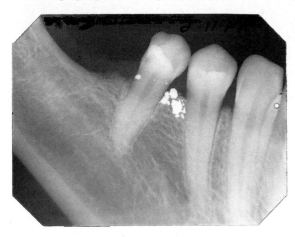

825 Amalgam particles. P.

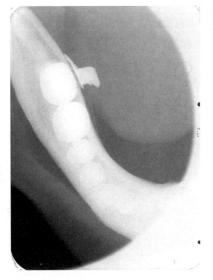

826 Retained impression material. LTO.

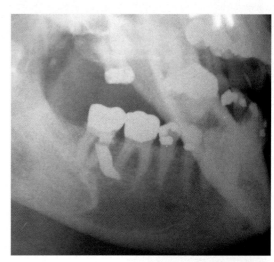

827 Retained impression material. OLM.

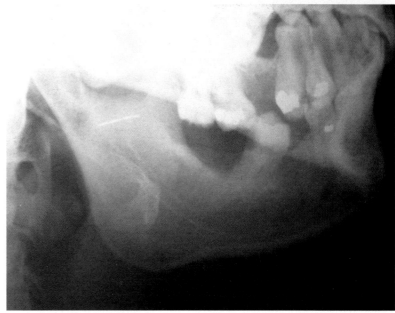

828 Fractured needle. OLM.

clearly demonstrated on the postero-anterior film (**829**). Less commonly, needle fractures occurred in other types of injection procedure, as in the next example (**830**, **831**) of a needle which broke into three separate pieces during the administration of a left posterior superior alveolar nerve block. The three fragments are slightly separate from each other (**831**), the smallest one being at the distal end of the needle (arrow).

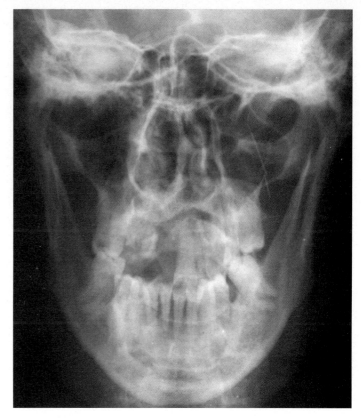

830 Fractured needle. PA.

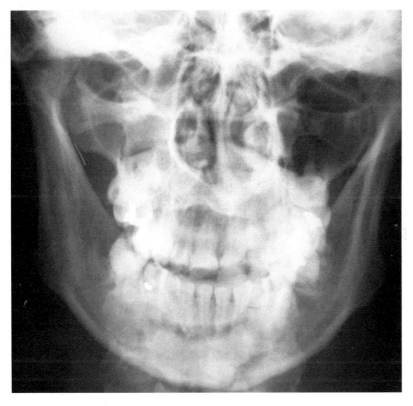

829 Fractured needle. PA.

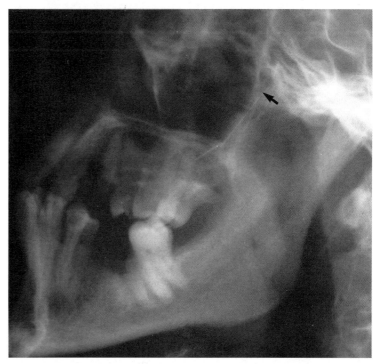

831 Fractured needle. L.

In the example (**832**) of a disposable needle, which fractured at the hub during the administration of an inferior alveolar nerve block in a ten-year-old, the needle is bent upwards approximately a third of the way along its length. It is shown superimposed upon the ramus of the mandible.

Retained contrast medium

Another unusual type of foreign body is contrast medium previously used for investigative procedures. In the example (**833**), globules of the radio-opaque medium, Myelodil, persist in the basilar system in the middle cranial fossa following a myelogram several years before.

Radium needles

One method of irradiating soft tissues is by the direct implantation of radioactive needles. Here (**834**), fine metallic needles are present in the tongue.

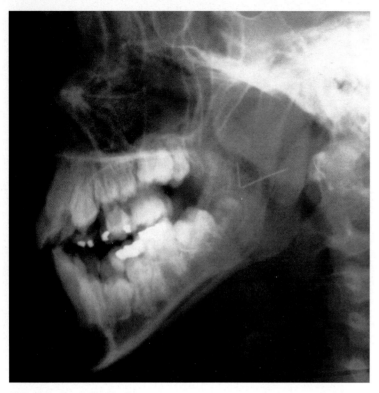

832 Fractured needle. L.

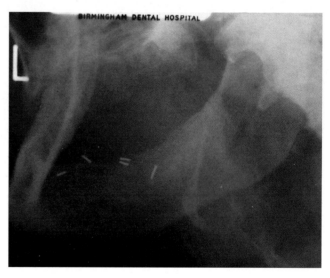

834 Radium needles. OLM.

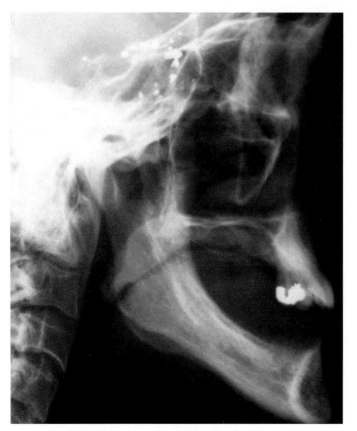

833 Retained radio-opaque medium (Myelodil). L.

Index